Derived from T
Edition, a b
The Merck
isn't over your
standards. Here
The Merck Manual—Home Edition.

"[A] very valuable resource . . . for any home."
—*Publishers Weekly*

"Doctors should encourage their patients to own [the Home Edition]."
—Dr. Sherwin Nuland, Clinical Professor of Surgery, Yale School of Medicine; author of *How We Die, Doctors,* and *The Wisdom of the Body*

"Essential for all medical, consumer health and public libraries."
—*Library Journal*

"Anyone interested in health should have this book."
—Ellen Levine, Editor-in-Chief, *Good Housekeeping*

"Devoid of doctor double talk . . . it should help put you and your doctor on the same wavelength."
—*USA Today*

"Well written and comprehensive, this book makes the patient a better partner."
—American Lung Association

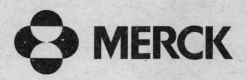

The Merck Manual of Children's Health

Justin L. Kaplan, MD
Robert S. Porter, MD
Editors

Peter G. Szilagyi, MD, MPH
Consulting Editor

Mark H. Beers, MD
Editor Emeritus

POCKET BOOKS

NEW YORK   LONDON   TORONTO   SYDNEY

POCKET BOOKS, a division of Simon & Schuster, Inc.
1230 Avenue of the Americas, New York, NY 10020

Copyright © 2003, 2007, by Merck & Co., Inc.

Published by arrangement with Merck & Co., Inc.

A previous version of this work was published as part of *The Merck Manual of Medical Information, Second Home Edition*.

ISBN-13: 978-1-4165-3610-9
ISBN-10:   1-4165-3610-8

This Pocket Books paperback edition January 2007

10 0 8 7 6

POCKET and colophon are registered trademarks of
Simon & Schuster, Inc.

Manufactured in the United States of America

For information regarding special discounts for bulk purchases, please contact Simon and Schuster Special Sales at 1-800-456-6798 or business@simonandschuster.com.

Preface

Information about children's health and medical care can be found easily on the web, in magazines, and in the many books that include the topic. Does the world need another book about children's health? What makes this book different from the others?

One difference is in the quality of information. *The Merck Manual of Children's Health* is adapted from the best-selling *The Merck Manual of Medical Information—Second Home Edition*. This book, written in everyday language, is a translation of *The Merck Manual of Diagnosis and Therapy*, commonly referred to as *The Merck Manual*. *The Merck Manual* is the oldest continuously published general medical textbook in the English language and the most widely used medical textbook in the world. Building on that tradition, *The Merck Manual of Children's Health* has been reviewed extensively and includes contributions from more than 45 experts. The material reflects the most widely accepted medical knowledge and practice.

The Merck Manual of Children's Health is comprehensive and detailed. All aspects of children's health are discussed, with topics ranging from finding and communicating with a health care practitioner to normal growth and development, well-child care, common problems such as excessive crying and separation anxiety, age-related disorders, disorders related to specific organ systems, accidents and emergencies, social and psychologic aspects of children's health, and much more. This book explains what a disorder is, who is likely to get it, what its symptoms are, how it is diagnosed, what its prognosis is, and how it can be prevented and treated. Medical terms are defined so that parents can more easily understand their children's doctors. Also included are bullet points that summarize topics and "Did You Know" boxes that describe particularly interesting, important, or surprising facts. The many illustrations, sidebars, and tables and the comprehensive index aid in locating and understanding the material.

No book can replace the expertise of an experienced heath care practitioner. This book is meant to supplement that relationship, not replace it. As a source of reliable information, *The Merck Manual of Children's Health* can help parents communicate better with the health care practitioners who care for their children.

The strength of this book ultimately derives from the efforts of the contributors, whose names are included following the table of contents, and the consulting editor. They deserve a degree of thanks that cannot be adequately expressed here.

We welcome all comments and suggestions.

Justin L. Kaplan, MD
Robert S. Porter, MD

Special Note to Readers

The contributors, reviewers, editors, and publisher have made extensive efforts to ensure that the information is accurate and conforms to the standards accepted at the time of publication. However, constant changes in information resulting from continuing research and clinical experience, reasonable differences in opinions among authorities, unique aspects of individual situations, and the possibility of human error in preparing such an extensive text require that the reader exercise judgment when making decisions and consult and compare information from other sources. In particular, the reader is advised to discuss information obtained in this book with a doctor, pharmacist, nurse, or other health care practitioner.

Contents

Part II Emergencies

Part III Medical Problems

EDITORS

Justin L. Kaplan, MD
Merck & Co., Inc. and Adjunct Clinical Associate Professor, Department of Emergency Medicine, Jefferson Medical College

Robert S. Porter, MD
Merck & Co., Inc. and Clinical Assistant Professor, Department of Emergency Medicine, Jefferson Medical College

---

CONSULTING EDITOR

Peter G. Szilagyi, MD, MPH
Professor of Pediatrics and Chief of General Pediatrics, University of Rochester Medical Center

---

EDITORIAL AND PRODUCTION STAFF

Executive Editor	Keryn A.G. Lane
Senior Staff Writer	Susan T. Schindler
Senior Staff Editor	Susan C. Short
Staff Editor	Michelle A. Steigerwald
Textbook Operations Manager	Diane C. Zenker
Senior Project Manager	Diane Cosner-Bobrin
Manager, Electronic Publications	Barbara Amelia Nace
Executive Assistant	Jean Perry
Merck Publisher	Gary Zelko
Merck Publishing Group Staff	Pamela J. Barnes-Paul, Leta Bracy, Jeanne Nilsen

---

ACKNOWLEDGMENTS

We thank Yasmin Suzanne N. Senturias, MD, and Francoise Thierfelder, MD, who assisted with the initial preparation of the chapter "Normal and School-Aged Children." We also thank Matthew J. Stiller, MD, who assisted with the initial preparation of the topic "Acne."

Contributors

Richard W. Besdine, MD
Professor of Medicine, Greer Professor of Geriatric Medicine, and Director, Division of Geriatrics (Medicine) and of Center for Gerontology and Healthcare Research, Brown Medical School

Ann S. Botash, MD
Professor of Pediatrics, State University of New York, Upstate Medical University

Thomas G. Boyce, MD
Assistant Professor of Pediatrics, Mayo Clinic College of Medicine; Consultant in Pediatric Infectious Diseases, Mayo Clinic

J. Raymond Buncic, MD
Professor of Ophthalmology, University of Toronto; Ophthalmologist-in-Chief, Hospital for Sick Children

Mary T. Caserta, MD
Associate Professor of Pediatrics, University of Rochester School of Medicine & Dentistry; Attending Physician, Golisano Children's Hospital at Strong

Robert B. Cohen, DMD
Clinical Assistant Professor, Tufts University School of Dental Medicine

Eve R. Colson, MD
Associate Professor of Pediatrics, Yale University School of Medicine; Director of Well Newborn Nursery, Yale-New Haven Children's Hospital

Norman L. Dean, MD
Pulmonologist, Internal Medicine, Geriatrics, North Carolina Department of Corrections; Director of Airway Clinics, North Carolina Correctional Institution for Women

Elizabeth A. Erwin, MD
Fellow, University of Virginia

E. Dale Everette, MD
Professor of Medicine, University of Missouri-Columbia

Eugene P. Frenkel, MD
Professor of Medicine and Radiology, Patsy R. and Raymond D. Nasher Distinguished Chair in Cancer Research; Elaine Dewey Sammons Distinguished Chair in Cancer Research in honor of Eugene P. Frenkel, MD; and A. Kenneth Pye Professorship in Cancer Research, Harold C. Simmons Comprehensive Cancer Center, The University of Texas Southwestern Medical Center at Dallas

Mitchell H. Friedlaender, MD
Adjunct Professor, The Scripps Research Institute, Head of Ophthalmology, Scripps Clinic

John P. Glazer, MD
Director, Pediatric Psychiatry Consultation-Liaison Service, Department of Psychiatry and Psychology, Cleveland Clinic

Barry Steven Gold, MD
Associate Professor of Medicine, Johns Hopkins University School of Medicine; Assistant Professor, Division of Emergency Medicine, Department of Surgery, University of Maryland School of Medicine

Nicholas Jospe, MD
Professor of Pediatrics, Department of Pediatrics, University of Rochester School of Medicine and Dentistry

Justin L. Kaplan, MD
Clinical Associate Professor of Emergency Medicine, Jefferson Medical School; Senior Assistant Editor, The Merck Manuals, Merck & Co., Inc.

Cheryl M. Kodjo, MD, MPH
Senior Instructor in Pediatrics and Adolescent Medicine, University of Rochester

Arthur E. Kopelman, MD
Professor of Pediatrics and Neonatology, The Brody School of Medicine at East Carolina University

David N. Korones, MD
Associate Professor of Pediatrics, Oncology, and Neurology, University of Rochester School of Medicine and Dentistry

Nancy Ebbesmeyer Lanphear, MD
Associate Professor of Pediatrics; Developmental and Behavioral Pediatrician, Cincinnati Children's Hospital Medical Center

Ruth A. Lawrence, MD
Professor of Pediatrics, Obstetrics and Gynecology, University of Rochester School of Medicine and Dentistry; Director of Normal Newborn Nursery, Strong Memorial Hospital

Gregory S. Liptak, MD, MPH
Professor of Pediatrics, Upstate Medical University; Chief, Center for Neurodevelopmental Pediatrics

John T. McBride, MD
Professor and Interim Chair of Pediatrics, Northeast Ohio College of Medicine; Interim Chair, Department of Pediatrics, Akron Children's Hospital

Daniel L. Menkes, MD
Associate Professor of Neurology, University of Tennessee, Health Sciences Center at Memphis

Joel L. Moake, MD
Professor of Medicine, Baylor College of Medicine; Associate Director, Biomedical Engineering Laboratory, Rice University

John D. Norante, MD
Associate Professor of Otolaryngology, University of Rochester Medical Center

J. D. Overton, DDS
Private Dental Practice, Biloxi

Elizabeth J. Palumbo, MD
Private Practice, The Pediatric Group, Fairfax

Richard D. Pearson, MD
Professor of Medicine and Pathology; Senior Associate Dean for Education, University of Virginia School of Medicine

Hart Peterson, MD
Clinical Professor of Neurology in Pediatrics (Retired), Cornell University Medical College; Attending Neurologist & Pediatrician (Retired), New York Hospital

Sidney F. Phillips, MD
Professor of Medicine (Emeritus), Mayo Clinic, Rochester

Thomas A.E. Platts-Mills, MD
Professor of Internal Medicine and Microbiology and Head of Asthma and Allergic Disease Center, University of Virginia

Douglas J. Pritchard, MD
Consultant of Orthopedic Surgery and Oncology, Mayo Foundation, Rochester

William O. Robertson, MD
Professor of Pediatrics, University of Washington; Medical Director, Washington Poison Center

Beryl J. Rosenstein, MD
Professor of Pediatrics, Johns Hopkins University School of Medicine; Johns Hopkins Hospital, Cystic Fibrosis Center

Thomas M. Rossi, MD
Professor of Pediatrics, Division of Gastroenterology and Nutrition, University of Rochester School of Medicine and Dentistry

Michael Rubin, MD
Professor of Clinical Neurology, Weill Cornell College of Medicine; Director, Neuromuscular Service & EMG Laboratory, New York Presbyterian Hospital-Cornell Medical Center

Charles A. Schiffer, MD
Professor of Medicine and Oncology, Wayne State University School of Medicine

H. Ralph Schumacher, Jr., MD

Professor of Medicine, University of Pennsylvania School of Medicine

E. Richard Stiehm, MD

Professor of Pediatrics, David Geffen School of Medicine at University of California, Los Angeles, Division of Immunology, Allergy, Rheumatology, Mattel Children's Hospital at University of California

Albert J. Stunkard, MD

Professor of Psychiatry, University of Pennsylvania

Stephen Brian Sulkes, MD

Professor of Pediatrics, Strong Center for Developmental Disabilities, Golisano Children's Hospital at Strong, University of Rochester School of Medicine and Dentistry

Moira Szilagyi, MD

Associate Professor of Pediatrics, University of Rochester; Medical Director of Foster Care, Monroe County Health Department

Geoffrey A. Weinberg, MD

Professor of Pediatrics, University of Rochester School of Medicine and Dentistry; Director, Pediatric HIV Program, Golisano Children's Hospital at Strong

Barbara Braunstein Wilson, MD

Edward P. Cawley Associate Professor of Dermatology, University of Virginia

Committed to Providing Medical Information: Merck and The Merck Manuals

In 1899, the American drug manufacturer Merck & Co. first published a small book titled *Merck's Manual of the Materia Medica*. It was meant as an aid to physicians and pharmacists, reminding doctors that "Memory is treacherous." Compact in size, easy to use, and comprehensive, *The Merck Manual* (as it was later known) became a favorite of those involved in medical care and others in need of a medical reference. Even Albert Schweitzer carried a copy to Africa in 1913, and Admiral Byrd carried a copy to the South Pole in 1929.

By the 1980s, the book had become the world's largest selling medical text and was translated into more than a dozen languages. While the name of the parent company has changed somewhat over the years, the book's name has remained constant, known officially as *The Merck Manual of Diagnosis and Therapy* but usually referred to as *The Merck Manual* and sometimes "The Merck."

In 1990, the editors of *The Merck Manual* introduced *The Merck Manual of Geriatrics*. This new book quickly became the best-selling textbook of geriatric medicine, providing specific and comprehensive information on the care of older people. The 3rd edition was published in five languages. The creation of this book reflects Merck's commitment to the world's aging population and the company's desire to improve geriatric care globally.

In 1997, *The Merck Manual of Medical Information–Home Edition* was published. In this revolutionary book, the editors translated the complex medical information in *The Merck Manual* into plain language, producing a book meant for all those people interested in medical care who did not have a medical degree. The book received critical acclaim and sold over 2 million copies. *The Second Home Edition* was released in 2003 and continued Merck's commitment to providing comprehensive, understandable medical information to all people.

The Merck Manual of Health & Aging, published in 2004, continued Merck's commitment to education and geriatric care, providing information on aging and the care of older people in words understandable by the lay public.

As part of its commitment to ensuring that all who need and want medical information can get it, Merck provides the content of these Merck Manuals on the web (visit www.merckmanuals.com) for free. Registration is not required, and use is unlimited. The web publications are continuously updated to ensure that the information is as up-to-date as possible.

Merck also supports the community of chemists and others with the need to know about chemical compounds with *The Merck Index*. First published in 1889, this publication actually predates *The Merck Manual* and is the most widely used text of its kind. *The Merck Veterinary Manual* was first published in 1955. It provides information on the health care of animals and is the pre-eminent text in its field.

The Merck Manual of Children's Health, published in 2007, is the latest book in the venerable tradition of The Merck Manuals. Adapted from *The Second Home Edition*, *The Merck Manual of Children's Health* is a complete resource for information about child growth and development and the common problems and medical disorders that affect children.

Merck & Co., Inc. is one of the world's largest pharmaceutical companies. Merck is committed to providing excellent medical information and, as part of that effort, continues to proudly provide all of The Merck Manuals as a service to the community.

Part I

Growth, Development, and Age-Related Problems

CHAPTER 1

Children's Health— An Introduction

Health care practitioners often consider the health care of children by age-specific groups. A newborn, or neonate, is up to 1 month old. An infant is age 1 month to 1 year. Young children are 1 to 4 years old. Older children are 5 to 10 years old. Adolescence usually encompasses age 10 through 21 years. Society uses additional and sometimes different terms. A toddler is usually considered to be about 15 months to about 3 years of age. A tween is an older child who has not yet become a teenager (age 13). Most people consider adolescence to end when a child turns 18.

Children develop physically, intellectually, behaviorally, emotionally, and socially at different rates. They go through growth spurts and plateaus. Intellectual, emotional, or social development almost never keeps strict pace with physical development, and vice versa. Although a child's development is usually continuous, temporary pauses may occur in a specific area or particular function, such as speech. In addition, children can temporarily regress developmentally if they undergo significant stress.

Choosing a Health Care Practitioner

Choosing a health care practitioner is an important decision. There are four basic types of qualified practitioners: pediatricians, family practice doctors, nurse practitioners, and physician assistants.

Doctors who specialize in the care of children are pediatricians. Pediatrics is the medical specialty fully focused on the physical, emotional, and social health of children from birth through adolescence or 21 years. Pediatricians complete 4 years of medical school followed by 3 years of pediatric residency. To be board-certified, a pediatrician must pass an examination given by the American Board in Pediatrics and recertify by passing an examination every 7 years. Some pediatricians complete additional training (usually 3 years) in a subspecialty area, for example, hematology or emergency medicine. Pediatricians who specialize in the care of newborns, usually premature newborns, are called neonatologists. Pediatricians who specialize may still provide some general care for children.

Family practice doctors complete 3 years of residency after medical school. The training includes several months in many areas of medicine, such as internal medicine, orthopedics, and pediatrics. After residency, most take an examination to be board-certified by the American Board of Family Medicine. To maintain their certification, they must pass periodic recertification examinations. Family practice doctors are qualified to care for patients of all ages, so a child would be able to see the same doctor from birth through adulthood. A family practice doctor who cares for all family members knows the family's medical history and may be aware of family issues that can affect the child's health. Some family practice doctors limit the number of children they see or have a policy of not taking newborns or infants as patients.

Pediatric nurse practitioners generally have a master's degree in nursing and training in taking medical histories, performing physical examinations on children, making medical diagnoses, and providing counseling and treatment. Pediatric nurse practitioners sometimes spend more time discussing health and child care issues with parents than doctors do. Pediatric nurse practitioners work closely with doctors in hospitals, clinics, and private practices. If nurse practitioners encounter a complex medical problem, they consult a doctor.

Physician assistants (PAs) practice medicine under the supervision of a physician. They complete a full-time education program (usually 2 years in length) and must pass a national certification examination to obtain a license. Every 6 years, they must pass a

SOME CONSIDERATIONS WHEN CHOOSING A PRACTICE

Office hours: Are evening or weekend hours offered?

Solo vs. group practice: If it is a solo practice, who provides back-up coverage (for example, when the usual doctor is on vacation or otherwise unavailable)? If it is a group practice, who are the other doctors?

Hospital affiliation: Will the doctor come to the hospital to examine the baby after birth? Who will care for a hospitalized child?

Questions: How does the office handle questions during and after hours? Are routine questions answered only during certain restricted hours? Is an advice line or web site available? How quickly does the doctor on call return phone calls? Is email an option?

Emergencies: Does the practice handle emergencies, or will the child be referred to an emergency department or urgent care center? Does it depend on whether the emergency occurs during office hours?

Testing: Can office personnel take blood and urine samples for laboratory tests in the office, or does the child need to be referred to a special center? How are test results communicated? Are parents told to assume results are normal if office personnel do not contact a parent?

Payment: What is the practice policy about payment? What are the fees for services? Do office personnel have difficulty working with some insurance plans?

Referrals: How are referrals to specialists handled? For example, does the practitioner call the specialist, or do the parents?

Personality: Does the health care practitioner view parents as partners in the child's care? Does the practitioner seem patient and willing to explain things carefully?

Office staff: Is the staff polite and friendly to people in the waiting room and on the phone? Are there special experts within the office, such as psychologists, nutritionists, or social workers?

Environment: Are there many children waiting to be seen? Is the waiting area clean and child-friendly? Are there separate sick and well child waiting areas?

recertification examination. They receive training to take medical histories, examine and treat patients, order and interpret laboratory tests and x-rays, and make diagnoses. They also can treat minor injuries that require suturing, splinting, and casting. In nearly all states, PAs may prescribe drugs.

A good time to begin searching for a health care practitioner is about 3 months before a baby is expected. An obstetrician or other doctor, nurse-midwife, relatives, friends, neighbors, and coworkers may have a recommendation. Parents new to a geographic area may want to contact area hospitals or medical schools for recommendations or ask nurses or doctors where they take their children. The American Academy of Pediatrics and the American Academy of Family Physicians can provide lists of board-certified pediatricians and family doctors.

Choosing a health care practitioner before the baby is born is ideal. Parents must feel comfortable with the practitioner's personality, office staff, location, and environment. Many practitioners allow prenatal appointments to allow parents to ask questions and get acquainted with the office staff. Some schedule group appointments so that many new parents can learn about their practice at the same time.

Visits to a Health Care Practitioner

Visits to a child's health care practitioner are usually classified as "sick child" or "well child." Sick-child visits involve some sort of illness or injury and, increasingly, management of a chronic developmental, behavioral, or mental health problem. Appointments for sick or injured children are usually available fairly quickly.

Well-child visits, also called preventive health care visits, involve periodic regular check-ups to make sure the child is developing and growing normally. These visits also aim to provide certain kinds of preventive care, such as counseling, screening for certain disorders, and providing vaccinations. Well-child visits are scheduled as far in advance as possible. Typically, well-child visits are frequent during the first year of life, taking place several days after birth, at 1 or 2 weeks of age, and at 2, 4, 6, 9, and 12 months. After that, visits are recommended at 15, 18, and 24 months of age, then yearly throughout childhood and adolescence.

Using a graph, the doctor plots the child's height, weight, and, for the first 18 months, head circumference measurements. Where the child's growth falls on the graph compared to that of other children is discussed as a "percentile." For example, if the child is in the 75th percentile for height that means that, out of a typical group of 100 children, the child would be taller than about 75 of them. Normally, percentiles for height and weight are reasonably similar. A high percentile for weight and a low percentile for height might mean that the child is overweight. Doctors also look to see if children consistently stay in a percentile as they grow. A sudden change, especially a significant movement down, might mean that the child is not growing or gaining weight as expected.

During a well-child visit, the doctor conducts a complete physical examination and assesses whether the child is developing appropriately by noting speech, fine motor skills, gross motor skills, and other developmental milestones. For example, to assess fine motor skills, the doctor may ask an 18-month-old to make a tower with 4 blocks. To assess flexibility and balance, which are gross motor skills, the doctor may ask a 4-year-old to hop on one foot. Age-appropriate questions are asked about the child's behavior and sleep patterns. Nutrition and exercise are discussed, and guidance is given if needed. Well-child visits are also key times for communication. In addition to receiving information about normal development, nutrition, sleep, and safety, parents have an opportunity to discuss their specific concerns. Concerns about behavior and discipline are common.

Communicating With the Health Care Practitioner

Actively participating in a child's health care helps ensure that the child receives the best care possible. The health care practitioner should be a good listener who is responsive to the parents' concerns. Parents should not feel too intimidated to ask questions. Also, parents should be open to what the practitioner recommends, even if it is contrary to a parent's expectations. For example, some parents expect antibiotics to be prescribed for infectious illnesses. However, for a common cold or mild ear infection, an antibiotic may not be recommended because antibiotics may not help, may make future infections more difficult to treat, and always carry some risk. Similarly, for infants and very young children who have colds, use of drugs, even those available over the counter, to treat symptoms may not be worth the risks of serious side effects. As another example, the practitioner may be concerned about the child becoming overweight before the parent becomes concerned about it. These visits are excellent opportunities to improve the health of the child through prevention and early detection of problems or potential problems.

Preparation for all doctor visits is important. For a well-child visit, having questions and concerns written down ahead of time makes them more likely to be asked or expressed. Although a doctor appreciates having an informed parent, the doctor's time is somewhat limited, so long discussions or evaluations of magazine articles or web printouts may not be possible. Many doctors can provide informational brochures about specific topics or can recommend some reliable health resources and web sites. The American Academy of Pediatrics (www.aap.org) is one reliable resource. For a sick-child visit, specific information about the child's condition before the visit is important. Details about symptoms—for example, how many times the child vomited, whether the child had a fever and what the temperature was, or whether diarrhea occurred—help the doctor assess the child's condition.

To get the most out of the time with a doctor, distractions such as cell phone calls should be avoided. Other children should be left with a spouse, babysitter, or relative, if possible. Generally, a parent should stick with the reason for the visit. For example, a sick-child visit is not the time to seek advice about discipline or behavior problems.

Adolescents become more and more responsible for their own health. They may prefer to speak to the practitioner privately when dealing with topics such as puberty and sexuality. A common and recommended practice is for health care practitioners to speak privately with adolescents about health care topics, so the parent may be asked to leave the examination room.

Childhood Dental Care

Parents also need to choose a dentist. Many general dentists care for children. However, some dentists specialize in children's dental care. These pediatric dentists receive 2 or 3 years of training in children's dental problems after completing 4 years of dental school. Children need to visit a dentist twice a year for routine care, beginning when the first tooth appears (usually between 6 and 12 months of age). Routine visits are for preventive care, which usually includes examinations, instructions on dental health, cleaning the teeth, and, at certain times, x-rays. Many children need to take supplemental fluoride, have fluoride applied to the teeth in the dental office (topical fluoride, usually applied using gels or foams), or have a coating applied to the teeth that helps prevent cavities (sealants). The web site of the American Academy of Pediatric Dentistry (www.aapd.org) has useful information and instructions on how to find a pediatric dentist.

Drug Treatment in Children

Drug treatment in children differs from that in adults, most obviously because it is usually based on the child's weight. Also, doses (and dosing intervals), even when adjusted for weight, differ because of age-related variations in drug absorption, distribution, metabolism, and elimination. Thus, parents cannot assume that a child's dose is proportional to an adult's; for example, that a 15-pound child requires 1/10 the dose of a 150-pound adult.

Adverse Drug Reactions

Adverse drug reactions are uncomfortable or dangerous side effects of drugs. Most adverse drug reactions in children are mild. Common mild reactions include digestive disturbances, fatigue, malaise (a general feeling of illness or discomfort), and changes in sleep patterns. Many disappear when the drug is stopped or the dose is changed. Some gradually subside as the body adjusts to the drug. Severe reactions may be life threatening and are relatively rare.

Infants and very young children are at high risk of adverse drug reactions because their capacity to metabolize and sometimes eliminate drugs is not fully developed. For example, newborns cannot metabolize and eliminate some anticonvulsants, pain relievers, and antibiotics. Doses may need to be much lower than in adults, or sometimes the drug cannot be taken at all. If tetracycline antibiotics are given to infants and young children during the period when their teeth are being formed (up to about age 8), tooth enamel may become permanently discolored. Children under age 18 are at risk of Reye's syndrome if they are given aspirin while they have influenza or chickenpox.

Drug Allergies

In contrast to other types of adverse drug reactions, the number and severity of allergic reactions do not correlate with the amount of drug taken. For a child who is allergic to a drug, even a small amount of the drug can trigger an allergic reaction. These reactions range from minor and simply annoying to severe and life threatening and may include some of the following:

- Skin rashes and itching
- Constriction of the airways and wheezing
- Swelling of tissues (such as the larynx and glottis), which impairs breathing
- A fall in blood pressure, sometimes to dangerously low levels

Drug allergies cannot be anticipated because reactions occur after a child has been previously exposed to the drug one or more times without any allergic reaction. Before prescribing a new drug, doctors usually ask if the child has any known drug allergies.

Drug Poisoning

Drug poisoning (see page 225), also called overdose toxicity, refers to serious, often harmful, and sometimes fatal toxic reactions to an accidental overdose of a drug (because of a doctor's, pharmacist's, or parent's error or because of a young child's curiosity).

Adherence to Drug Treatment

Taking drugs as prescribed is called adherence (compliance). Adherence is often poor for various reasons. Sometimes parents do not understand a doctor's instructions. Also, parents forget, on average, about half the information 15 minutes after meeting with a doctor. They remember the first third of the discussion best and remember more about diagnosis than about the details of treatment. Some drugs are very expensive. The more doses needed per day and the longer a drug needs to be taken, the less likely is adherence. For example, adherence is much more likely when a drug needs to be taken once per day than when a drug needs to be taken 4 times per day. In a study of children who had streptococcal infections and who were supposed to take a 10-day course of penicillin, 56% had stopped taking the drug by the third day, 71% by the sixth day, and 82% by the ninth day.

Young children may have difficulty swallowing pills and may resist taking liquid medicine that tastes bad. Older children often resist drugs or regimens (for example, insulin for diabetes or a metered-dose inhaler for asthma) that require them to leave their classes or activities or that make them appear different from their peers. Adolescents may express rebellion and assert independence from parents by not taking their drugs.

To improve the chances of adherence, parents can ask health care practitioners to try to keep the treatment plan simple and provide written instructions. When a drug is too expensive, a parent can request that the practitioner consider using a less expensive drug. A parent should repeat the dosing instructions to the practitioner to make sure that the instructions have been understood. The parent can ask the practitioner whether a drug prescribed for a young child tastes good and whether a liquid preparation or chewable tablet can be used. The practitioner or parent should ask older children and adolescents whether they will adhere to treatment and then discuss ways to minimize barriers to adherence.

Alternative Medicine and Children

While alternative medicine generally falls outside the conventional medical system of doctors and hospitals, alternative medicine varies widely. Few studies have been done to prove the effectiveness of alternative therapies, and the majority of alternative medicine practices are not covered by health insurance. The lack of scientific studies means that some potential problems associated with the alternative therapy may be difficult to identify. The few studies that have been conducted have used adults as subjects. Little or no research has been conducted on children.

Unlike prescription and over-the-counter drugs, herbal remedies are not subjected to extensive tests before they are marketed, and they do not have to adhere to quality standards. The amount of herb can vary, with some capsules containing much less of the active herb than stated on the label. Depending on where the herb originated, there might also be other plants mixed in or contaminants such as pesticides or heavy metals. Some herbal remedies can cause health problems, such as high blood pressure, liver damage, or allergic reactions, in children.

However, not all alternative medicine involves ingestion of a product. For example, one major group of therapies involves relaxation, meditation, and self-regulation. There is some evidence for the effectiveness of such therapies and little evidence for their harm as long as necessary traditional therapies are not excluded. Anxiety-related health problems are common among children and adolescents, and these types of alternative therapies can be quite helpful. Therefore, many experts are increasingly calling such therapies complementary medicine since they complement traditional health care. Studies have shown that a large number of families, including children, use some type of complementary therapy.

Although many states license certain alternative medicine specialists, such as acupuncturists or massage therapists, other alternative medicine practitioners may have no oversight and no standards of treatment. Using an alternative therapy for a serious chronic or acute condition can jeopardize the child's health, particularly if the alternative therapy is used instead of a traditional therapy with proven effectiveness. Parents who want to try alternative medicine should first discuss the proposed treatment with their child's doctor to make sure that it is not dangerous and that it will not conflict with traditional care. The child's doctor may have helpful information about alternative treatment options. Discussion with a health care practitioner helps ensure the best possible care for each child.

CHAPTER 2

Normal Newborns and Infants

The successful transition of a fetus, immersed in amniotic fluid and totally dependent on the placenta for nutrition and oxygen, to a squalling, air-breathing baby is a source of wonder. Healthy newborns (age birth to 1 month) and infants (age 1 month to 1 year) need good care to ensure their normal development and continued health.

Initial Care

Immediately after a baby is born, the doctor or nurse gently clears mucus and other material from the mouth, nose, and throat with a suction bulb. The newborn is then able to take a breath. Two clamps are placed on the newborn's umbilical cord, side by side, and the umbilical cord is then cut between the clamps. The newborn is dried and laid carefully on a sterile warm blanket or on the mother's abdomen.

The newborn is then weighed and measured. The doctor examines the newborn for any obvious abnormalities or signs of distress; a full physical examination comes later. The newborn's overall condition is recorded at 1 minute and at 5 minutes after birth using the Apgar score. A low Apgar score is a sign that the newborn is having difficulty and may need extra assistance with breathing or blood circulation. However, contrary to what people may think, babies with

DID YOU KNOW?

- Breastfeeding can be attempted shortly after birth.
- A newborn with a low Apgar score is not more likely to develop cerebral palsy or permanent disabilities.
- All babies are born with low levels of vitamin K and thus are given an injection of vitamin K.

low Apgar scores are not more likely to develop certain problems, such as cerebral palsy or permanent disabilities.

Keeping the newborn warm is critical. As soon as possible, the newborn is wrapped in lightweight clothing (swaddled), and the head is covered to reduce the loss of body heat. A few drops of an antibiotic are placed into the eyes to prevent infection from any harmful organisms that the newborn may have had contact with during delivery.

The mother, father, and newborn usually recover together in the delivery room. If the delivery is in a birth center, the mother, father, and newborn remain together in the same room. If the mother is

Cutting the Umbilical Cord

Soon after a baby is born, two clamps are placed on the umbilical cord, and the cord is cut between the clamps. The clamp on the cord's stump is removed within 24 hours after birth. The stump should be kept clean and dry. Some doctors recommend applying an alcohol solution to the stump daily. The stump falls off on its own in a week or two.

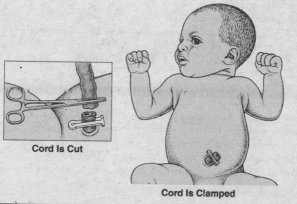

Cord Is Cut

Cord Is Clamped

breastfeeding, she can put the infant to her breast within the first 30 minutes. Because all babies are born with low levels of vitamin K, a doctor or nurse administers an injection of vitamin K to prevent bleeding (hemorrhagic disease of the newborn).

About 6 hours or more after birth, the newborn is bathed.

Physical Examination

The doctor usually gives the newborn a thorough physical examination within the first 12 to 24 hours of life. The examination begins with a series of measurements, including weight, length, and head circumference. The average weight at birth is 7 pounds, and the average length is 20 inches. Then the doctor examines the baby's skin, head and face, heart and lungs, nervous system, abdomen, and genitals.

The skin is usually reddish, although the fingers and toes may have a bluish tinge because of poor blood circulation during the first few hours. Rarely, the skin has several hard lumps (subcutaneous fat necrosis) where pressure from bones destroyed some fatty tissue. Such lumps are most common on the head, cheek, and neck—particularly if forceps were used during delivery. The lumps may break through to the skin surface, releasing a clear yellow fluid, but they usually heal fairly quickly.

A normal head-first delivery leaves the head slightly misshapen for several days. The bones that form the skull overlap, which allows the head to become compressed for delivery. Some swelling and bruising of the scalp is typical. Sometimes bleeding from one of the bones of the skull and its outer covering causes a small bump on the head that disappears in a few weeks. When the baby is delivered buttocks first (breech delivery), the head usually does not become misshapen; however, the buttocks, genitals, or feet may become swollen and bruised instead.

DID YOU KNOW?

- A head that is misshapen because of passage through the birth canal regains its typical appearance after a few days.
- All states require some blood tests to detect diseases in the newborn, but the required tests vary by state.

Pressure during a vaginal delivery may bruise the newborn's face. In addition, compression through the birth canal may make the face initially appear asymmetrical. This asymmetry sometimes results when one of the nerves supplying the face muscles is damaged during delivery. Recovery is gradual over the next few weeks.

The doctor listens to the heart and lungs through a stethoscope to detect any abnormality. The doctor inspects the newborn's skin color and general condition for any sign of a problem. The strength of the pulse is checked.

The doctor looks for any abnormalities of the nerves and tests the baby's reflexes. Three commonly identified reflexes are the Moro, rooting, and sucking reflexes.

Many serious disorders that are not apparent at birth can nonetheless be detected by blood tests in newborns. Because of this, all states require a number of blood tests in newborns. Early diagnosis and prompt treatment can reduce or prevent disorders that may interfere with an infant's healthy development.

The doctor examines the general shape of the abdomen and also checks the size, shape, and position of internal organs, such as the kidneys, liver, and spleen. Enlarged kidneys may indicate an obstruction to the outflow of urine.

The doctor examines the flexibility and mobility of the arms, legs, and hips, and checks to see if the newborn has dislocated hips.

The doctor examines the genitals to ensure the urethra is open and in the proper location. In a boy, the testes should be present in the scrotum. In a girl, the labia are prominent; exposure to the mother's hormones causes them to be swollen for the first few weeks. The doctor examines the anus to make sure the opening is not sealed shut.

THREE COMMON REFLEXES OF NEWBORNS

In the **Moro reflex,** when the newborn is startled, the arms and legs swing out and forward in a slow movement with fingers outstretched. In the **rooting reflex,** when either side of the mouth is touched, the newborn turns his head toward that side. This reflex enables the newborn to find the nipple. In the **sucking reflex,** when an object is placed in the newborn's mouth, sucking begins immediately.

First Few Days

Immediately after a normal birth, the mother and father are encouraged to hold their newborn. Breastfeeding may be initiated at this time if the mother plans to breastfeed. Some experts believe that early physical contact with the newborn helps establish bonding. However, parents can bond well with their newborn even when the first hours are not spent together (for example, if the newborn is ill). Mother and baby spend a day or two in the hospital during which time new parents are taught to feed, bathe, and dress the baby and become familiar with the baby's activities and sounds. In the United States, discharge from the hospital within 24 hours is common.

The plastic cord clamp on the umbilical cord is removed within 24 hours after birth. Some doctors recommend that the stump be moistened daily with an alcohol solution to speed drying and reduce the chance of infection; an antibiotic ointment should not be used because it can prolong the drying process. The stump falls off on its own in a week or two.

Circumcision, if desired, generally is performed within the first few days of life before the newborn is discharged. The decision about having a newborn circumcised usually depends on the parents' religious beliefs or personal preferences. The main medical reason for circumcision is to remove an unusually tight foreskin that is obstructing the flow of urine. Although circumcised males also have a lower risk of cancer of the penis and urinary tract infections, these risks can be minimized with proper hygiene. Circumcision can result in infection, excessive bleeding, scarring, and very rarely in accidental amputation of the penis tip. About 2 to 20 boys per 1,000 require a minor surgical procedure later to correct various problems resulting from circumcision. An equal number of uncircumcised males require a circumcision later in life.

DID YOU KNOW?

- Most newborns have a mild skin rash.
- Every newborn should pass meconium (a sticky greenish black bowel movement) within the first 24 hours.
- In most boys, there is no compelling medical reason for circumcision.

Circumcision should not be performed if the boy has not voided, or if the penis is abnormal in any way, because the foreskin may be needed for any plastic surgical repair that may be needed later. Circumcision must be delayed if, during the pregnancy, the mother had been taking drugs that increase the risk of bleeding, such as anticoagulants or aspirin; the doctor waits until all such drugs have been eliminated from the newborn's circulation.

Most newborns have a mild skin rash sometime during the first week after birth. The rash usually appears in areas of the body rubbed by clothing—the arms, legs, and back—and rarely on the face. It tends to disappear on its own without treatment. Applying lotions or powders, using perfumed soaps, and putting plastic pants over the diapers are likely to make the rash worse, especially in hot weather. Dryness and some skin peeling often occur after a few days, especially in the creases at the wrists and ankles.

Newborns who are otherwise normal may develop a yellow color to their skin (jaundice) after the first day. Jaundice that appears before 24 hours of age is of particular concern.

The first urine produced by a newborn is concentrated and often contains chemicals called urates, which can turn the diaper pink. If a newborn does not urinate within the first 24 hours of life, the doctor tries to find out why. Delay in starting to urinate is more common in boys.

The first bowel movement is a sticky greenish black substance (meconium). Every baby should pass meconium within the first 24 hours after birth. Failure to pass a bowel movement is usually caused by a hardened plug of meconium inside the baby's intestine, which can usually be removed by one or more gentle enemas. A birth defect may cause a more serious blockage.

After a few days in the hospital, the newborn is able to go home. Having a new baby in a household requires a great deal of adjustment for all involved. For a household that has had no children, changes in lifestyle may be dramatic. When other children are present, jealousy can be a problem. Preparing other children for the newcomer and being careful to pay attention to them and include them can ease the transition. Pets may also need some extra attention to help them adjust to the baby. In some cases, keeping pets away from the baby may be necessary.

Feeding

A normal newborn has active rooting and sucking reflexes and can start eating immediately after birth. If the baby has not been placed at the mother's breast immediately after birth, feedings are ordinarily begun within 4 hours after birth.

DID YOU KNOW?

- A newborn can begin eating immediately after birth.
- Most babies swallow air as they are feeding; burping the baby helps expel the air.

Most babies swallow air along with their milk. Because they cannot usually burp on their own, parents help the baby expel the air by holding him upright leaning against the parent's chest with his head against the shoulder and patting gently on his back. The combination of patting and pressure against the shoulder usually leads to an audible burp, often accompanied by spitting up of a small amount of milk. Many experts recommend exclusive breast or formula feeding for 6 months.

BREASTFEEDING

Breast milk is the ideal food for newborns. Besides providing the necessary nutrients in the most easily digestible and absorbable form, breast milk contains antibodies and white blood cells that protect the baby against infection. Breast milk favorably changes the pH of the stool and intestinal flora, thus protecting the baby against bacterial diarrhea. Because of the protective qualities of breast milk, many types of infections occur less often in babies who are breastfed rather than bottle-fed. Breastfeeding offers many advantages to the mother as well; for example, it helps her to bond and feel close to her baby in a way that bottle-feeding cannot. About 60% of mothers in the United States breastfeed their babies, and this proportion is steadily increasing. Mothers who work may breastfeed while at home and have the baby bottle-feed pumped breast milk or formula during the hours they are away. Most doctors recommend giving daily vitamin D supplements to breastfed infants after 2 months of age.

A thin yellow fluid, called colostrum, flows from the nipple before breast milk is produced. Colostrum is rich in calories, protein,

Positioning a Baby to Breastfeed

The mother settles into a comfortable, relaxed position. She may sit or lie almost flat, and she may hold the baby in several different positions. A mother should find the position that works best for her and her baby. She may wish to alternate among different positions.

A common position is holding the baby on the lap so that the baby is stomach to stomach with the mother. The mother supports the baby's neck and head with her left arm when the baby is feeding on the left breast. The baby is brought to the level of the breast, not the breast to the baby. Support for the mother and the baby is important. Pillows can be placed behind the mother's back or under her arm. Placing her feet on a footstool or coffee table may help keep her from leaning over the baby. Leaning over may strain her back and result in sore nipples. A pillow or folded blanket may be placed under the baby for added support.

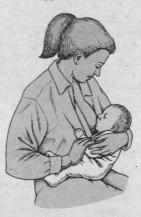

and antibodies. The antibodies are absorbed directly into the body from the stomach, protecting the baby against many infections.

To begin breastfeeding, the mother settles into a comfortable, relaxed position, either seated or lying almost flat, and turns from one side to the other to offer each breast. The baby faces the mother. The mother supports her breast with her thumb and index finger on top and other fingers below and brushes her nipple against the middle of the baby's lower lip. This stimulates the baby to open his mouth—the rooting reflex—and grasp the breast. As the mother eases the nipple and areola into the baby's mouth, she makes sure the nipple is centered, which helps keep the nipple from becoming sore. Before removing the baby from the breast, the mother breaks the suction by inserting her finger into the baby's mouth and gently pressing the baby's chin down. Sore nipples result from poor positioning and are easier to prevent than to cure.

Initially, the baby tends to feed for several minutes at each breast. The resulting reflex (let-down reflex) in the mother triggers milk production. The production of milk depends on sufficient suckling time, so feeding times should be long enough for milk production to be fully established. During the first few weeks, the infant should be encouraged to nurse on both breasts with each feeding; however, some infants fall asleep while feeding at the first breast. The breast used last should be used first for the next feeding. For a first baby, full milk production is usually established in 72 to 96 hours. Less time is needed for subsequent babies. If the mother is particularly tired during the first night, one middle of the night feeding may be replaced with water. However, no more than 6 hours should elapse between feeding sessions during the first few days in order to stimulate the production of breast milk. Feeding should be on demand (the baby's, that is) rather than by the clock. Similarly, the length of each breastfeeding session should be adjusted to meet the baby's needs. Babies often nurse 8 to 12 times in a 24-hour period, but the frequency of breastfeeding varies widely.

DID YOU KNOW?

- Breast milk is the best food for infants.
- Exclusively breastfeeding for the first 6 months may be ideal.
- Most doctors recommend giving daily vitamin D supplements to breastfed infants after 2 months of age.

The mother should take the baby, especially a first baby, to the doctor 3 to 5 days after delivery so that the doctor can find out how breastfeeding is going and answer any questions. A doctor may need to see the baby earlier if the baby was discharged within 24 hours, is not feeding well, or if the parents have a particular concern. Because mothers cannot tell exactly how much milk a baby takes, doctors use frequency of feeding and weight gain to tell whether milk production is adequate. Babies that are hungry and feed every hour or two but fail to gain weight appropriately for their age and size are probably not getting enough milk.

When to stop breastfeeding (wean the infant) depends on the needs and desires of both mother and baby. Breastfeeding exclusively for at least 6 months and breastfeeding along with solid foods until age 12 months are considered most desirable. Gradual weaning over weeks or months is easier for both the baby and mother than stopping suddenly. Mothers initially replace one to three breastfeeding sessions a day with a bottle or cup of fruit juice, expressed breast milk, or formula. Some feedings, particularly those at mealtimes, should be replaced by solid food. Learning to drink from a cup is an important developmental milestone, and weaning to a cup can be completed by age 10 months. Mothers gradually replace more and more breastfeedings, although many infants continue one or two breastfeedings daily until the age of 18 to 24 months or longer. When breastfeeding continues longer, the child should also be eating solid foods and drinking from a cup.

BOTTLE-FEEDING

In the hospital, newborns are usually fed shortly after delivery, then ideally on demand thereafter. During the first week after birth, babies take 1 or 2 ounces at a time, gradually increasing to 3 or 4 ounces about 6 to 8 times a day by the second week. Parents should not urge newborns to finish every bottle but, rather, allow them to take as much as they want whenever they are hungry. As infants grow, they drink larger amounts, consuming up to 6 to 8 ounces at a time by the third or fourth month. The proper position for babies who are bottle-feeding is semi-reclining or sitting up. Babies should not bottle-feed lying flat on their backs because milk may flow into the nose or the eustachian tube. Older infants who are able to hold their own bottles should not be put to sleep holding the bottle because the continuous exposure to milk or juice can damage their teeth and lead to cavities.

DID YOU KNOW?

- Infants who are bottle feeding should be semi-reclining or sitting up, not lying on their back.
- Parents should not encourage infants to finish every bottle.
- Formula can be warmed before feeding, but only to body temperature.

Commercial baby formulas containing a proper balance of nutrients, calories, and vitamins are available in ready-to-feed, sterile bottles, cans of concentrated formula that must be diluted with water, and powder. Formulas are available both with and without an iron supplement; most doctors recommend a formula that contains iron. Parents who use concentrated formula or powders must carefully follow the directions for preparation on the container. Formulas are usually made from cow's milk, although soy-based formulas—which are of benefit to infants who cannot tolerate cow's milk—are also available. There are no long-term health differences in infants fed either type of formula. Plain cow's milk, however, is not an appropriate food during the first year of life.

To minimize the infant's exposure to microorganisms, formula must be fed from a sterile container. Disposable plastic liners eliminate the need to sterilize bottles. Nipples for the bottles should be sterilized in a pot of boiling water for 5 minutes. Parents should warm formula feedings to body temperature. Filled bottles—or formula containers, if disposable liners are used—are placed in a *warm* water bath and allowed to come to body temperature. Babies may be seriously burned if formula is too hot, so parents need to shake the bottle gently to even out the temperature and then check the temperature by placing a few drops on the sensitive skin inside their wrist. Formula at body temperature should feel neither warm nor cold to the touch. Microwave ovens may dangerously overheat formula and are not recommended for warming formula or baby food.

The size of the nipple opening is important. In general, formula should drip slowly out of a bottle held upside down. Larger, older infants want larger volumes of liquid and can tolerate a larger nipple opening.

STARTING SOLID FOODS

The time to start solid food depends on the infant's needs and readiness. Generally, infants need solids when they are large enough to need a more concentrated source of calories than formula. This is recognized when an infant takes a full bottle and is satisfied, but then is hungry again in 2 or 3 hours. This typically occurs by the age of 6 months. Infants younger than this cannot easily swallow solid food, although some can swallow solids at younger ages if the food is placed on the back of the tongue. Some parents coax very young infants to eat large amounts of solid food so that they will sleep through the night. This is unlikely to work, and forcing an infant to eat early can cause aspiration pneumonia and feeding problems later. Many infants take solids after a breastfeeding or bottle-feeding, which both satisfies their need to suck and quickly relieves their hunger.

Infants develop food allergies or intolerance easier than older children or adults. If many different foods are given in a brief period, it is difficult to tell which one may have been responsible for a reaction. Because of this, parents should introduce new foods one at a time, no more than one new food a week. Once it is clear a food is tolerated, another one may be introduced.

DID YOU KNOW?

- Typically solids are introduced when an infant is about 6 months old.
- Infants should not be coaxed to eat large amounts of solid foods.
- Foods should be introduced one at a time so that food allergies or intolerance can be identified.
- Infants can begin to learn to self-feed by about 6 to 9 months.
- Small, hard foods (such as peanuts, raw carrots, candies, and small crackers) can cause choking in the first year of life and should be avoided.
- Honey can cause botulism in the first year of life and should be avoided.

Single-grain cereals are begun first, followed by fruits and vegetables. Meats, which are a good source of protein, should be introduced later, after about 7 months. Many infants initially reject meat.

The food should be offered on a spoon so that the infant learns the new feeding technique. By age 6 to 9 months, infants are able to grasp food and bring it to their mouths, and they should be encouraged to help feed themselves. However, babies easily choke on food in small, hard bits (such as peanuts, raw carrots, candies, and small crackers), so these foods should be avoided. Pureed home foods are less expensive than commercial baby foods and offer adequate nutrition.

Although infants enjoy sweet foods, sugar is not an essential nutrient and should be given only in small quantities, if at all.

Sweetened dessert baby foods have no benefit for babies. Honey must be avoided during the first year because it may contain the spores of Clostridium botulinum, which are harmless to older children and adults but can cause botulism in infants.

Stools and Urine

Infants typically urinate 15 to 20 times per day. The urine varies in color from nearly clear to dark yellow. Stools vary a great deal from infant to infant in frequency, color, and consistency depending on the nature of the individual infant and the contents of his diet. The number of times infants defecate varies—from once every other day to 6 or 8 times a day. Stool consistency ranges from firm and formed to soft and runny. Stool color ranges from mustard yellow to dark brown. The stool of breastfed babies tends to be softer and of lighter color than that of formula-fed babies.

DID YOU KNOW?

- Infants may defecate as infrequently as once every other day and as often as eight times per day.
- Baby powders that contain talcum should be avoided.

Diapers must be changed often to keep the underlying skin dry. Wet skin chafes more easily than dry skin and is more likely to develop diaper rash. Modern, super-absorbent disposable diapers contain a layer of gel that absorbs liquid and keeps it away from the skin. These diapers keep skin drier than cloth diapers after small to moderate amounts of urine, but diapers of any type should be changed when the skin is exposed to wetness. Bacteria normally present in stool can break down urea, a substance in urine, resulting in an alkaline pH that irritates the skin, so diapers should be checked frequently for stool and changed immediately. There are several environmental considerations related to diapers. Disposable diapers consume larger amounts of material than cloth and contribute a significant volume of landfill waste. Cloth diapers consume large amounts of energy and chemicals in the laundering process.

Baby powders help keep skin dry when the baby is sweating slightly, but they do not help keep the skin dry from urine or stool and are not essential. Powder made of talcum may cause lung problems if inhaled by infants, so parents should purchase baby powders that contain cornstarch instead.

Sleeping

Because the nervous system of newborns is immature, newborns sleep a great deal, but often only for an hour or two at a time, independent of day or night. By 4 to 6 weeks of age, many infants are on a cycle of waking for 4 hours and sleeping for 4 hours. Only by 2 to 3 months of age are infants capable of adopting a pattern of nighttime sleeping. By 1 year of age, most infants sleep 8 to 9 hours continuously through the night.

DID YOU KNOW?

- Infants should sleep on their back.
- Newborns sleep only an hour or two at a time.
- So that they can eventually sleep alone, infants should be encouraged from an early age to fall asleep on their own, not in a parent's arms.

Parents can assist infants to sleep at night by handling and stimulating the child less in the late evening and keeping the child's room dark at night, which is important in the development of normal vision. Infants should be encouraged at an early age to fall asleep on their own and not in a parent's arms. In this way, they will be able to quiet themselves when they wake in the middle of the night.

To minimize the risk of sudden infant death syndrome (SIDS), infants should sleep on their back, rather than on their stomach. This recommendation has helped reduce the incidence of SIDS in recent years. Also, infants should not sleep with soft pillows, toys, or heavy blankets, which may obstruct their breathing.

Physical Development

An infant's physical development depends on heredity, nutrition, and environment. Physical and psychologic abnormalities can also influence growth. Optimal growth requires optimal nutrition and health.

DID YOU KNOW?

- Infants normally regain their birth weight by 2 weeks of age, then gain about an ounce per day for the next 6 weeks, followed by a pound per month.

A newborn normally loses 5 to 7% of his birth weight during the first few days of life. Newborns who are breastfeeding can lose up to 7% of their birth weight. This weight is regained by the

An Infant's First Year: Physical Development

During the first year of life, an infant's weight and length are charted at each doctor's visit to make sure that growth is proceeding at a steady rate. Percentiles are a way of comparing infants of the same age. For an infant at the 10th percentile for weight, 10% of infants weigh less and 90% weigh more. For an infant at the 90th percentile, 90% of infants weigh less and 10% weigh more. For an infant at the 50th percentile, 50% of infants weigh less and 50% weigh more. Of more significance than the actual percentile is any significant change in percentile between doctor's visits.

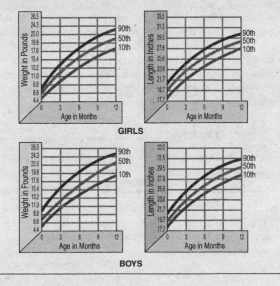

GIRLS

BOYS

end of the first 2 weeks as the newborn starts to eat more. After this, an infant typically gains around one ounce per day during the first two months, and a pound per month after that. This generally results in a doubling of birth weight by age 5 months and a tripling by 1 year. An infant's length increases about 30% by age 5 months and more than 50% by 1 year.

Different organs grow at different rates. For example, the reproductive system has a brief growth spurt just after birth, then changes very little until just before puberty. In contrast, the brain grows almost exclusively during the early years of life. At birth, the brain is one fourth of its future adult size. By 1 year, the brain is three fourths of its adult size. The kidneys function at the adult level by the end of the first year.

Lower front teeth begin to appear at the age of 5 to 9 months. Upper front teeth begin to appear at 8 to 12 months.

Behavioral, Social, and Intellectual Development

The rate of behavioral, social, and intellectual development varies considerably from infant to infant. Some infants develop faster, although certain patterns may run in families, such as late walking or talking. Environmental factors, such as lack of sufficient stimulation, can slow development; conversely, stimulation can hasten development. Physical factors, such as deafness, can also slow development. Although a child's development is usually continuous, temporary pauses may occur in the development of a particular function, such as speech.

DID YOU KNOW?

- Temporary pauses may occur in the development of a particular function.

Crying is one means of communication. Infants cry because they are hungry, uncomfortable, distressed, and for many other reasons that may not be obvious. Infants cry most—typically 3 hours a day—at 6 weeks of age, usually decreasing to an hour a day by 3 months of age. Parents generally offer a crying baby

An Infant's First Year: Developmental Milestones

AGE	MILESTONE
1 month	Brings hands toward eyes and mouth
	Moves head from side to side when lying on stomach
	Follows an object moved in an arch about 6 inches above face to the midline (straight ahead)
	Responds to a noise in some way, such as startling, crying, or quieting
	May turn toward familiar sounds and voices
	Focuses on a face
3 months	Raises head 45 degrees (possibly 90 degrees) when lying on stomach
	Opens and shuts hands
	Pushes down when feet are placed on a flat surface
	Swings at and reaches for dangling toys
	Follows an object moved in an arch above face from one side to the other
	Watches faces intently
	Smiles at sound of mother's voice
	Begins to make speechlike sounds
5 months	Holds head steady when upright
	Rolls over one way, usually from stomach to back
	Reaches for objects
	Recognizes people at a distance
	Listens intently to human voices
	Smiles spontaneously
	Squeals in delight
7 months	Sits without support
	Bears some weight on legs when held upright
	Transfers objects from hand to hand
	Looks for dropped object
	Responds to own name
	Responds to being told "no"
	Babbles, combining vowels and consonants
	Wiggles with excitement in anticipation of playing
	Plays peekaboo
9 months	Works to get a toy that is out of reach
	Objects if toy is taken away
	Crawls or creeps on hands and knees
	Pulls self up to standing position
	Stands holding on to someone or something
	Says "mama" or "dada" indiscriminately

(Continued)

An Infant's First Year: Developmental Milestones (Continued)

AGE	MILESTONE
12 months	Gets into a sitting position from stomach
	Walks by holding furniture; may walk one or two steps without support
	Stands for a few moments at a time
	Says "dada" and "mama" to the appropriate person
	Drinks from a cup
	Claps hands and waves bye-bye

food, change the diaper, and look for a source of pain or discomfort. If this does not work, holding or walking with the baby sometimes helps. Occasionally nothing works. Parents should not force food on a crying infant, who will readily eat if hunger is the cause of his distress.

Promoting Optimal Development

Babies obviously require appropriate food and shelter for their physical growth. If their physical needs are met regularly and consistently, infants quickly learn that their caretaker is a source of satisfaction, creating a firm bond of trust and attachment.

In addition to their physical needs, babies need affection and stimulation to develop emotionally and intellectually. Some parents provide a highly organized, structured environment for their infant using a variety of toys and gadgets. However, the particular content of the environment is less important than the existence of a pleasant, positive interaction enjoyed by both parent and baby. Parents who provide smiling faces, frequent amiable speech, physical contact, and love but who do not buy a variety of toys and gadgets are not shortchanging their baby's development.

Preventive Health Care Visits

Healthy infants should be seen by their doctor often during the first year of life. Visits typically take place within a few days of birth if the newborn is discharged within 24 hours and is breastfeeding, by 1 to 2 weeks, and at 2, 4, 6, 9, and 12 months of age. During these visits, the doctor monitors the child's growth and development by measuring the child's length, weight, and head circumference, and asking the parents questions about various developmental milestones. The doctor also examines the child for various abnormalities, including signs of hereditary disorders. Hearing and vision are tested. An infant who was born prematurely (after spending less than 37 weeks in the uterus) is regularly examined for retinopathy of prematurity, an eye disease (see page 59). Finally, on many visits, the doctor vaccinates the child against various illnesses.

Preventive health care visits also allow the doctor to educate the parents about eating, sleeping, behavior, child safety, and good health habits. In addition, the doctor advises the parents what changes to expect in their child by the next visit.

Vaccinations

Children should be vaccinated to protect them against infectious diseases. Vaccination has eliminated smallpox and nearly eliminated other infections, such as polio and measles, that were once common childhood scourges in the United States. Despite this success, it is important for health care professionals to continue to vaccinate children. Many of the diseases prevented by vaccination are still present in the United States and remain common in other parts of the world. These diseases can spread rapidly among unvaccinated children, who will also be at particular risk when traveling to other countries.

DID YOU KNOW?

- All evidence indicates that benefits of vaccination outweigh the risks.
- Evidence indicates that vaccination does not produce autism.
- Vaccination need not be delayed if the infant has a mild illness.

No vaccine is 100% effective and 100% safe. A few vaccinated children fail to become immune, and a few develop side effects. Most often, the side effects are minor, such as pain at the injection site, an itchy rash, or a mild fever. Very rarely, there are more serious problems. The oral polio vaccine, which is made of a live, weakened virus, can cause polio if the weakened virus mutates, which happens once in every 2.4 million children. Although this is an extremely small chance, it led doctors in the

United States to recommend completely switching to an inactivated, injectable polio vaccine. Also, the pertussis component of the older whole-cell diphtheria, tetanus, and pertussis vaccine (DTP) occasionally led to febrile seizures (see page 152) in about 1 in 10,000 children, and more rarely confusion and fainting. Although these episodes do not leave any lasting damage, they are distressing to parents. Doctors now recommend a newer version of the vaccine using *acellular* pertussis (DTaP), which has a much lower chance of these reactions. Similarly, febrile seizures have occurred in about 3 in 10,000 children following the measles, mumps, rubella vaccine. Although the public press has reported concerns that the measles, mumps, rubella vaccine may produce autism, scientific evidence shows that this does not happen.

To help people evaluate the risks of vaccination, the federal government requires doctors to give parents a *Vaccine Information Statement* each time a child is vaccinated. Also, a federal Vaccine Injury Compensation Program was established to compensate anyone suffering permanent consequences of vaccination. This program was established because doctors and health authorities want as many children as possible to be protected from life-threatening diseases. When considering the risks of vaccination, parents must remember that their child is at much greater risk from the diseases that vaccinations prevent.

Recommended Immunization Schedule for Children*

AGE	VACCINES RECOMMENDED	DOSE NUMBER AND TOTAL NUMBER OF DOSES
Birth to 2 months	Hepatitis B	1 of 3
1 to 4 months	Hepatitis B	2 of 3
2 months	Diphtheria, tetanus, acellular pertussis (DTaP)	1 of 5
	Haemophilus influenzae type b (Hib)	1 of 4
	Inactivated poliovirus (IPV)	1 of 4
	Pneumococcal conjugate vaccine (PCV)	1 of 4

Recommended Immunization Schedule for Children* (Continued)

AGE	VACCINES RECOMMENDED	DOSE NUMBER AND TOTAL NUMBER OF DOSES
4 months	DTaP	2 of 5
	Hib	2 of 4
	IPV	2 of 4
	PCV	2 of 4
6 months	DTaP	3 of 5
	Hib	3 of 4
	PCV	3 of 4
6 to 18 months	Hepatitis B	3 of 3
	IPV	3 of 4
6 to 23 months	Influenza†	Given annually
12 to 15 months	Hib	4 of 4
	Measles, mumps, rubella	1 of 2
	PCV	4 of 4
	Varicella (chickenpox)	1 of 1
12 to 23 months	Hepatitis A	1 of 2
15 to 18 months	DTaP	4 of 5
18 to 30 months	Hepatitis A	2 of 2
4 to 6 years	DTaP	5 of 5
	IPV	4 of 4
	Measles, mumps, rubella	2 of 2
	Meningococcal conjugate vaccine‡	1 of 1
	Tetanus toxoid, reduced diphtheria toxoid, acellular pertussis (Tdap)	Follow-up doses are needed every 10 years

*Changes to this schedule that are under consideration include giving rotavirus vaccine, giving a second dose of varicella (chickenpox) vaccine, and, for girls, giving human papillomavirus vaccine.

†Given to children with heart or lung disease (including asthma), diabetes, kidney failure, or sickle cell disease and to those children whose immune system is compromised (including children with HIV infection and those undergoing chemotherapy).

‡Unvaccinated adolescents who are entering high school (about age 15) or college should also receive this vaccine

Most doctors follow the vaccination schedule recommended by the American Academy of Pediatrics, which begins during the first week after birth with the hepatitis B vaccine. The recommended ages for vaccinations should not be construed as absolute. For example, 2 months can mean 6 to 10 weeks. Although parents should try to have their children vaccinated according to the schedule, a slight delay does not interfere with the final immunity achieved nor does it entail restarting the series of injections from the beginning. Vaccination need not be delayed, however, if the infant has a slight fever from a mild infection such as an ordinary cold. Some vaccines are recommended only under special circumstances.

More than one vaccine may be given during a visit to the doctor's office, but several vaccines are often combined into one injection, for example, pertussis, diphtheria, tetanus, and *Haemophilus influenzae* type b vaccines. A combination vaccine reduces the number of injections needed but does not reduce the safety or effectiveness of the vaccines.

CHAPTER 3

Problems in Newborns

After birth, a newborn may have a number of problems. Some problems may be due to difficulties during the birthing process; many of these problems affect the newborn's ability to breathe properly. A newborn may be bigger or smaller than usual or suffer from problems affecting blood, such as the levels of sugar (glucose) in the blood being too high or too low. Birth defects may be present (see page 76). A newborn may have problems due to the mother's health and health habits, such as smoking or use of alcohol or drugs (especially those given immediately before birth. Infection may pass from mother to child, either during pregnancy or during delivery.

DID YOU KNOW?

- When newborns must be kept in incubators, the sound of their mother's voice, which they heard before birth, can comfort them.

Doctors may be able to anticipate many problems by monitoring fetal growth and development, particularly using ultrasound. Many newborns with problems are cared for in a neonatal intensive care unit (NICU).

WHAT IS A NEONATAL INTENSIVE CARE UNIT?

Often referred to as the "NICU," this specialized facility brings together the medical team and technology needed to care for newborns with a variety of disorders. The largest group of newborns needing such care is those born very prematurely. Other newborns need care because of sepsis or pneumonia, respiratory disorders, and birth defects that require surgery. These newborns are cared for in incubators to keep them warm or they are placed under overhead radiant warmers, which provide warmth while allowing increased access to the newborn by the staff. Newborns are attached to monitors that can continuously measure their heart rate, breathing, blood pressure, and oxygen levels in the blood. They may have catheters placed inside the artery and vein running inside the umbilical cord to permit continuous blood pressure monitoring, to allow repeated blood sampling, and to administer intravenous fluids and drugs.

The NICU tends to be a very busy place. This is sometimes at odds with the parents' need for time and space to become acquainted with their newborn, to learn the newborn's personality, likes and dislikes, and ultimately to learn any special care that they will need to provide at home. A trend to make the NICU quieter and to design units to allow families increased privacy has helped. Visiting hours have been greatly extended so that families can spend much more time with their newborns, and often hospitals arrange for nearby sleeping facilities for the parents.

Sometimes, parents feel that they have little to offer to a newborn in a NICU. However, their presence, including stroking, speaking, and singing, is very important. The newborn has heard his mother's voice even before birth and is accustomed to it, and he often responds better to his own parents' attempts to calm him. Skin-to-skin contact (also termed kangaroo care), in which the newborn is allowed to lie directly on the mother or father's chest, is comforting to the newborn and enhances bonding. Increasing evidence indicates that premature newborns fed breast milk are significantly protected from developing necrotizing enterocolitis and infections and that breastfeeding is otherwise beneficial.

Parents need to be kept informed of their newborn's condition and the doctor's plans, as well as the expected course and time of discharge. Regular meetings with the doctors and nurses are essential. Many NICUs have a social worker who can help to see that parents are kept informed.

Birth Injury

Birth injury is damage sustained during the birthing process, usually occurring during transit through the birth canal.

- Many newborns have minor injuries.
- Rarely, nerves are damaged or bones are broken.
- Most injuries resolve on their own.

A difficult delivery, with the risk of injury to the fetus, may occur if the birth canal is too small or the fetus is too large (as sometimes occurs when the mother has diabetes). Injury is also more likely if the fetus is lying in an abnormal position before birth. Overall, the rate of birth injuries is much lower now than in previous decades.

Many newborns experience minor injuries from the birthing process, with swelling or bruising only in certain areas.

Head Injury: In most births, the head is the first part to enter the birth canal and experiences much of the pressure during the delivery. Swelling and bruising are not serious and resolve within a few days. Cephalohematoma is a bleeding injury in which a soft lump forms over the surface of one of the skull bones but below its thick fibrous covering. A cephalohematoma does not need treatment and disappears over weeks to months.

Very rarely, one of the bones of the skull may fracture. Unless the fracture forms an indentation (depressed fracture), it heals rapidly without treatment.

Nerve Injury: Rarely, nerve injuries may occur. Pressure to the facial nerves caused by forceps can result in weakness of the muscles on one side of the face. This injury is evident when the newborn cries and the face appears asymmetric. No treatment is needed, and the newborn usually recovers within a few weeks.

In a difficult delivery of a large infant, some of the larger nerves to one or both of the newborn's arms can be stretched and injured. Weakness (paralysis) of the newborn's arm or hand results. Occasionally, the nerve going to the diaphragm (the muscle that separates the organs of the chest from those of the abdomen) is damaged, resulting in paralysis of the diaphragm on the same side. In this case, the newborn may have difficulty breathing. Injury of the nerves to the newborn's arm and diaphragm usually resolves completely within a few weeks. Extreme movements at the shoulder should be avoided to allow the nerves to heal. Very rarely, the arm and possibly the diaphragm remain weak after several months. In this case, surgery may be needed to reattach torn nerves.

COMMON BIRTHMARKS AND MINOR SKIN CONDITIONS IN THE NEWBORN

There are a number of skin conditions that are considered normal in the newborn. There may be bruises or marks from forceps on the newborn's face and scalp, or bruising of the feet following a breech delivery, all of which resolve within just a few days. Pink marks that are due to dilated capillaries under the skin may be seen on the forehead just above the nose, in the upper eyelids, or at the back of the neck (where it is called "stork-bite"). This type of birthmark fades as the infant grows but in some people remains as a faint mark that becomes brighter when the person becomes excited or upset. Some newborns have a few acne pimples, especially over the cheeks and forehead. These go away, and the only recommended action is to keep the skin clean and not to use creams or lotions.

Milia are tiny, pearly white cysts that are normally found over the nose and upper cheeks. Milia become smaller or disappear over a period of weeks. Similar white cysts are sometimes found on the gums in the midline of the roof of the mouth (Epstein's pearls) and are also of no consequence.

Mongolian spots are bluish gray, flat areas that usually occur over the lower back or buttocks. At first glance they appear to be bruises but are not. They are usually seen in black or Asian newborns and are of no consequence.

A **"strawberry hemangioma"** is a common birthmark. It is a flat, slightly pink or red area anywhere on the skin. Over a period of weeks, it becomes darker red and also becomes raised up over the surface of the skin, appearing much as a strawberry. After several years, strawberry hemangiomas shrink and become fainter, so that by the time the child reaches school age, most are no longer visible. For this reason, surgery is not needed.

Injuries to the spinal cord due to overstretching during delivery are extremely rare. These injuries can result in paralysis below where the injury occurred. Damage to the spinal cord is often permanent.

Bone Injury: Rarely, bones may be broken (fractured) during a difficult delivery. A fracture of the collarbone is most common and generally heals without complications. Fractures of other bones in the newborn are splinted and almost always heal completely and rapidly.

Prematurity

A premature newborn is a newborn delivered before 37 weeks in the uterus; such a newborn has underdeveloped organs.

- Early prenatal care reduces the risk of a premature birth.
- Because many organs are underdeveloped, premature newborns have difficulty breathing and feeding and are prone to bleeding in the brain, infections, and other problems.
- Premature newborns may need to be hospitalized for days, weeks, or months.
- Premature labor can sometimes be delayed by giving the mother drugs to slow or stop contractions.
- Most premature newborns grow up without any permanent problems.

About 8% of newborns are born prematurely (preterm). Many of these newborns are born just a few weeks early and do not experience problems related to their prematurity. However, the more prematurely newborns are born, the more they are prone to a number of serious and even life-threatening complications. Very premature birth is the single most common cause of death in the newborn. Also, newborns born very prematurely are at high risk for chronic problems, especially delayed development and learning disorders. Such disorders occur because the internal organs have not had time to develop adequately before birth.

The reason for a premature birth cannot usually be determined. However, the risk of premature birth is higher in women who are poor, have little education, and have poor nutrition or health or untreated illnesses or infections during pregnancy. The risk is lower in women who had early prenatal care. For unknown reasons, black women are significantly more likely than women of other racial groups to have a premature delivery. Other women at increased risk for premature delivery are those carrying more than one fetus and those who have serious or life-threatening disorders, including severe high blood pressure or kidney disease, preeclampsia or eclampsia, or infection of the uterus (chorioamnionitis).

DID YOU KNOW?

- Very premature birth is the most common cause of death in newborns.

Symptoms

Premature newborns usually weigh less than $5\frac{1}{2}$ pounds. Physical features help doctors determine the newborn's gestational age (length of time spent in the uterus after the egg is fertilized).

Underdeveloped Lungs: The lungs of the premature newborn may not have had enough time to develop fully before birth. Such newborns are likely to have respiratory distress syndrome. Respiratory distress syndrome occurs if the lungs are not mature enough to produce surfactant, a mixture of lipids (fats) and proteins that allows the air sacs of the lungs to remain open (see page 47).

Underdeveloped Brain: The part of the brain that controls regular breathing may be so immature that the newborn has inconsistent breathing, with short pauses in breathing or periods during which breathing stops for 20 seconds or longer (apnea). The parts of the brain that control the mouth and throat are immature so the newborn cannot suck and swallow normally and will have difficulty coordinating feeding with breathing.

Brain Hemorrhage: Newborns born very prematurely are at increased risk of bleeding (hemorrhage) in the brain. Bleeding typically begins in an area called the germinal matrix and may extend into spaces within the brain called the ventricles. This form of hemorrhage is most likely to occur in those born very prematurely (before 32 weeks of pregnancy) and if there were problems during labor or delivery or breathing problems (such as respiratory distress syndrome) after birth. Depending on the size of the hemorrhage, newborns may have no symptoms or may experience lethargy, seizures, or even persistent unconsciousness (coma). Newborns with small or moderate-sized hemorrhages usually develop normally. Those with very large hemorrhages are at higher risk of dying or of having learning disorders or other brain-related problems later in life.

Abnormal Blood Sugar: Because premature newborns have difficulty maintaining normal blood sugar (glucose) levels, they are often treated with intravenous glucose solutions or given small frequent feedings. Without regular intake of sugar, a newborn may develop low blood sugar levels (hypoglycemia). Most newborns with hypoglycemia do not develop symptoms. Others may become listless with poor muscle tone, feed poorly, or become jittery. Rarely, seizures may develop. These newborns are also prone to developing high blood sugar levels (hyperglycemia) if they receive too much sugar intravenously. Most newborns with hyperglycemia do not develop symptoms.

Underdeveloped Immune System: Newborns who are born very prematurely have low levels of antibodies, which cross the placenta from mother to the fetus during the latter part of pregnancy and offer protection from infection. Therefore, the risk of developing infections, especially infection in the blood (sepsis), is higher in premature newborns. The use of special devices for treatment, such as catheters and ventilators, further increases the newborn's risk of developing serious infections.

Underdeveloped Kidneys: Before delivery, waste products produced in the fetus are removed by the placenta and then excreted by the mother's kidneys. After delivery, the newborn's kidneys must take over these functions. Kidney function is poor in newborns who are born very prematurely but improves as the kidneys mature. A newborn with underdeveloped kidneys is likely to have difficulty regulating the amount of salt and water in the body.

Underdeveloped Digestive Tract and Liver: Initially premature newborns may have difficulty with feedings. Not only do they have immature sucking and swallowing reflexes, but also their small stomach empties slowly. Very premature newborns may develop a serious injury to the inner surface of the intestines (necrotizing enterocolitis—see page 60).

In premature newborns, the excretion of bilirubin may be impaired. Thus, premature newborns, even more than term new-

---

PHYSICAL FEATURES OF A PREMATURE NEWBORN

- Small size
- Large head relative to rest of the body
- Little fat under the skin
- Thin, shiny, pink skin
- Veins visible beneath the skin
- Few creases on soles of feet
- Scant hair
- Soft ears, with little cartilage
- Underdeveloped breast tissue
- Boys: Small scrotum with few folds. Testicles may be undescended in very premature newborns
- Girls: Labia majora not yet covering labia minora
- Rapid breathing with brief pauses (periodic breathing), often apnea spells (pauses lasting greater than 20 seconds)
- Weak, poorly coordinated sucking and swallowing reflexes
- Reduced physical activity (a premature newborn tends not to draw up the arms and legs as does a full-term newborn)
- Sleeping for most of the time

borns, tend to become jaundiced in the first few days after birth because of the build-up of bilirubin in their blood. Usually, the jaundice is mild and resolves as the newborn takes larger amounts of feedings and has more frequent bowel movements. Rarely, very high levels of bilirubin accumulate and put the newborn at risk for developing kernicterus, a form of brain damage caused by deposits of bilirubin in the brain.

Difficulty Regulating Body Temperature: Because premature newborns have a large skin surface area relative to their weight, they tend to lose heat rapidly, especially if they are in a cool room or if there is a draft. A lowering of body temperature results in a markedly increased rate of the body's metabolism, as the newborn attempts to maintain normal body temperature.

Prevention

The best way for premature birth to be prevented is for the expectant mother to take good care of her own health. She should eat a nutritious diet and avoid cigarettes, alcohol, and drugs. Ideally, she should receive early and regular prenatal care so that any complications of pregnancy can be recognized and treated. Any infection, such as a urinary tract infection, should be treated promptly. If it seems probable that early labor is about to start, an obstetrician may administer drugs (such as magnesium sulfate or ritodrine) to the mother to slow or stop contractions. Corticosteroids such as betamethasone or dexamethasone may also be given to the mother to accelerate maturation of the fetus's lungs. Corticosteroids also significantly reduce the risk of brain hemorrhage if the newborn is born prematurely.

Treatment and Prognosis

Treatment involves managing the complications, such as respiratory distress syndrome and high bilirubin levels. Very premature newborns are fed intravenously until they can tolerate tube feedings and finally feedings by mouth. A premature newborn may need to be hospitalized for days, weeks, or months. Over recent decades, the survival of premature newborns has improved dramatically. For most premature newborns, the long-term prognosis is very good, and they develop normally. However, those born extremely early (often before 28 weeks of pregnancy) are at an increased risk of death and of serious problems, including mental retardation, cerebral palsy, epilepsy, or blindness. Fortunately, only a minority of extremely premature newborns who survive have these problems. A larger percentage have normal intelligence, but many have learning disorders that eventually require special help.

Postmaturity

A postmature newborn is a newborn delivered after more than 42 weeks in the uterus.

- Near the end of a term pregnancy, the placenta shrinks, providing fewer nutrients and less oxygen to the fetus.
- A postmature fetus may not get enough oxygen during labor, sometimes causing fetal distress.
- Postmature newborns have dry, peeling, loose skin and may appear emaciated.
- Some newborns need resuscitation, but generally, treatment focuses on providing good nutrition and general care.

Postmature (postterm) delivery is much less common than premature (preterm) delivery. The reason for a pregnancy to continue beyond term is usually unknown.

Reduced function of the placenta is the greatest risk to fetuses who go beyond term. Near the end of a term pregnancy, the placenta begins to shrink. As it shrinks, the placenta becomes less able to provide adequate nutrients to the fetus. To compensate, the fetus begins to use its own fat and carbohydrates to provide energy. As a result, its growth rate slows, and occasionally its weight may decrease. If the placenta shrinks sufficiently, it may not provide adequate oxygen to the fetus, particularly during labor. A lack of adequate oxygen may result in fetal distress and, in extreme cases, may result in injury to the fetal brain and other organs. Fetal distress may cause the fetus to pass stools (meconium) into the amniotic fluid. The fetus may also take deep, gasping breaths triggered by the distress and thereby inhale the meconium-containing amniotic fluid into the lungs before or during birth. As a result, the newborn may have difficulty breathing after delivery (meconium aspiration syndrome).

Symptoms

A postmature newborn has dry, peeling, loose skin and may appear emaciated, especially if the function of the placenta was severely reduced. The newborn often appears alert. The skin and nail beds may be stained green if meconium was present in the amniotic fluid. A postmature newborn is prone to developing low blood sugar levels (hypoglycemia) after delivery, especially if oxygen levels were low during labor.

Treatment

The postmature newborn who experienced low oxygen levels and fetal distress may need resuscitation at birth. If meconium has been breathed into the lungs, a ventilator may be needed. Intravenous glucose solutions or frequent breast milk or formula feedings are given to prevent hypoglycemia.

If these problems do not occur, the major goal is to provide good nutrition and supportive care.

Small for Gestational Age

A newborn, whether delivered preterm, term, or postterm, whose weight is less than that of 90% of babies of the same gestational age at birth (below the 10th percentile) is considered small for gestational age.

- Newborns may be small because the parents are small or because the mother had a disorder, smoked cigarettes, used illicit drugs, or consumed alcohol during pregnancy.

There are several causes for this condition. In many cases, the newborn may be small simply because of genetic factors, such as having small parents (less commonly, a specific genetic syndrome associated with small stature may be involved). In other cases, the placenta may have functioned poorly, so that the fetus did not receive adequate nutrients and growth was impaired. This may happen if the mother has high blood pressure, preeclampsia, kidney disease, or long-standing diabetes. A viral infection, such as cytomegalovirus acquired before birth, may be responsible. Fetal growth may also have been impaired if the mother smoked or used alcohol or illicit drugs during the pregnancy. Unless they have a genetic syndrome or viral infection, most small-for-gestational-age newborns have no symptoms. If the fetal growth was impaired because of poor placental function and inadequate nutrition, the newborn's growth may accelerate when provided with good nutrition after delivery. Some small-for-gestational-age newborns remain small as children and adults.

Large for Gestational Age

A newborn, whether delivered preterm, term, or postterm, whose weight is above that of 90% of babies of the same gestational age at birth (above the 90th percentile) is considered large for gestational age.

- Newborns may be large because the parents are large or because the mother has diabetes.
- Delivery by cesarean section may be needed.
- These newborns may have low levels of glucose, requiring frequent feedings and sometimes intravenous glucose.

Some newborns are large for gestational age because of genetic factors, such as having large parents. Another cause is diabetes in the mother.

If the mother has diabetes during pregnancy, a large amount of glucose (sugar) crosses the placenta and results in high levels of glucose in the fetus's blood, with the release of increased amounts of insulin. The result is accelerated growth of the fetus, including almost all organs with the exception of the brain, which grows normally. Vaginal delivery of a very large-for-gestational-age fetus may be problematic, increasing the risk of injury. Therefore, such a fetus may have to be delivered by caesarean section.

The large-for-gestational-age newborn born to a diabetic mother typically has a florid (reddish) complexion and appears obese and sometimes lethargic. Large-for-gestational-age newborns born to mothers who do not have diabetes are large, but not reddish or lethargic. After birth, when the supply of glucose from the placenta stops, the continuing rapid production of insulin leads to low levels of glucose (hypoglycemia). Often hypoglycemia produces no symptoms. Sometimes, the newborn is listless, limp, or jittery. Despite their large size, newborns of diabetic mothers often do not feed well for the first few days. Occasionally, newborns born to diabetic mothers have an abnormally high red blood cell count. As the red blood cells are broken down, bilirubin is formed, and these newborns tend to have high bilirubin levels, resulting in jaundice (see page 62).

Large-for-gestational-age newborns born prematurely to diabetic mothers are also more likely to have immature lungs and to develop respiratory distress syndrome, even when born only a few weeks before full term. They also have a higher rate of birth defects than other newborns.

Testing the amniotic fluid in mothers with diabetes before delivery can be performed to determine lung maturity and the likelihood of the newborn developing respiratory distress syndrome after birth. If labor appears imminent, a corticosteroid may be given to increase lung maturity.

To treat hypoglycemia in the newborn, intravenous glucose or frequent feedings by mouth or by tube into the stomach are often needed. Treatment of other complications, such as respiratory distress syndrome, is needed.

Large-for-gestational-age newborns born to diabetic mothers are likely to be significantly overweight later in childhood and as adults, which puts them at risk for type 2 diabetes.

Respiratory Distress Syndrome

Respiratory distress syndrome is a breathing disorder of premature newborns in which the air sacs (alveoli) in a newborn's lungs do not remain open because the production of surfactant is absent or insufficient.

- Breathing is visibly labored or may not begin after birth.
- The skin turns blue, and without treatment, the syndrome may cause brain damage or death.
- The diagnosis is based on symptoms and chest x-ray results.
- If premature birth is imminent, doctors give the mother drugs to help the fetus's lungs mature.
- Newborns may be given supplemental oxygen or assistance breathing and a surfactant preparation.

For a newborn to be able to breathe easily, the air sacs in the lungs must be able to remain open and filled with air. Normally, the lungs produce a mixture of lipids (fats) and proteins called surfactant. Surfactant acts as a wetting agent and lines the surface of the air sacs, where it lowers the surface tension and allows the air sacs to remain open throughout the respiratory cycle. Usually, production of surfactant begins after about 34 weeks of pregnancy. The more premature the newborn, the greater the likelihood that respiratory distress syndrome will develop after birth. Respiratory distress syndrome occurs almost exclusively in premature newborns and is more common in those whose mother has diabetes.

Symptoms and Diagnosis

In an affected newborn, the lungs are stiff and the air sacs tend to collapse completely, emptying the lungs of air. In some very premature newborns, the lungs may be so stiff that the newborn is unable to begin breathing at birth. More commonly, the newborn tries to breathe, but because the lungs are so stiff, severe respiratory distress occurs. Respiratory distress is manifested by visibly labored breathing, including retractions of the chest below the rib cage, flaring of the nostrils during breathing in, and "grunting" during breathing out. Because a good portion of the lung is airless, the newborn has low blood oxygen levels, which cause a bluish discoloration to the skin (cyanosis). Over a period of hours, the respiratory distress tends to become more severe, as the small amount of surfactant in the lungs is used up and increasing numbers of air sacs collapse and also as the muscles used for breathing tire and become weak. Eventually, without treatment, the newborn may suffer damage to the brain and other organs from a lack of oxygen or may die.

Diagnosis of respiratory distress syndrome is based on the symptoms and on abnormal chest x-ray results in a premature newborn.

DID YOU KNOW?

- Newborns with lung problems may have bluish skin, breathe rapidly, draw the chest wall in when breathing in, and grunt when breathing out.
- Respiratory distress syndrome occurs almost exclusively in premature newborns.

Prevention and Treatment

The risk of respiratory distress syndrome is greatly reduced if delivery can be safely delayed until the fetal lungs have produced sufficient surfactant. The obstetrician can perform amniocentesis, in which some amniotic fluid is withdrawn into a syringe and analyzed for the adequacy of surfactant production. If production is not adequate but premature delivery cannot be avoided, the obstetrician may give the mother injections of a corticosteroid drug (betamethasone or dexamethasone). The corticosteroid crosses the placenta into the fetus and accelerates the production of surfactant. Within 48 hours of starting the injections, the fetal lungs mature to the point that respiratory distress syndrome will not develop after delivery or, if it does, is likely to be milder.

After delivery, a newborn with mild respiratory distress syndrome may require only supplemental oxygen, which is given through an oxygen hood or through a tube placed in the nose. A newborn with severe respiratory distress syndrome may require oxygen delivered by continuous positive airway pressure (CPAP—breathing spontaneously against positive pressure oxygen or air administered through tubes placed in both nostrils). In a very sick infant, a tube may need to be passed into the windpipe (intubation), and the infant's breathing supported with mechanical ventilation.

Use of a surfactant preparation can be lifesaving and reduces complications, such as rupture of the lungs (pneumothorax). The surfactant preparation acts in the same way that natural surfactant does. Surfactant may be given immediately after birth in the delivery room to attempt to prevent respiratory distress syndrome or in the early hours after birth to a premature newborn who already has symptoms of this disorder. A newborn who is intubated can receive surfactant through the tube in the windpipe.

Surfactant treatments may be repeated several times over the first days until respiratory distress syndrome resolves.

Transient Tachypnea

Transient tachypnea of the newborn (transient rapid breathing, neonatal wet-lung syndrome) is temporary difficulty with breathing and low blood oxygen levels due to excessive fluid in the lungs after birth.

- Affected newborns breathe rapidly and grunt when breathing out, and the skin may be bluish.
- Most of these newborns need supplemental oxygen, and some need assistance breathing.
- Most of these newborns recover completely in 2 to 3 days.

This disorder usually occurs in newborns born a few weeks before term or at term. It is more common after a caesarean section delivery. It is especially likely to occur if the mother has not been in labor before delivery (for example, a mother who has a scheduled caesarean section).

Before birth, the air sacs of the lungs are filled with fluid. Immediately after birth, the fluid must be cleared from the lungs so that the air sacs can fill with air and the newborn can establish normal breathing. Some of the fluid is squeezed out of the lungs by pressure on the chest during a vaginal delivery. More of the fluid is rapidly reabsorbed directly by the cells lining the air sacs and from which it is immediately transported into the bloodstream. If this fluid transfer does not occur rapidly, then the air sacs continue to be partially filled with fluid and the newborn has difficulty breathing.

A newborn with transient tachypnea has respiratory distress with rapid breathing, drawing in of the chest wall during breathing in and "grunting" during breathing out, and may develop a bluish discoloration of the skin (cyanosis) if the blood oxygen levels become low. A chest x-ray shows abnormal results.

Most newborns with transient tachypnea recover completely within 2 to 3 days. Treatment with oxygen is usually needed, although some newborns may need continuous positive airway pressure (CPAP—breathing spontaneously against positive pressure oxygen or air administered through tubes placed in the newborn's nostrils) or assistance with a ventilator.

Meconium Aspiration Syndrome

Meconium aspiration syndrome is respiratory distress in a newborn who has breathed (aspirated) meconium into the lungs before or around the time of birth.

- Affected newborns breathe rapidly and grunt when breathing out, and the skin may be bluish.
- The diagnosis is based on observing meconium in amniotic fluid at birth, respiratory distress in the newborn, and abnormal chest x-ray results.
- Immediate suctioning of the affected newborn's mouth, nose, and throat to remove meconium is followed by treatment with oxygen and sometimes use of a ventilator.

Meconium is the dark green fecal material that is produced in the intestines before birth. Normally, meconium is expelled after birth when a newborn starts to feed. However, in response to stress, such as an inadequate blood oxygen level, the fetus may pass meconium into the amniotic fluid. The same stress causes the fetus to take forceful gasps, so that the meconium-containing amniotic fluid may be breathed into the lungs. After delivery, the aspirated meconium may block the airways leading to portions of the newborn's lungs, which may cause them to collapse. Alternatively, when some airways are only partially blocked, air may be able to reach the parts of the lung beyond the block but may be prevented from being breathed out. Thus, the involved lung may become overexpanded. Progressive overexpansion of a portion of the lung can eventually result in rupture and then collapse of the lung. Air may then accumulate within the chest cavity around the lung (pneumothorax). Meconium breathed into the lungs may also cause inflammation of the lungs (pneumonitis).

Meconium aspiration syndrome is often most severe in post-mature newborns because the meconium is very concentrated in a smaller amount of amniotic fluid and it causes more irritation than in a term newborn (see page 44). Newborns with meconium aspiration syndrome are also at increased risk for developing persistent pulmonary hypertension.

An affected newborn suffers from respiratory distress, in which he breathes rapidly, draws in his lower chest wall while breathing in, and grunts during breathing out. The newborn's skin may be bluish (cyanotic) if the blood levels of oxygen are reduced.

A doctor makes the diagnosis based on the observation of thick meconium in the amniotic fluid at the time of birth, respiratory distress in the newborn, and abnormal chest x-ray results.

At delivery, if the newborn is covered with meconium, the newborn's mouth, nose, and throat are immediately suctioned to remove any meconium. If the newborn is lethargic or unresponsive, a tube may need to be passed into the windpipe to suction as much meconium as possible from the respiratory tract.

The newborn is treated with oxygen and placed on a ventilator if necessary. If the newborn needs intubation, then repeated suctioning is performed to try to remove more of the meconium. A newborn on a ventilator is observed closely for serious complications, such as pneumothorax or persistent pulmonary hypertension.

Most newborns with meconium aspiration syndrome survive. However, if the disorder is severe and especially if it leads to persistent pulmonary hypertension, it can be fatal.

Persistent Pulmonary Hypertension

Persistent pulmonary hypertension is a serious disorder in which the newborn's arteries to the lungs remain constricted after delivery, thus limiting the amount of blood flow to the lungs and therefore the amount of oxygen in the bloodstream.

- Causes include other lung disorders and certain drugs taken by the mother before delivery.
- Usually, breathing is rapid, and the skin is bluish.
- Diagnosis is by echocardiography.

- An environment with 100% oxygen, sometimes with a small amount of nitric acid, and possibly intravenous sodium bicarbonate help open the arteries.
- If these treatments are ineffective, extracorporeal membrane oxygenation (similar to using an artificial lung) can be used.

Normally, the blood vessels to the lungs are tightly constricted during fetal life. The lungs do not need much blood flow before birth because the placenta eliminates carbon dioxide and transports oxygen to the fetus. Immediately after birth, the umbilical cord is cut and the newborn's lungs must take over the role of oxygenating the blood and removing carbon dioxide. To achieve this, it is necessary not only that the fluid filling the air sacs be replaced by air, but that the arteries bringing blood to the lungs widen (dilate) so that an adequate amount of blood flows through the lungs.

In response to severe respiratory distress, or as a consequence of certain drugs taken by the mother before delivery (such as large doses of aspirin), the blood vessels to the lungs may not dilate as they normally should. As a result, there is insufficient blood flow to the lungs and not enough oxygen reaches the blood.

Persistent pulmonary hypertension is more common in newborns who are term or postterm and in newborns whose mothers were regular users of aspirin or indomethacin during pregnancy. In many newborns, the respiratory distress that initiates persistent pulmonary hypertension results from other lung diseases, such as meconium aspiration syndrome or pneumonia, but persistent pulmonary hypertension can also develop in newborns with no other lung disorder.

Symptoms and Diagnosis

Sometimes persistent pulmonary hypertension is present from birth; other times, it develops over the first day or two. Breathing is usually rapid, and there may be severe respiratory distress if the newborn has an underlying lung disease (see page 47). The most prominent feature is a bluish discoloration of the skin (cyanosis) due to low blood oxygen levels. Sometimes low blood pressure (hypotension) leads to symptoms such as weak pulses and a pale, grayish hue to the skin.

A doctor may suspect persistent pulmonary hypertension if the mother used aspirin or indomethacin during pregnancy or had a stressful delivery, or if the newborn has severe respiratory distress and measurement of oxygen levels is unexpectedly low. A chest x-ray is performed, but definitive diagnosis requires an echocardiogram.

Treatment

Treatment involves placing the newborn in an environment with 100% oxygen to breathe. Alternatively, a ventilator providing 100% oxygen may be needed. A high percentage of oxygen in the blood helps open the arteries going to the lungs. To make the blood slightly alkaline, which may also open these arteries, the newborn is often given intravenous sodium bicarbonate.

In more severe cases, a very small concentration of the gas nitric oxide may be added to the oxygen that the newborn is breathing. Inhaled nitric oxide opens the arteries in the newborn's lungs and reduces pulmonary hypertension. This treatment may be needed over several days. If all other treatments fail, extracorporeal membrane oxygenation (ECMO) can be used. In this procedure, blood from the newborn is circulated through a machine that adds oxygen and removes carbon dioxide and then returns the blood to the newborn. ECMO has been lifesaving, allowing many newborns to survive until the pulmonary hypertension resolves.

Pneumothorax

Pneumothorax is a collection of air within the chest (pleural) cavity surrounding a lung that develops when air leaks out of the lung.

- Pneumothorax is more likely to develop in newborns who have disorders that make the lungs stiff, who are treated with continuous positive airway pressure, or who must use a ventilator.
- The lung may collapse, breathing may be difficult, and blood pressure may decrease.
- Diagnosis is based on chest x-ray results.
- If symptoms occur, supplemental oxygen is given, or air is removed with a needle or another instrument inserted into the chest cavity.

Pneumothorax most often occurs in a newborn with stiff lungs, such as a newborn with respiratory distress syndrome or meconium aspiration syndrome. Occasionally, it occurs as a complication from the use of continuous positive airway pressure (CPAP) or a ventilator. If the pneumothorax is under pressure, it can result in collapse of the lung and in difficulty breathing. Also, if under pressure, the pneumothorax can compress the veins bringing blood to the heart. As a result, less blood fills the chambers of the heart, the output of the heart decreases, and the newborn's blood pressure decreases.

Air that leaks from the lungs into the soft tissues in front of the heart is called pneumomediastinum. Unlike pneumothorax, this condition usually does not affect breathing.

Diagnosis and Treatment

Pneumothorax is suspected when a newborn with underlying lung disease, or a newborn on continuous positive airway pressure (CPAP) or a ventilator, develops worsening respiratory distress or a drop in blood pressure. When examining the newborn, a doctor notices a diminished sound of air entering and leaving the lung on the side of the pneumothorax. In premature newborns, a fiberoptic light may be used to light up the affected side of the newborn's chest while in a darkened room (positive transillumination); this procedure is used to look for air in the chest cavity. A chest x-ray provides a definitive diagnosis.

No treatment is needed in newborns who do not have symptoms. A term newborn with mild symptoms may be placed in an oxygen hood. However, if the newborn's breathing is labored, and particularly if the circulation of blood is impaired, the air must be rapidly removed from the chest cavity, which can be done using a needle and syringe. If the newborn is in significant distress, is receiving CPAP, or is on a ventilator, a doctor may need to place a chest tube to continuously suction and remove air from the chest cavity. The tube can usually be removed after several days.

A pneumomediastinum can be seen on an x-ray; no treatment is needed.

Bronchopulmonary Dysplasia

Bronchopulmonary dysplasia (chronic lung disease) is a disorder due to repetitive lung injury.

- The disorder usually occurs in premature newborns who have a severe lung disease at birth or who use a ventilator for more than a few weeks.
- Breathing is rapid and may be labored, and the skin may be bluish.
- Diagnosis is based on the history, symptoms, oxygen levels in the blood, and chest x-ray results.
- Treatment may include ventilators (used as briefly and gently as possible), supplemental oxygen, good nutrition, restriction of fluids, and diuretics.

Bronchopulmonary dysplasia (commonly referred to as BPD) occurs most often in premature newborns who had severe lung disease at birth, such as respiratory distress syndrome, particularly in those who needed treatment with a ventilator for more than a few weeks after birth. The delicate tissues of the lungs can become injured when the air sacs are overstretched by the ventilation or by high oxygen levels. As a result, the lungs become inflamed and additional fluid accumulates within the lungs. Full-term newborns who have lung disease (such as pneumonia) occasionally develop bronchopulmonary dysplasia.

Symptoms and Diagnosis

Affected newborns usually breathe rapidly and may have respiratory distress, with drawing in of the lower chest while breathing in and low levels of oxygen in the blood, causing a bluish discoloration of the skin (cyanosis). Some newborns with severe cases exhale air from the lungs slowly and develop "air trapping," in which the chest appears to be overexpanded.

Although a few newborns with very severe bronchopulmonary dysplasia die even after months of care, most newborns survive. Over several years, the lung injury heals. However, later these children are at increased risk of developing asthma and viral pneumonia, such as that caused during winter months by respiratory syncytial virus (RSV).

The diagnosis of bronchopulmonary dysplasia is made in the premature newborn who has received ventilation for a prolonged time and who has signs of respiratory distress and a prolonged need for supplemental oxygen. Measurement of low levels of oxygen in the blood and results of a chest x-ray support the diagnosis.

> **DID YOU KNOW?**
>
> - Infants with bronchopulmonary dysplasia need to be protected from second-hand smoke, fumes from wood-burning stoves and some space heaters, and viral infections, even mild ones.

Prevention and Treatment

Ventilators are used only when absolutely necessary, and then as gently as possible to avoid injury to the lungs. The newborn is taken off the ventilator as early as is safe.

In a newborn with bronchopulmonary dysplasia, supplemental oxygen may be needed initially to prevent cyanosis.

Good nutrition is important to help the newborn's lungs grow and to keep the new lung tissue healthy. Thus, the damaged areas of lung become less and less important relative to the overall size of the newborn's lungs.

Because fluid tends to accumulate in the inflamed lungs, sometimes the daily intake of fluids is restricted, and diuretics may be used to increase the rate of excretion of fluid in the urine.

After discharge from the hospital, newborns with bronchopulmonary dysplasia should not be exposed to cigarette smoke or fumes from a space heater or wood-burning stove. They should be protected from exposure to people who have upper respiratory tract infections. In certain cases, doctors can give them partial immunity to RSV infection by administering doses of a specific antibody to that virus. This antibody must be injected monthly during the fall and winter.

Apnea of Prematurity

Apnea of prematurity is a pause in breathing that lasts for more than 20 seconds.

- Episodes occur because the respiratory center of the brain has not matured fully, and episodes end when the respiratory center matures.

- The skin may be bluish, and the heart rate may be slow.
- Premature newborns are monitored for long pauses in breathing and slowing of heart rate.
- Newborns may be given a drug that stimulates the respiratory center, or they may require assistance breathing.

Apnea of prematurity commonly occurs in newborns who are born before 34 weeks of pregnancy, increasing in frequency and severity among the most prematurely born. In these newborns, the part of the brain that controls breathing (respiratory center) has not matured fully. As a result, the newborns may have repeated episodes of normal breathing alternating with brief pauses in breathing. In very tiny premature newborns, apnea can be caused by temporary obstruction of the pharynx due to low muscle tone or a bending forward of the neck; this is called obstructive apnea. Over time, as the respiratory center matures, episodes of apnea become less frequent, and by the time the newborn approaches term, they no longer occur.

Symptoms and Diagnosis

Premature newborns are routinely attached to a monitor that sounds an alarm if the newborn stops breathing for a prolonged time or if the heart rate slows. Depending on the length of the episodes, stoppage of breathing may decrease the oxygen levels in the blood, which results in a bluish discoloration of the skin (cyanosis). Low levels of oxygen in the blood may slow the heart rate (bradycardia).

Apnea can sometimes be a sign of a disorder, such as infection of the blood (sepsis), low blood sugar (hypoglycemia), or a low body temperature (hypothermia). Therefore, the doctor evaluates the newborn to rule out these disorders when there is a sudden or unexpected increase in frequency of episodes.

DID YOU KNOW?

- Apnea in infants may be a sign of a blood infection, low blood sugar, a low body temperature, or another disorder.
- There is no proof that using a home apnea monitor decreases the risk of sudden infant death syndrome (SIDS).

Treatment

Treatment of apnea depends on the cause. Apnea caused by obstruction of the pharynx may be decreased by keeping the newborn lying on his back or side with his head in the midline position. If episodes of apnea become frequent, and especially if the newborn has cyanosis, the newborn may be treated with a drug that stimulates the respiratory center, such as caffeine or aminophylline. If these treatments fail to prevent frequent and severe episodes of apnea, the premature newborn may need treatment with continuous positive airway pressure (CPAP) or a ventilator.

Virtually all premature newborns stop having episodes of apnea several weeks before they reach term. Although a few infants are discharged from the hospital and placed on home monitors before they have completely outgrown their episodes of apnea, this practice is not standard or generally accepted. An association between apnea in the premature newborn and the risk for sudden infant death syndrome (SIDS) (see page 155), which usually occurs months after birth, has not been proven. Likewise, there is no proof that discharging an infant home on an apnea monitor decreases the risk of SIDS.

Retinopathy of Prematurity

Retinopathy of prematurity is a disease in which the small blood vessels in the back of the eye (retina) grow abnormally.

- The retina may scar or, in severe cases, become detached, causing loss of vision.
- No symptoms occur as retinopathy is developing.
- The retinas of premature newborns are checked by an ophthalmologist soon after delivery and regularly thereafter as needed.
- Supplemental oxygen is used as seldom as possible and at the lowest possible concentrations because high oxygen levels increase the risk of this disorder.
- Usually, the disorder resolves on its own, but in severe cases, laser treatment may be needed.

In newborns born very prematurely, growth of the blood vessels supplying the retina may stop for a period of time. When growth resumes, it occurs in a disorganized fashion. During disorganized rapid growth, the small blood vessels may bleed and eventually lead to scarring. In the most severe cases, this process may ultimately result in detachment of the retina from the back of the eye and loss of vision. High blood oxygen levels may also increase the risk of retinopathy of prematurity.

The newborn who is developing retinopathy of prematurity does not have symptoms, and diagnosis depends on careful examination of the back of the eyes by an eye specialist (ophthalmologist). Routinely, therefore, an ophthalmologist examines the eyes of premature newborns who weigh less than 1,500 grams at birth starting 4 or more weeks after delivery. Eye examinations are repeated every 1 to 2 weeks as needed, until growth of the blood vessels in the retina is complete. Infants who develop severe retinopathy must have eye examinations, at least yearly, for the rest of their lives. If detected early, retinal detachment can occasionally be treated to avoid complete loss of vision in the affected eye.

Prevention, Treatment, and Prognosis

In a premature newborn who needs oxygen, the oxygen use is monitored carefully to prevent excessive oxygen levels in the blood that would put the newborn at increased risk of retinopathy of prematurity. Alternatively, the oxygen levels can be indirectly monitored using a pulse oximeter, which measures the level of oxygen in the blood going through a finger or toe.

Retinopathy is usually mild and resolves spontaneously, but the eyes need to be monitored by an ophthalmologist until blood vessel growth is mature.

For very severe retinopathy of prematurity, laser treatment is applied to the outermost portions of the retina. This treatment stops the abnormal growth of blood vessels and decreases the risk of retinal detachment and loss of vision.

Necrotizing Enterocolitis

Necrotizing enterocolitis is injury to the inner surface of the intestine.

- Necrotizing enterocolitis occurs most commonly in premature newborns.

- Complications include infection of the abdominal cavity or bloodstream and, in severe cases, death.
- The abdomen may be swollen, stools may be bloody, and newborns may vomit up a greenish, yellow, or rust-colored fluid (stained with bile) and appear very sick.
- The diagnosis is confirmed by abdominal x-rays.
- Treatment involves stopping feedings, passing a suction tube into the stomach to relieve pressure, and giving antibiotics and intravenous fluids.
- In severe cases, drains are placed in the abdominal cavity, or part of the intestine is removed.

Necrotizing enterocolitis usually occurs in premature newborns. The cause is not understood. Diminished blood flow to the intestine in a sick premature newborn may result in injury to the inner layers of the intestine, allowing bacteria that normally exist within the intestine to invade the damaged intestinal wall. If the injury progresses through the entire thickness of the bowel wall and the intestinal wall perforates, intestinal contents leak into the abdominal cavity and cause peritonitis. Necrotizing enterocolitis can also lead to infection of the blood (sepsis). In the most severe cases, necrotizing enterocolitis can be fatal.

Newborns with necrotizing enterocolitis may develop swelling of the abdomen. They may vomit bile-stained intestinal fluid, and blood may be visible in the stools. These newborns soon appear very sick and lethargic and have low body temperature and repeated pauses of breathing (apnea spells). The diagnosis of necrotizing enterocolitis is confirmed by abdominal x-rays. Blood samples are taken for blood cultures to identify the bacteria responsible for the infection.

Prevention, Treatment, and Prognosis

Feeding the premature newborn breast milk rather than formula appears to provide some protection. In tiny or sick premature newborns, the risk may also be reduced by delaying feedings for several days and then increasing the amount of feedings slowly. Feedings are stopped if necrotizing enterocolitis is suspected. A suction tube is passed into the newborn's stomach to remove pressure from swallowed air and formula, thereby decompressing the intestine. Intravenous fluids are given to maintain hydration, and antibiotics are begun after blood cultures have been obtained.

About 70% of newborns with necrotizing enterocolitis do not need surgery. If the intestine perforates, then surgery is needed. Surgery may also be needed if the condition progressively worsens despite treatment.

In the tiniest and sickest newborns, "peritoneal drains" are placed into the abdominal cavity on each side of the lower abdomen. The drains allow stool and peritoneal fluid to drain from the abdominal cavity and, along with antibiotics, may allow symptoms to improve. The condition of many newborns treated with drains stabilizes, so that an operation can be performed more safely at a later time. In some cases, the newborns recover completely without needing additional surgery.

Larger infants need surgery in which portions of the bowel are removed and the ends of the healthy bowel are brought out to the skin surface to create a temporary opening for the excretion of bodily wastes (ostomy).

Intensive medical treatment and surgery when needed have improved the prognosis for newborns with necrotizing enterocolitis. More than two thirds of such newborns survive.

Hyperbilirubinemia

Hyperbilirubinemia is an abnormally high level of bilirubin in the blood.

- Causes include illnesses that interfere with feeding, serious disorders, and rapid break down of red blood cells (hemolysis).
- Occasionally, very high bilirubin levels cause brain damage (kernicterus).
- The skin and whites of the eyes are yellow (jaundiced), and newborns with kernicterus may become lethargic and feed poorly.
- An examination and blood tests to check for jaundice are routinely done soon after birth.
- When treatment is needed, phototherapy and, for very severe cases, exchange blood transfusion can help.

Aging red blood cells are removed by the spleen, and the hemoglobin from these red blood cells is broken down and recycled. The heme portion of the hemoglobin molecule is converted into a yellow pigment called bilirubin, which is carried in the blood to the liver where it is chemically modified and then excreted in the bile into the newborn's digestive tract. It is removed from the body when the newborn passes stools. Bilirubin in the stools of newborns gives them their yellow color.

In most newborns, the level of bilirubin in the blood increases in the first days after birth, causing the newborn's skin and the whites of the eyes to appear yellow (jaundice). If feedings are delayed for any reason, as occurs when newborns are sick or have a digestive tract problem, blood levels of bilirubin can become high. Also, breastfed newborns tend to have somewhat higher blood levels of bilirubin during the first week or two.

Hyperbilirubinemia may also occur when a newborn has a serious medical disorder, such as infection in the blood (sepsis). It may also be caused by hemolysis (rapid breakdown of red blood cells), as occurs with Rh incompatibility or ABO incompatibility.

DID YOU KNOW?

- Breastfed newborns tend to have slightly higher bilirubin levels, making their skin yellowish, during the first week or two after birth.
- Newborns discharged from the hospital early need to be assessed within a few days for hyperbilirubinemia.

In the large majority of cases, elevated levels of bilirubin in the blood are not serious. However, very high bilirubin levels can produce brain damage (kernicterus). Very premature and critically ill newborns are at higher risk for developing kernicterus. In almost all cases, moderately elevated blood levels of bilirubin due to breastfeeding are not of concern. However, newborns who are slightly premature and are breastfeeding, especially if discharged early from the hospital, must be monitored closely for hyperbilirubinemia because they can develop kernicterus if the bilirubin level becomes very high.

Symptoms and Diagnosis

Newborns with hyperbilirubinemia have a yellow color to their skin and the whites of their eyes (jaundice). It may be more difficult to recognize jaundice in dark-skinned newborns. Jaundice usually first appears on the newborn's face and then, as the bilirubin level increases, progresses downward to involve the chest, abdomen, and finally the legs and feet.

Newborns with hyperbilirubinemia who are showing symptoms of kernicterus may become lethargic and feed poorly; these newborns should be examined immediately by a doctor. The later stages of kernicterus involve irritability, muscle stiffening or seizures, and a fever.

It is important that a doctor assess the degree of jaundice in all newborns during the first days of life. Some newborns have developed dangerously high levels of bilirubin after being discharged from the hospital on the first day after birth before their blood level of bilirubin had risen. Therefore, it is very important that newborns discharged early be examined at home by a visiting nurse or in the doctor's office within a few days after discharge to assess their bilirubin levels. If the doctor or nurse is concerned about the level of jaundice, a blood test will be done to measure the amount of bilirubin in the blood. This is especially true for newborns born a few weeks prematurely and those breastfeeding.

A doctor first examines the newborn under good lighting and then measures the level of jaundice by holding a specialized piece of equipment (bilirubinometer) against the newborn's skin or by testing a small sample of blood.

Treatment

Treatment depends on the age of the child and the degree of bilirubin increase. Mild hyperbilirubinemia does not require special treatment. Offering frequent feedings accelerates the passage of stools, thus reducing the reabsorption of bilirubin from the intestinal contents and lowering the bilirubin level. Moderate hyperbilirubinemia can be treated with phototherapy, in which the newborn is placed without clothes under fluorescent bilirubin lights. The light exposure alters the composition of the bilirubin in the newborn's skin, changing it to a form that is more readily excreted by the liver and kidneys. The newborn's eyes are shielded with a blindfold. Newborns can also be treated at home by having them lie on a fiber-optic "bilirubin blanket," which exposes their skin to bright light. These newborns need to have their blood levels of bilirubin tested repeatedly until they decrease.

Rarely, it may be necessary for a mother to change from breastfeeding to formula feeding temporarily to ensure that the newborn is obtaining adequate volumes with each feeding. The mother should resume breastfeeding as soon as the bilirubin levels start to decrease. Moderate hyperbilirubinemia sometimes continues for weeks in infants who are breastfed, a normal phenomenon that poses no problems for the infant and that does not usually require withholding of breastfeeding.

If the newborn's blood level of bilirubin approaches a dangerous level, it can be lowered rapidly by performing an exchange blood transfusion. In this procedure, a sterile catheter is placed into the umbilical vein located in the cut surface of the umbilical cord. The newborn's bilirubin-containing blood is removed and replaced with equal volumes of fresh blood.

Anemia

Anemia is a disorder in which there are too few red blood cells in the blood.

- Anemia can occur when red blood cells are broken down too rapidly or when too much blood is lost.
- If red blood cells are broken down too rapidly, the skin and whites of the eyes appear yellow (jaundiced).
- If too much blood is lost, newborns may appear pale and lethargic, with rapid, shallow breathing,
- Treatment may involve intravenous fluids followed by a blood transfusion or exchange blood transfusion.

Normally, the newborn's bone marrow does not produce new red blood cells between birth and 3 or 4 weeks of age. Anemia can occur when red blood cells are broken down too rapidly, too much blood is lost, or more than one of these processes occurs at the same time.

Any process that leads to red blood cell destruction, if sufficiently severe, results in anemia and high levels of bilirubin (hyperbilirubinemia). Hemolytic disease of the newborn may cause the newborn's red blood cells to be destroyed rapidly. The red blood cells may also be rapidly destroyed if the newborn has a hereditary abnormality of the red blood cells. An example is hereditary spherocytosis, in which the red blood cells appear small and spherical in shape when viewed under a microscope.

DID YOU KNOW?

- A pregnant woman who has Rh-negative blood may produce antibodies that destroy red blood cells in a fetus whose blood is Rh-positive.

Infections acquired before birth, such as toxoplasmosis, rubella, cytomegalovirus, herpes simplex, or syphilis, may also rapidly destroy red blood cells, as can bacterial infections of the newborn acquired during or following birth.

Another cause of anemia is blood loss. Blood loss can occur in many ways, for example, if there is a large transfusion of the fetal blood across the placenta and into the mother's circulation (fetal-maternal transfusion) or if too much blood gets trapped in the placenta at delivery, when the umbilical cord is clamped. The placenta may separate from the uterine wall before delivery (placental abruption), leading to hemorrhage of the fetal blood. Rarely, anemia may result from a failure of the fetal bone marrow to produce red blood cells. One example of this is a genetic disorder called Fanconi's anemia. Another rare example is that due to exposure of the mother and fetus to certain drugs used during pregnancy.

Symptoms and Treatment

A newborn who has suddenly lost a large amount of blood during labor or delivery may appear pale and have a rapid heart rate and low blood pressure, along with rapid, shallow breathing. Milder anemia may result in lethargy, poor feeding, or no symptoms. When the anemia is a result of rapid breakdown of red blood cells, there is also increased production of bilirubin, and the newborn's skin and the whites of the eyes appear yellow (jaundice).

A newborn who has rapidly lost a large amount of blood, often during labor and delivery, is treated with intravenous fluids followed by a blood transfusion. Very severe anemia caused by hemolytic disease may also require a blood transfusion, but the anemia is more often treated with an exchange blood transfusion, in which part of the newborn's blood is gradually removed and replaced with equal volumes of fresh donor blood. The exchange transfusion also removes bilirubin in the circulation and thus treats the hyperbilirubinemia.

WHAT IS HEMOLYTIC DISEASE OF THE NEWBORN?

Hemolytic disease of the newborn (also called erythroblastosis fetalis) is a condition in which red blood cells are broken down or destroyed more rapidly than is normal. The newborn's red blood cells are destroyed by antibodies that were produced by the mother and crossed the placenta from the mother's circulation into the fetal circulation before delivery. A mother who is Rh-negative may have produced antibodies against Rh-positive blood cells after she was exposed to red blood cells of a previous fetus that was Rh-positive. Such exposure may occur during pregnancy or labor, but may also occur if the mother had been accidentally transfused with Rh-positive blood at any time earlier in life.

The mother's body responds to the "incompatible blood" by producing antibodies to destroy the "foreign" Rh-positive cells. These antibodies cross the placenta during a subsequent pregnancy. If the fetus she is carrying is Rh-negative, there is no consequence. However, if the fetus has Rh-positive red blood cells, the mother's antibodies attach to, and start to destroy, the fetal red blood cells, leading to anemia of varying degrees. This anemia begins in the fetus and continues after delivery.

Sometimes other blood group incompatibilities may lead to similar hemolytic diseases. For example, if the mother is blood type O and the fetus has blood type A or B, then the mother's body produces anti-A or anti-B antibodies that can cross the placenta, attach to fetal red blood cells, and lead to their breakdown (hemolysis). Rh incompatibility usually leads to more severe anemia than ABO incompatibility.

(Continued)

WHAT IS HEMOLYTIC DISEASE OF THE NEWBORN? (Continued)

Prevention of hemolytic disease due to Rh incompatibility involves injecting the mother with a $Rh_0(D)$ immune globulin preparation at about 28 weeks of pregnancy and again immediately after delivery. Injection of this immune globulin rapidly destroys any Rh-positive fetal red blood cells that have entered the mother's circulation before they stimulate the mother's body to produce antibodies.

Severe anemia caused by hemolytic disease of the newborn is treated in the same way as any other anemia. The doctor also observes the newborn for jaundice, which is likely to occur because hemoglobin from the red blood cells that are being rapidly broken down is converted to the yellow pigment, bilirubin, giving the newborn's skin and whites of the eyes a yellow appearance. Jaundice can be treated by exposing the newborn to bright lights (phototherapy) or by having the newborn undergo an exchange blood transfusion. Very high levels of bilirubin in the blood can lead to brain damage (kernicterus).

Polycythemia

Polycythemia is an abnormally high concentration of red blood cells.

- The high concentration of red blood cells makes the blood thick and slows blood flow.

A markedly increased concentration of red blood cells may result in the blood being too thick, which slows the flow of blood through small blood vessels and interferes with the delivery of oxygen to tissues. A newborn who is born postmaturely or whose mother has severe high blood pressure, smokes, or lives at a high altitude is more likely to have polycythemia. Polycythemia may also result if the newborn receives too much blood from the placenta at birth, as may occur if the newborn is held below the level of the placenta for a period of time before the umbilical cord is clamped.

The newborn with polycythemia may have a ruddy or dusky color. Most such newborns do not have other symptoms. However, the newborn may be sluggish, feed poorly, have rapid heart and respiratory rates, and, rarely, may have seizures. If the newborn has such symptoms and a blood test indicates too many red blood cells (high hematocrit), a partial exchange blood transfusion is performed, in which the newborn's blood is removed and replaced with equal volumes of albumin solution or saline, thus diluting the remaining red blood cells and correcting the polycythemia.

Thyroid Disorders

- Blood tests to measure levels of thyroid hormone help confirm the diagnosis of a thyroid disorder.
- Producing too little thyroid hormone (hypothyroidism) slows growth and mental development, sometimes resulting in mental retardation.
- Early treatment with thyroid hormone can prevent mental retardation.
- Producing too much thyroid hormone (hyperthyroidism) is rare, usually occurring in newborns of women with Graves' disease.
- Newborns with hyperthyroidism may have bulging eyes, an enlarged thyroid gland, and a very rapid heart rate.
- Drugs, such as propylthiouracil, are needed for only a few months to slow the production of thyroid hormone.

These disorders occur if the thyroid gland produces too little thyroid hormone (hypothyroidism) or too much thyroid hormone (hyperthyroidism).

Hypothyroidism: If untreated, hypothyroidism in the newborn results in poor growth and mental delay, eventually resulting in mental retardation. The most common cause of hypothyroidism in the newborn is complete absence or underdevelopment of the thyroid gland. Initially, the newborn has no symptoms. Later, the newborn may have lethargy, poor appetite, constipation, a hoarse cry, umbilical hernia (a bulging of the abdominal contents where the umbilicus penetrates the abdominal wall), and slow growth. Eventually, the infant may develop coarse facial features and an enlarged tongue.

Early treatment can prevent mental retardation. For this reason, a blood test is performed in the hospital after birth on all newborns to measure thyroid hormone levels. Treatment is with thyroid hormone.

DID YOU KNOW?

- Without treatment, newborns who produce too much thyroid hormone (hyperthyroidism) may develop heart failure and die.

Hyperthyroidism: Rarely, a newborn may have hyperthyroidism, or neonatal Graves' disease. This generally occurs if the mother has Graves' disease during pregnancy or has been treated for it before pregnancy. In Graves' disease, the woman's body produces antibodies that stimulate the thyroid gland to produce increased blood levels of thyroid hormone. These antibodies cross the placenta and similarly affect the fetus. The result in an affected newborn is too high a metabolic rate, with rapid heart rate and breathing, irritability, and excessive appetite with poor weight gain.

The newborn, like the mother, may have bulging eyes (exophthalmos). If the newborn has an enlarged thyroid gland (goiter), the gland may press against the windpipe and interfere with breathing. A very rapid heart rate can lead to heart failure. Graves' disease is potentially fatal if not recognized and treated.

Doctors suspect hyperthyroidism by the typical symptoms and confirm the diagnosis by measuring elevated levels of thyroid hormone and the thyroid-stimulating antibodies from the mother in the newborn's blood.

Newborns with hyperthyroidism are treated with drugs, such as propylthiouracil, that slow the production of thyroid hormone by the thyroid gland. Treatment is needed for only a few months because the antibodies that cross the placenta from the mother only last in the infant's bloodstream for this long.

Sepsis

Sepsis is bacterial infection in the blood.

- Newborns are at higher risk of sepsis because their immune system is immature.
- Newborns with sepsis are usually listless, do not feed well, and often have a low body temperature.
- Sepsis can lead to other infections, including meningitis.
- As soon as sepsis is suspected, a blood sample is taken for culture, and intravenous antibiotics are given.
- Doctors may perform a spinal tap to check for meningitis.

Newborns, especially premature ones, are at much higher risk of sepsis than are children and adults because of their immature immune system. Premature newborns also lack certain antibodies against specific bacteria; these antibodies usually cross the placenta from the mother late in pregnancy. Another important risk factor for sepsis is the use of intravenous lines and ventilators.

The most common type of bacteria causing sepsis in the newborn around the time of birth is Group B streptococcus. Sepsis that occurs later while the newborn is being cared for in the neonatal intensive care unit (NICU) is most likely to be caused by a type of staphylococcus (coagulase negative).

Some Infections of Newborns

INFECTION	MODE OF INFECTION	SYMPTOMS	TREATMENT/ PREVENTION
Herpes	Usually, the virus (herpes simplex) infects the fetus after rupture of the membranes during labor and delivery	Usually, a skin rash of small fluid-filled blisters appears; infection may be widespread, affecting many organs, such as eyes, lungs, liver, brain, and skin	Antiviral drugs are given intravenously; eye infections are treated with trifluridine drops

(Continued)

Some Infections of Newborns (Continued)

INFECTION	MODE OF INFECTION	SYMPTOMS	TREATMENT/ PREVENTION
Hepatitis B	Usually, the virus infects the fetus after rupture of the membranes during labor and delivery	Chronic liver infection (chronic hepatitis) develops but usually does not produce symptoms until young adulthood	A newborn born to an infected mother is given both hepatitis B virus vaccine and hepatitis B immune globulin within 24 hours of birth
Cytomegalovirus infection	The virus is thought to cross the placenta from the mother during pregnancy or during delivery (a risk of 1%); after birth, a newborn may become infected from infected breast milk or contaminated blood from a transfusion	Most newborns do not have symptoms; about 10% have low birth weight, a small head, jaundice, small bruises, and an enlarged liver and spleen; deafness may occur	The infection cannot be cured; ganciclovir may help some symptoms; newborns should have repeated hearing evaluations during the first year
Rubella	The virus may cross the placenta during pregnancy (rare because vaccination is now routine); infection is more severe if the fetus is infected early in pregnancy	Effects on the fetus range from death before birth to birth defects or hearing loss without other symptoms; newborns may have low birth weight, brain inflammation, cataracts, damage to retina, heart defects, an enlarged liver and spleen; bruising, bluish red skin lesions, enlarged lymph nodes, and pneumonia	No specific treatment is available; to prevent infection in the mother, all women of childbearing age should be vaccinated before pregnancy; immune globulin is sometimes injected if a pregnant woman who has not been immunized comes into close contact with an infected person early in pregnancy

Some Infections of Newborns (Continued)

INFECTION	MODE OF INFECTION	SYMPTOMS	TREATMENT/ PREVENTION
Toxoplasmosis	The parasite (*Toxoplasma gondii*) may cross the placenta during pregnancy; infection is more severe if the fetus is infected early in pregnancy	The fetus may grow slowly and be born prematurely; the newborn may have a small head, brain inflammation, jaundice, an enlarged liver and spleen, and inflammation of the heart, lungs, or eyes; rashes may occur	Women should avoid handling cat litter during pregnancy; transmission from the mother to the fetus may be prevented if the mother takes spiramycin; pyrimethamine and sulfonamides may be taken later in pregnancy if the fetus is infected; infected newborns with symptoms are treated with pyrimethamine, sulfadiazine, and leucovorin; corticosteroids can be used for inflammation of heart, lungs, or eyes
Syphilis	The bacterium (*Treponema pallidum*) crosses the placenta during pregnancy if the mother acquires syphilis during pregnancy or if she has been inadequately treated for syphilis in the past	Stillbirth or premature birth may occur. The newborn may have no symptoms; in the first month of life, the newborn may develop large fluid-filled blisters or flat copper-colored rash on palms and soles, with raised bumps around the nose and mouth and in the diaper area; usually lymph nodes, liver, and spleen are enlarged; the newborn may not grow well and have a characteristic "old man" look, with cracks around the mouth; mucus, pus, or blood may run from the nose; rarely, meningitis occurs	Before birth, the mother is treated with penicillin. After birth, if still infected, the mother and newborn are treated with penicillin

(Continued)

Some Infections of Newborns (Continued)

INFECTION	MODE OF INFECTION	SYMPTOMS	TREATMENT/ PREVENTION
Conjunc- tivitis	The bacteria (most com- monly *Chlamydia* or *Neisseria gonorrhoeae*) infects the fetus after rupture of the membranes during labor or delivery	When caused by *Chlamydia*: Conjunctivitis usu- ally begins 5 to 12 days after delivery but sometimes 6 weeks after, as watery discharge from eyes contain- ing increasing amounts of pus When caused by *Neisseria gonor- rhoeae*: Conjunc- tivitis begins usually 2 to 3 days after, but some- times up to 7 days after, delivery, as discharge of pus from eyes	When caused by *Chlamydia*: Erythromycin is given as eye oint- ment and also as tablets by mouth When caused by *Neisseria gonorrhoeae*: An eye ointment con- taining polymyxin and bacitracin eryth- romycin, or tetracy- cline is used. An antibiotic such as ceftriaxone is also given intravenously
Human papilloma- virus infec- tion	Usually new- borns become infected dur- ing delivery	Symptoms are an altered cry; some- times difficulty breathing or even significant obstruc- tion of the airways due to warts that grow inside the windpipe; lung infection	Warts are removed surgically; recur- rence can be reduced by use of interferon

Symptoms and Diagnosis

A newborn with sepsis is usually listless, does not feed well, and often has a low body temperature. Other symptoms may include pauses in breathing (apnea), fever, pale color, and poor skin circula- tion, with cool extremities, abdominal swelling, and jaundice.

Because newborns have decreased immunity against infection, bacteria in the bloodstream may invade and infect various organs. One of the most serious complications of sepsis is infection of the membranes surrounding the brain (meningitis). A newborn with meningitis may have extreme lethargy, coma, seizures, or bulging of the fontanelle (the soft spot between the skull bones). A doctor

DID YOU KNOW?

- Sepsis is the most common cause of death in premature newborns who are more than 1 week old.

can rule out or diagnose meningitis by performing a spinal tap (lumbar puncture), examining the cerebrospinal fluid, and culturing a sample of this fluid. Infection of a bone (osteomyelitis) may cause pain and swelling of an arm or leg, often suspected because the newborn does not move that extremity. Infection of a joint may cause swelling, warmth, redness, and tenderness over the joint, again with little or no movement of that joint. If joint infection is suspected, a sample of fluid from the infected site is removed by needle and cultured.

Treatment and Prognosis

While awaiting blood culture results, a doctor gives intravenous antibiotics to a newborn with suspected sepsis. Once the specific organism has been identified, the type of antibiotic can be adjusted. In addition to antibiotic therapy, other treatments may be needed, such as use of a ventilator, intravenous fluids, and support of the blood pressure and circulation.

Sepsis is the major cause of mortality in premature newborns after the first week. Newborns who recover from sepsis should not have long-term problems, except those with meningitis, who may have mental delay, cerebral palsy, seizures, or hearing loss later in life.

CHAPTER 4

Birth Defects

Birth defects, also called congenital anomalies, are physical abnormalities that occur before a baby is born; they are usually obvious at birth or by 1 year of age.

DID YOU KNOW?

- Birth defects are the leading cause of death in infants in the United States.
- Many birth defects develop before a woman knows she is pregnant.
- Increasingly, birth defects are being diagnosed before the baby is born.
- Taking folic acid before pregnancy and through the 1st trimester of pregnancy reduces the risk of cleft lip and cleft palate and can reduce the risk of neural tube defects by as much as 70%.

Birth defects can involve any part of any organ in the body. Some birth defects are more common than others. Birth defects are the leading cause of death in infants in the United States. A birth defect is evident in about 7.5% of all children by age 5 years, although many of these are minor. Major birth defects are evident in about 3 to 4% of newborns. Several birth defects can occur together in the same infant.

Examples of Some Birth Defects

MAJOR SYSTEM	BIRTH DEFECT	WHAT HAPPENS	TREATMENT
Heart	Hypoplastic left heart syndrome	Underdevelopment of the left ventricle, leading to inability to pump blood to the body	Separate operations to rebuild the left ventricle
Digestive tract	Omphalocele and gastroschisis	Hole or weakening of abdominal muscles, allowing internal abdominal organs to protrude externally	Surgery to close the abdomen
Musculo-skeletal	Congenital torticollis	Abnormal twisting of the head and neck	Physical therapy, surgery, or injections of botulinum toxin
	Prune-belly syndrome	Missing layers of abdominal muscles, causing the abdomen to bulge; urinary system defects often develop	Surgery if a urinary system defect blocks urine flow
Neurologic	Porencephaly	Brain tissue is missing and is replaced with fluid-filled sacs	No treatment is available; ventricular shunt may decrease pressure
	Hydranencephaly	Severe porencephaly with little remaining brain tissue	No treatment is available .
Genital	Vanishing testes (bilateral anorchia; testicular regression)	Both testes are absent at birth	Supplemental male hormone (testosterone) beginning before puberty

(Continued)

Examples of Some Birth Defects (Continued)

MAJOR SYSTEM	BIRTH DEFECT	WHAT HAPPENS	TREATMENT
Eye	Congenital glaucoma	Glaucoma is present at birth; pressure is raised in the eyeball (usually both); the eye may enlarge, and its normal appearance may be distorted	Surgery usually performed soon after birth; eye drops used until surgery; if the glaucoma is not treated, blindness can result
	Congenital cataracts	Cataracts (cloudy areas) in the lens of the eye are present at birth; usually vision is impaired	Surgery to remove the cataract as soon as possible is the best chance of normal vision

Causes and Risks

It is not surprising that birth defects are fairly common, considering the complexities involved in the development of a single fertilized egg into the millions of specialized cells that constitute a human being. Although the cause of most birth defects is unknown, certain genetic and environmental factors increase the chance of birth defects developing. These factors include exposure to radiation, certain drugs (for example, isotretinoin, which is used to treat severe acne), alcohol, nutritional deficiencies, some infections in the mother, injuries, and hereditary disorders. Some risks are avoidable. Others occur no matter how strictly a pregnant woman adheres to healthful living practices.

Exposure to Harmful Substances (Teratogens): A teratogen is any substance that can cause or increase the chance of a birth defect. Radiation (including x-rays), certain drugs, and toxins (including alcohol) are teratogens. Most pregnant women who are exposed to teratogens have newborns without abnormalities. Whether or not a birth defect occurs depends on when, how much, and how long the pregnant woman was exposed to the teratogen. Exposure to a teratogen most commonly affects the fetal organ that is developing at the time of exposure. For example, exposure to a teratogen during the time that certain parts of the brain are developing is more likely to cause a defect in those areas than exposure before or after this critical period. Many birth defects develop before a woman knows she is pregnant.

Nutrition: Keeping a fetus healthy requires maintaining a nutritious diet. For example, insufficient folic acid (folate) in the diet increases the chance that a fetus will develop spina bifida or other abnormalities of the brain or spinal cord known as neural tube defects (see page 108). Maternal obesity also increases the risk of a neural tube defect.

Genetic and Chromosomal Factors: Chromosomes and genes may be abnormal. These abnormalities may be inherited from the parents, who can be affected by the condition or who can be carriers without symptoms. However, many birth defects are caused by seemingly random and unexplained changes (mutations) in the genes of the child. Most birth defects caused by genetic factors include more than just the obvious malformation of a single body part.

Infections: Certain infections in pregnant women can cause birth defects. Whether an infection causes a birth defect depends on the age of the fetus. The infections that most often cause birth defects are cytomegalovirus, herpesvirus, parvovirus (fifth disease), rubella (German measles), varicella (chickenpox), toxoplasmosis (which can be transmitted in cat litter), and syphilis. A woman can have such an infection and not know it, because these infections can produce few or no symptoms in adults.

Diagnosis: During pregnancy, doctors assess whether a woman is at increased risk of having a baby with a birth defect. The chance is higher for women who are older than 35 years, have had frequent miscarriages, or have had other children with chromosomal abnormalities, birth defects, or who died for unknown reasons. These women may need special tests to find out if their baby is normal.

A prenatal ultrasound can often detect specific birth defects. Sometimes blood tests can also help; for example, a high level of alpha-fetoprotein in the mother's blood may indicate a defect of the brain or spinal cord. Amniocentesis (removing fluid from around the fetus) or chorionic villus sampling (removing tissue from the sac around the developing baby) may be necessary to confirm a suspected diagnosis. Increasingly, birth defects are being diagnosed before the baby is born.

Heart Defects

- Usually, blood flow in the heart is altered, or the heart cannot pump enough blood to the rest of the body, often because of a blockage or narrowing.
- When blood flow is altered, the blood pumped to the body does not contain enough oxygen.
- The skin is bluish (cyanotic) because of lack of oxygen.
- Children may not grow or be able to exercise normally, have difficulty breathing, or develop heart failure.
- Echocardiography helps identify almost all heart defects.
- Treatment includes open-heart surgery for severe defects, use of a catheter with a balloon at its tip to open or widen valves or blood vessels, or the drug prostaglandin E_1.

One of 120 babies is born with a heart defect. Some are severe, but many are not. Defects may involve abnormal formation of the heart's walls or valves or of the blood vessels that enter or leave the heart.

Before birth, a fetus uses oxygen obtained from the mother's blood through the placenta. The fetus does not breathe. Also, the path by which blood circulates through the heart and lungs is different in a fetus. After birth, a newborn must obtain oxygen using his own lungs. Therefore, many changes occur in the heart and blood vessels soon after birth.

Before birth, blood that has not yet traveled to the lungs (venous blood) mixes with blood that has already traveled to the lungs (arterial blood). Such mixing occurs in the foramen ovale, a hole between the right and left atria (the upper chambers of the heart that receive blood), and the ductus arteriosus, a blood vessel connecting the pulmonary artery and the aorta. In the fetus, both venous and arterial blood contain oxygen, so mixing arterial and venous blood does not affect how much oxygen gets pumped to the body. After birth, arterial blood and venous blood do not normally mix. The foramen ovale and ductus arteriosus normally close within days to a couple of weeks after birth.

Two general processes account for most of the symptoms resulting from heart defects. One is that blood flow gets altered or rerouted (shunting). Another is that not enough blood gets pumped to the body, usually because of a blockage.

Shunting can cause oxygen-poor blood to mix with oxygen-rich blood that is pumped to the body tissues (right-to-left shunt). The more oxygen-poor blood (which is blue) that flows to the body, the more blue the body appears, particularly the skin and lips. Many heart defects are characterized by a bluish discoloration of the skin (called cyanosis); cyanosis indicates that not enough oxygen-rich blood is reaching the tissues where it is needed.

Shunting can also mix oxygen-rich blood, which is pumped under high pressures, with oxygen-poor blood being pumped through the pulmonary artery to the lungs (left-to-right shunt). This deprives the body of oxygen-rich blood and increases the pressure in the pulmonary artery. The high pressure damages the pulmonary artery and lungs. The shunt also eventually leads to an insufficient amount of blood being pumped to the body (heart failure).

DID YOU KNOW?

- One of 120 babies is born with a heart defect.
- Most heart murmurs in children are not caused by heart defects and are not cause for concern.
- Most children with significant heart defects need to take antibiotics before certain treatments and procedures.

In heart failure, blood also backs up, often in the lungs. Heart failure can also develop when the heart pumps too weakly (for example, when a baby is born with a weak heart muscle) or when blood is blocked from flowing to the baby's body.

Blockages may develop in the valves of the heart or in the blood vessels leading away from the heart. Blood may be impeded from flowing to the lungs because of narrowing of the pulmonary valve (pulmonary valve stenosis) or narrowing within the pulmonary artery itself (pulmonary artery stenosis). Blood may be impeded from flowing through the aorta to the body because of narrowing of the aortic valve (aortic valve stenosis) or blockage within the aorta itself (coarctation of the aorta).

Symptoms and Diagnosis

Often, heart defects produce few or no symptoms and are not detectable even during a physical examination of the child. Some mild defects produce symptoms only later in life. However, many heart defects do result in symptoms during childhood. Because oxygen-rich blood is necessary for normal growth, development, and activity, infants and children with heart defects may fail to grow or gain weight normally. They may not be able to exercise fully. In more severe cases, cyanosis may develop, and breathing or eating may be difficult. Abnormal blood flow through the heart usually produces an abnormal sound (murmur) that can be heard using a stethoscope; however, the vast majority of heart murmurs that occur during childhood are not caused by heart defects and are not indicative of any problems. Heart failure makes the heart beat rapidly and often causes fluid to collect in the lungs or liver.

Many heart defects can be diagnosed before birth using ultrasound. After birth, heart defects are suspected when symptoms develop or when particular heart murmurs are heard.

Diagnosing heart defects in children involves the same techniques used for diagnosing heart problems in adults. A doctor may be able to diagnose the defect after asking the family specific questions and performing a physical examination, electrocardiography (ECG), and a chest x-ray. Ultrasound (echocardiography) is used to diagnose almost all of the specific defects. Cardiac catheterization often can show small abnormalities that are not detected with echocardiography or can further illuminate the details of the abnormality.

Treatment

Many significant heart defects are effectively corrected using open-heart surgery. When to perform the operation depends on the specific defect, its symptoms, and severity. For example, it may be better to postpone surgery until the child is a little older. However, severe symptoms resulting from a heart defect are most effectively relieved with immediate surgery.

A narrowing can sometimes be relieved by passing a thin tube (catheter) through a blood vessel in the arm or leg into the narrowed area. A balloon attached to the catheter is inflated and widens the narrowing, usually in a valve (a procedure called balloon valvuloplasty) or blood vessel (a procedure called balloon angioplasty. These balloon procedures spare the child from general anesthesia and open-heart surgery. However, balloon procedures are not usually as effective as surgery.

If the aorta or pulmonary artery is severely blocked, a temporary shunt can sometimes be created to keep an adequate amount of blood flowing. A shunt can be created with a catheter balloon (for example, between the right and left atria—balloon septostomy). Or the drug prostaglandin E_1 (alprostadil) can be given to keep the ductus arteriosus open, shunting blood between the aorta and pulmonary artery. In rare cases, when no other treatment helps, a heart transplant is performed, but the lack of donor hearts limits the availability of this procedure.

Most children who have significant heart defects are at increased risk for developing life-threatening bacterial infections of the heart and its valves (endocarditis). They need to take antibiotics before certain treatments and procedures.

PATENT DUCTUS ARTERIOSUS

- The blood vessel that connects the pulmonary artery and aorta does not close shortly after birth as it usually does.

In patent ductus arteriosus, the blood vessel connecting the pulmonary artery and the aorta (ductus arteriosus) fails to close as it usually does within the first 2 weeks after birth; a left-to-right shunt causes extra blood flow, and pressure in the lungs may damage the lung tissue. Premature newborns are especially susceptible to patent ductus arteriosus and lung damage.

Most often, the defect causes no symptoms. When symptoms do occur, they are usually difficulty breathing or cyanosis, which may be present at birth or not for several weeks after birth. When

Patent Ductus Arteriosus: Failure to Close

The ductus arteriosus is a blood vessel that connects the pulmonary artery and aorta. In the fetus, it enables blood to bypass the lungs. The fetus does not breathe air, and thus blood does not need to pass through the lungs to be oxygenated. After birth, blood needs to be oxygenated in the lungs, and normally, the ductus arteriosus closes quickly, usually within days up to 2 weeks. In patent ductus arteriosus, this connection does not close, allowing some oxygenated blood, intended for the body, to return to the lungs. As a result, the blood vessels in the lungs may be overloaded and the body may not receive enough oxygenated blood.

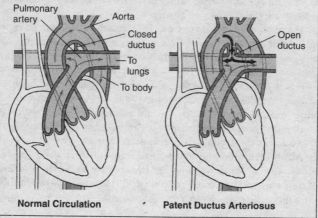

Normal Circulation   **Patent Ductus Arteriosus**

the infant has no symptoms, doctors most often suspect the defect when they hear a heart murmur.

Use of indomethacin, a drug that inhibits the production of chemicals called prostaglandins, closes the defect in 80% of infants. Indomethacin is most effective if given in the first 10 days after birth and is more effective in premature newborns than in full-term newborns. If the defect does not close after several doses of indomethacin, it is closed surgically.

ATRIAL AND VENTRICULAR SEPTAL DEFECTS

- Holes occur in the walls (septa) that separate the heart into right and left sides.
- Many defects are small, cause no symptoms, and close on their own.

- Some atrial septal defects do not cause symptoms until middle age.
- Some large septal defects must be closed surgically.

Atrial and ventricular septal defects are holes in the walls (septa) that separate the heart into the left and right sides. Atrial septal defects are located between the heart's upper chambers (atria), which receive blood. Ventricular septal defects are located between the lower chambers (ventricles), which pump blood. These holes typically cause left-to-right shunting of blood. Many atrial septal defects close by themselves, especially in the first year of life; many ventricular septal defects close within the first 2 years.

Infants and most older children with atrial septal defects have no symptoms, and this defect is often not detected until adulthood. In more severe cases, children may develop heart murmurs, fatigue, and difficulty breathing. The symptoms caused by atrial septal defects increase as the person ages. For example, heart failure may develop during middle age.

Ventricular septal defects can vary from small holes, which may cause a heart murmur but no symptoms and usually close by themselves, to larger holes that cause symptoms in infants. Significant ventricular septal defects usually cause more severe symptoms than atrial septal defects, because there is more shunting of blood. Because of the way lungs develop, shunting increases during the first 6 weeks after birth. Usually the murmur becomes louder, and symptoms, typically rapid breathing, sweating, and difficulty feeding, worsen. Mild symptoms of a ventricular septal defect may be treated with diuretics (such as furosemide) or drugs that decrease resistance to the flow of blood to the body (such as captopril). If atrial and ventricular septal defects are large or use symptoms, they are closed, usually surgically.

TETRALOGY OF FALLOT

- Children have four defects: (1) a hole in the wall between ventricles, (2) a displaced aorta, and a right ventricle with (3) a narrowed outflow passage and (4) a thickened wall.
- Infants have mild to severe cyanosis (a bluish discoloration of the skin) because not enough oxygen-rich blood reaches the tissues.

Septal Defect: A Hole in the Heart's Wall

A septal defect is a hole in the wall (septum) that separates the heart into the left and right sides. Atrial septal defects are located between the heart's upper chambers (atria). Ventricular septal defects are located between the lower chambers (ventricles). In both types, some oxygenated blood, intended for the body, is shortcircuited. It is returned to the lungs rather than pumped to the rest of the body.

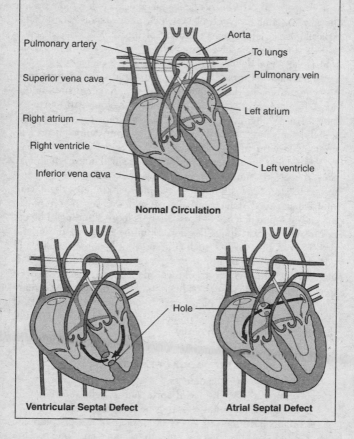

Pulmonary artery

Superior vena cava

Right atrium

Right ventricle

Inferior vena cava

Aorta

To lungs

Pulmonary vein

Left atrium

Left ventricle

Normal Circulation

Hole

Ventricular Septal Defect

Atrial Septal Defect

- Some infants have life-threatening attacks and turn blue or lose consciousness during crying or other activity.
- Oxygen, morphine, intravenous fluids, or phenylephrine may help relieve attacks, and propranolol may help prevent them.
- Eventually, surgery is required.

In tetralogy of Fallot, four specific heart defects occur together. The defects are a large ventricular septal defect, displacement of the aorta that allows oxygen-poor blood to flow directly from the right ventricle to the aorta (causing a right-to-left shunt), a narrowing of the outflow passage from the right side of the heart, and a thickening of the wall of the right ventricle.

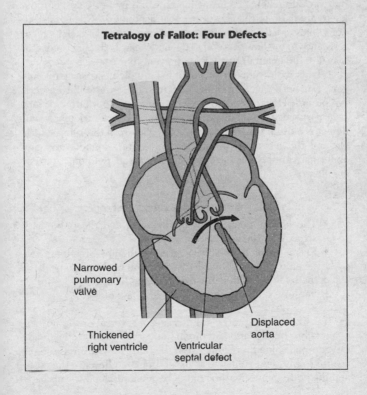

Tetralogy of Fallot: Four Defects

Narrowed pulmonary valve

Thickened right ventricle

Ventricular septal defect

Displaced aorta

In infants with tetralogy of Fallot, the narrowed passage from the right ventricle restricts blood flow to the lungs. The restricted blood flow causes the oxygen-poor blood in the right ventricle to pass through the septal defect to the left ventricle and into the aorta (right-to-left shunt). The most important symptom is cyanosis, which can be mild or severe. Some infants have life-threatening attacks (hypercyanosis or "tet" spells), in which cyanosis suddenly worsens in response to activity, such as crying or having a bowel movement. The infant becomes very short of breath and may lose consciousness. Infants with tetralogy of Fallot usually have a heart murmur. Echocardiography confirms the diagnosis.

When an infant has a hypercyanotic spell, oxygen and morphine may provide relief. The infant may breathe more easily when the knees are close to the chest (knee-chest position). Giving intravenous fluids or a drug such as phenylephrine, both of which increase resistance to the flow of blood to the body, may be helpful. A doctor may give the infant propranolol to prevent future spells.

Infants with tetralogy of Fallot eventually need surgery. Surgery can be delayed until later in infancy if the child has few symptoms. However, if the symptoms develop often or are severe, surgery should be performed soon. The ventricular septal defect is closed, the narrowed passageway from the right ventricle and the narrowed pulmonary valve are widened, and any abnormal connections between the aorta and pulmonary artery are closed.

TRANSPOSITION OF THE GREAT ARTERIES

- The normal connections of the aorta and the pulmonary artery with the heart are reversed.
- From birth, infants have great difficulty breathing and severe cyanosis (a bluish discoloration of the skin) because the body does not receive oxygenated blood.
- Surgery is done during the first few days of life.

Transposition of the great arteries is a reversal of the normal connections of the aorta and the pulmonary artery with the heart. Oxygen-poor blood returning from the body flows from the right atrium to the right ventricle as usual, but then flows to the aorta and the body, bypassing the lungs. Oxygenated blood travels back and forth between the heart and lungs (from the lungs to the pulmonary vein, then left atrium and ventricle, then the pulmonary artery) but is not transported to the body. The body cannot survive without oxygen. However, infants with this defect may survive briefly after birth because the foramen ovale (a hole between the right and left atria) and the ductus arteriosus (a blood vessel connecting the pulmonary artery with the aorta) (see page 83) are still open at birth. These openings allow oxygen-rich blood to mix with oxygen-poor blood, sometimes supplying enough oxygen to the body to keep the infant alive. Transposition of the great arteries is often accompanied by a ventricular septal defect.

Transposition of the great arteries usually results in severe cyanosis and difficulty breathing, beginning at birth. A doctor performs a physical examination, x-ray, electrocardiography, and echocardiography to confirm the diagnosis. Usually, surgery is performed within the first few days of life. Surgery consists of attaching the aorta and pulmonary artery to the appropriate ventricles and reimplanting the heart's coronary arteries in the aorta after the aorta is repositioned. Giving alprostadil or performing a balloon septostomy can shunt the blood, which can keep the infant alive until surgery can be performed.

AORTIC VALVE STENOSIS

- The heart valve between the left ventricle and aorta is narrowed.
- In most children, the only symptom is a heart murmur.
- Sometimes, surgery to replace or widen the valve is needed.

Aortic valve stenosis is a narrowing of the valve that opens to allow blood to flow from the left ventricle into the aorta and then to the body. To propel blood through the narrowed aortic valve, the left ventricle must pump under very high pressures. Sometimes, not enough blood is pumped to supply the body with oxygenated blood.

Most children with aortic valve stenosis do not develop symptoms other than a heart murmur. In some older children, the defect causes fatigue, chest pain, shortness of breath, or fainting.

In adolescents, severe aortic valve stenosis may lead to sudden death, presumably because of an erratic heart rhythm caused by poor blood flow through the coronary arteries to the heart. A few infants who have aortic valve stenosis develop irritability, an unnatural lack of color to the skin (pallor), low blood pressure, sweating, rapid heartbeat, and severe shortness of breath.

A doctor suspects aortic valve stenosis after detecting a particular murmur or if the child develops symptoms. Cardiac catheterization is often used to determine the severity of the narrowing.

For older children with severe narrowing or symptoms, the aortic valve must be replaced or widened. Usually the valve is opened surgically (using a procedure called balloon valvulotomy) or replaced with an artificial one. Children with an artificial valve must take an anticoagulant drug, such as warfarin, to prevent blood clots from forming. Infants with heart failure must have emergency treatment, usually including drugs and emergency surgery or balloon valvoplasty.

PULMONARY VALVE STENOSIS

- The heart valve between the right ventricle and the artery to the lungs is narrowed.
- In most children, the only symptom is a heart murmur.
- Balloon valvuloplasty to open the valve or surgery to reconstruct it is sometimes needed.

Pulmonary valve stenosis is a narrowing of the pulmonary valve, which opens to allow blood to flow from the right ventricle to the lungs. In most children with pulmonary valve stenosis, the valve is mildly to moderately narrowed, making the right ventricle pump harder and at a higher pressure to propel blood through the valve. Severe narrowing increases pressure in the right ventricle and prevents almost any blood from reaching the lungs. When pressure in the right ventricle becomes extremely high, oxygen-poor blood is forced through abnormal paths (usually a hole in the atrial wall [atrial septal defect]) instead of the pulmonary artery, causing right-to-left shunting.

Most children with pulmonary valve stenosis have no symptoms other than a heart murmur. However, severe cyanosis or heart failure is possible. Moderate symptoms, such as difficulty breathing with exertion and fatigue, may develop as the child gets older. Occasionally, cardiac catheterization is needed to assess the severity of the narrowing.

If the valve is moderately narrowed, it may be opened with balloon valvuloplasty. If the valve is not well formed, it can be surgically reconstructed.

Severe disease that causes cyanosis in newborns is treated by giving alprostadil, which opens the ductus arteriosus, until a surgeon can create another way to open or bypass the pulmonary valve. For some of these newborns, more surgery is needed when they are older.

COARCTATION OF THE AORTA

- The aorta narrows, usually just before the ductus arteriosus joins the aorta.
- Blood flow to the lower half of the body is reduced.
- Most infants have no symptoms or have a heart murmur.
- Severe coarctation can cause heart failure and high blood pressure.
- Severe symptoms require emergency treatment, including drugs and surgery, but otherwise, surgery is usually done when children are 3 to 5 years old.

Coarctation of the aorta is a narrowing of the aorta, usually just before the ductus arteriosus joins the aorta. Coarctation reduces blood flow to the lower half of the body; therefore, the blood pressure is lower than normal in the legs and tends to be higher than normal in the arms. Coarctation can cause heart murmurs. Without treatment, coarctation eventually strains and enlarges the heart, causing heart failure; it also causes high blood pressure. It predisposes the child to rupture of the aorta, bacterial endocarditis, and bleeding in the brain. Children with coarctation often have other heart defects, such as aortic valve stenosis or an atrial or ventricular septal defect.

For most infants, mild or moderate coarctation does not cause symptoms. Rarely, children with coarctation have headaches or nosebleeds because of high blood pressure in the arms, or leg pains during exercise because of insufficient blood and oxygen to the legs.

With a severe coarctation in infancy, blood can flow only to the lower portion of the aorta (at a point past its narrowing) through the open connection between the aorta and the pulmonary artery, the ductus arteriosus. Symptoms usually do not occur until the ductus closes, usually when the newborn is a few days to about 2 weeks old. After the closure, the blood supplied through the ductus disappears, sometimes causing sudden loss of almost the entire blood supply to the lower body. Sudden, catastrophic heart failure and low blood pressure can result.

Coarctation is usually suspected only when a doctor notices a heart murmur or differences in pulses or blood pressures between the arms and legs when performing a physical examination. X-rays, electrocardiography, and echocardiography are usually used to confirm the diagnosis.

Coarctation that does not cause severe symptoms should be surgically repaired in early childhood, usually when the child is about 3 to 5 years old. Infants with severe symptoms from coarctation require emergency treatment, including giving alprostadil to reopen the ductus arteriosus, other drugs to strengthen the heart's pumping, and emergency surgery to widen the narrowing. Some infants who undergo emergency surgery need more surgery when they are older. Sometimes, instead of surgery, doctors use balloon angioplasty to relieve coarctation.

Urinary Tract Defects

- Any part of the urinary tract may be affected: kidneys, ureters, bladder, or urethra.
- Most children have no symptoms but may be more likely to have blood in the urine, urinary tract infections, or kidney stones.
- Defects may damage kidneys over time, usually causing symptoms only when little kidney function remains.
- Ultrasound, computed tomography (CT), nuclear scanning, intravenous urography, and cystoscopy may aid in the diagnosis.
- If symptoms occur or pressure on the kidneys increases, surgery is usually needed.

Birth defects are more common in the kidney and urinary system than in any other system of the body. Defects can develop in the kidneys, the tubes that transport urine from the kidneys to the bladder (ureters), the bladder, or the tube that expels urine from the bladder (urethra). Any birth defect that blocks or slows the flow of urine can cause urine to stagnate, which can result in infections or formation of kidney stones. Blockage also causes urine pressure to increase, which damages the kidneys and ureters over time.

DID YOU KNOW?

- More birth defects occur in the kidneys and urinary tract than in any other system in the body.
- Many kidney defects do not cause symptoms and are never detected.

Symptoms

Many urinary tract defects cause no symptoms. Some, such as kidney defects, may cause blood in the urine after minor injuries. Infections due to defects can develop anywhere in the urinary system and cause symptoms. Kidney damage results from blockage, but it usually causes symptoms only when very little kidney function remains. Then, kidney failure develops. Kidney stones may develop and cause severe, crampy pain in the side between the ribs and the hip (flank) or groin, or blood in the urine.

Diagnosis and Treatment

The techniques used to diagnose abnormalities of the urinary tract include physical examination, ultrasound, computed tomography (CT), nuclear scans, intravenous urography, and rarely, cystoscopy. Defects that cause symptoms or those that lead to increased pressure on the kidneys usually need to be surgically corrected.

KIDNEY AND URETER DEFECTS

A number of defects may result in abnormal formation of the kidneys. The kidneys may be in the wrong place (ectopia), in the wrong position (malrotation), joined together (horseshoe kidney), or missing (kidney agenesis). In Potter's syndrome, which causes death, both kidneys are missing. Kidney tissue may also develop abnormally. For example, a kidney may contain many cysts (fluid-filled sacs), as in polycystic kidney disease. If an abnormality blocks an infant's urine flow, the affected kidney may swell so that it becomes visible and can be felt by a doctor.

Many birth defects involving the kidney do not cause symptoms and are never detected. Some defects may interfere with the function of the kidneys, leading to kidney failure, which can require dialysis or kidney transplantation.

Abnormalities of the tubes that connect the kidneys to the bladder (ureters) include formation of extra ureters, misplaced ureters, and narrowed or widened ureters. A narrowed ureter prevents urine from passing normally from the kidney to the bladder.

BLADDER AND URETHRA DEFECTS

The bladder may not close completely, so that it opens out onto the surface of the abdomen (exstrophy). The wall of the bladder may develop outpouchings (diverticula) where urine can stagnate, sometimes causing urinary tract infections. The bladder outlet (the passageway from the bladder to the urethra) may be narrowed, causing the bladder to empty incompletely. In this case, the urine stream is weak.

The urethra may be abnormal or missing altogether. In posterior urethral valves, abnormal tissue blocks (usually partially) the flow of urine from the bladder. Affected infants have a weak urinary stream and urinary tract infections; they may fail to gain weight normally or may have anemia. Less severe defects may not cause symptoms until childhood. In this case, the symptoms that develop are also milder. Surgery to open the blockage must be performed in infants.

In boys, the opening of the urethra may be in the wrong place, such as on the underside of the penis (hypospadias). In boys with hypospadias, the penis may bend downward (chordee). Both hypospadias and chordee can be repaired surgically. The urethra in the penis may lie open as a channel rather than closed as a tube (epispadias). In both boys and girls, a narrowed urethra may obstruct the flow of urine.

Genital Defects

- Genital defects may result from abnormal levels of sex hormones, a metabolic disorder called congenital adrenal hyperplasia, or chromosomal abnormalities in the fetus.
- Sometimes the genitals are not clearly male or female (ambiguous).
- To determine the sex of an infant with ambiguous genitals, a physical examination and blood tests to analyze chromosomes and check hormone levels are done.
- Sex is then assigned, and hormones, surgery, or both may be needed.

Defects of the external genital organs (penis, testes, or clitoris) usually result from abnormal levels of sex hormones in the blood before birth. Congenital adrenal hyperplasia (a metabolic disorder) and chromosomal abnormalities commonly cause genital defects.

A child may be born with genitals that are not clearly male or female (ambiguous genitals, or intersex state). Most children with ambiguous genitals are pseudohermaphrodites—that is, they have ambiguous external genital organs but either ovaries or testes (not both). Pseudohermaphrodites are genetically male or female.

Diagnostic evaluation of a child with ambiguous genitals includes physical examination and blood tests to analyze the chromosomes (the XY chromosome pattern is male and XX is female) and hormone levels (pituitary hormones and male sex hormones, or androgens, such as testosterone). X-rays and ultrasound of the pelvis may help identify internal sex organs. Treatment with testosterone may help enlarge the penis so that assignment to a male sex is more realistic.

Most experts believe that the child's sex must be assigned quickly. Otherwise, bonding by the parents to the child may become more difficult and the child may develop a gender identity disorder. Surgery to correct the ambiguous genitals can be performed later, especially if the defect is complex. The underlying problem causing pseudohermaphroditism may also need treatment.

MALE GENITAL DEFECTS

Pseudohermaphroditism in the male is usually caused by a deficiency of male sex hormones (androgens) or a chromosomal abnormality. The penis and testes may be absent if androgen deficiency develops before the 12th week of pregnancy. If androgen deficiency develops later in pregnancy, a male fetus may have an abnormally small penis (microphallus) or testes that do not descend fully into the scrotum (see page 148). Pseudohermaphroditism may also result from an inability to respond to androgens. After they develop, the testes produce most of the male body's androgens. Absent or underdeveloped testes causes androgen deficiency.

Androgen deficiency during childhood causes incomplete sexual development. An affected boy retains a high-pitched voice and has poor muscle development for his age. The penis, testes, and scrotum are underdeveloped. Pubic and underarm hair is sparse, and the arms and legs are abnormally long.

Androgen deficiency can be treated with testosterone. The testosterone is usually given by injection or through a skin patch. Injection and skin application cause fewer side effects than taking testosterone by mouth. Testosterone stimulates growth, sexual development, and fertility.

FEMALE GENITAL DEFECTS

Female pseudohermaphroditism (also called virilization) is caused by exposure to high levels of male hormones. The most common cause is enlarged adrenal glands (congenital adrenal hyperplasia) that overproduce male hormones because an enzyme is missing. The male hormones cannot be converted to female hormones as occurs in normal females. Sometimes, male hormones enter the placenta from the mother's blood; for example, the mother may have been given drugs such as progesterone to prevent a miscarriage, or she may have had a hormone-producing tumor, although this is much less common.

A female pseudohermaphrodite has female internal organs but has an enlarged clitoris that resembles a small penis.

If the child is assigned to the female gender, surgery is performed to create female-appearing genitals. This surgery can include reduction of the clitoris, formation or repair of a vagina (vaginoplasty), and repair of the urethra.

Congenital adrenal hyperplasia can be life-threatening because it can cause serious abnormalities of electrolytes (sodium and potassium) in the blood. These are diagnosed with blood tests and treated with corticosteroids.

Digestive Tract Defects

- The digestive organs may be incompletely developed or abnormally positioned, causing blockages, or the muscles or nerves of the digestive tract may be defective.
- Crampy abdominal pain, abdominal swelling, and vomiting are common.
- Surgery is usually required.

A birth defect can occur anywhere along the length of the digestive tract—in the esophagus, stomach, small intestine, large intestine, rectum, or anus. In many cases, an organ is not fully developed or is abnormally positioned, which often causes narrowing or blockage (obstruction). The internal or external muscles surrounding the abdominal cavity may weaken or develop holes. The nerves to the intestines may also fail to develop (Hirschsprung disease, or congenital megacolon).

Blockages (obstructions) that develop in the intestines, rectum, or anus can cause rhythmic, crampy abdominal pain, abdominal swelling, and vomiting.

Most digestive tract defects require surgery. Generally, obstructions are surgically opened. Weakenings or holes in the muscles surrounding the abdominal cavity are sewn shut.

ESOPHAGEAL ATRESIA AND TRACHEOESOPHAGEAL FISTULA

- In newborns with atresia, the esophagus narrows or ends without connecting to the stomach.
- In newborns with a fistula, the esophagus connects with the windpipe (trachea).

Normally, the esophagus, a long tubelike organ, connects the mouth to the stomach. In esophageal atresia, the esophagus narrows or comes to a blind end; food is delayed or prevented from going from the esophagus to the stomach. Most newborns with esophageal atresia also have a tracheoesophageal fistula, an abnormal connection between the esophagus (below the narrowing) and the trachea. Swallowed food and saliva travel through the fistula to the lungs, leading to coughing, choking, difficulty breathing, and possibly pneumonia. Food or fluid in the lungs may impair oxygenation of blood, leading to a bluish discoloration of the skin (cyanosis). Characteristically, a newborn with esophageal atresia coughs and drools after attempting to swallow. Many children with esophageal atresia and tracheoesophageal fistula have other abnormalities, such as heart defects.

Atresia and Fistula: Defects in the Esophagus

In esophageal atresia, the esophagus narrows or comes to a blind end. It does not connect with the stomach as it normally does. A tracheoesophageal fistula is an abnormal connection between the esophagus and the trachea (which leads to the lungs).

Trachea
Esophagus
Stomach

Atresia

Fistula

| Normal Anatomy | Atresia Only | Fistula Only | Atresia Plus Fistula |

To detect a blockage, x-rays are taken as a tube is passed down the esophagus.

The first steps in treatment are withholding oral feedings and placing a tube in the upper esophagus to suction out saliva continuously before it can reach the lungs. The infant is fed intravenously. Surgery needs to be performed soon to establish a normal connection between the esophagus and stomach and to close the connection between the esophagus and the trachea.

ANAL ATRESIA

Anal atresia is narrowing or blockage of the anus. Most infants with anal atresia develop some type of abnormal connection (fistula) between the anus and either the urethra, the area between the urethra and anus (the perineum), the vagina, or the bladder.

Infants with anal atresia fail to defecate normally after birth. Eventually, intestinal obstruction develops. However, doctors often detect the abnormality by looking at the anus when they first examine the baby after birth, before symptoms develop.

Using x-rays, a radiologist can see the path of a fistula. Anal atresia usually requires immediate surgery to open a passage for feces and to close the fistula. Sometimes, a temporary colostomy (making a hole in the abdomen and connecting it to the colon to allow stool to flow into a plastic bag on the abdominal wall) may be necessary.

INTESTINAL MALROTATION

- The intestines develop incompletely or abnormally, sometimes causing them to twist.

Intestinal malrotation (abnormal rotation of the intestines) is a potentially life-threatening defect in which the intestines develop incompletely or abnormally. Malrotation can cause the intestines to later twist (volvulus), cutting off their blood supply. Infants with intestinal malrotation can suddenly develop symptoms of vomiting, diarrhea, and abdominal swelling; these symptoms can also come and go. If the blood supply to the middle of the intestine is completely cut off (mid-gut volvulus), sudden, severe pain and vomiting develop. Bile, a substance formed in the liver, may be vomited and appear yellow, green, or rust-colored. Eventually, the abdomen swells. X-rays may help the doctor determine the diagnosis. However, the volvulus can be seen only on x-rays taken after placing barium, a substance visible on the x-ray, in the rectum (barium enema).

Treatment, including intravenous fluids and usually emergency surgery, must begin within hours. If not treated rapidly, the defect can result in loss of intestinal tissue or death.

BILIARY ATRESIA

- The bile ducts are partially or completely destroyed, causing yellowing of the skin (jaundice).
- The urine is dark, stools are pale, and the liver enlarges, leading to scarring by age 2 months if the defect is not corrected.

- Blood tests and sometimes ultrasound aid in the diagnosis.
- Surgery to construct replacement bile ducts can be done in almost half of infants, and the rest require liver transplantation.

Bile, a fluid secreted by the liver, carries away the liver's waste products and helps digest fats in the small intestine. Bile ducts within the liver collect the bile and carry it to the intestine. In biliary atresia, the bile ducts are destroyed—either partially or completely—so bile cannot reach the intestine. Eventually, the bile accumulates in the liver and then escapes into the blood, causing a yellowish discoloration of the skin (jaundice). Progressive, irreversible scarring of the liver, called biliary cirrhosis, starts by the age of 2 months if the defect is not treated.

In infants with biliary atresia, the urine becomes dark, the stools become pale, and the skin becomes increasingly jaundiced. These symptoms and an enlarged, firm liver are usually first noticed about 2 weeks after birth. By the time the infant is 2 to 3 months old, he may have stunted growth, be itchy and irritable, and have large veins visible on his abdomen, as well as a large spleen.

To prevent biliary cirrhosis, the diagnosis of biliary atresia must be made before the age of 2 months. To make the diagnosis, a doctor performs a series of blood tests. Ultrasound may be helpful. If the defect is still suspected after these tests, surgery (which consists of examination of the liver and bile ducts and a liver biopsy) is performed to diagnose the defect.

Surgery is needed to create a path for bile to drain from the liver. Constructing replacement bile ducts that flow into the intestine is best, and this kind of operation is possible in 40 to 50% of infants. Most of the infants with replacement bile ducts can lead normal lives. Infants who cannot have replacement bile ducts constructed usually require liver transplantation by age 2 years.

DIAPHRAGMATIC HERNIA

A diaphragmatic hernia is a hole or weakening in the diaphragm that allows some of the abdominal organs to protrude into the chest. Diaphragmatic hernias occur on the left side of the body 90% of the time. The stomach, loops of intestine, and even the liver and spleen can protrude through the hernia. If the hernia is large, the lung on the affected side is usually incompletely developed. Many children with diaphragmatic hernias also have heart defects.

After delivery, as the newborn cries and breathes, the loops of intestine quickly fill with air. This rapidly enlarging structure pushes against the heart, compressing the other lung and causing severe difficulty breathing, often right after birth. A chest x-ray usually shows the defect. The defect can also be detected before birth using ultrasound. Diagnosis before birth allows the doctor to prepare for treatment of the defect. Surgery is required to repair the diaphragm. Measures to deliver oxygen, such as a breathing tube and ventilator, may be needed.

HIRSCHSPRUNG DISEASE

- Some of the nerves that control the rhythmic contractions of the large intestine are missing.
- Children may vomit, refuse to eat, and be constipated, and the abdomen may be swollen.
- Toxic enterocolitis, a life-threatening disorder, can develop.
- Doctors perform a barium enema or rectal biopsy and measure pressure inside the rectum to make the diagnosis.
- Surgery to bypass the affected part of the intestine is usually done.

The large intestine depends on a network of nerves within its wall to synchronize rhythmic contractions and move digested material toward the anus, where the material is expelled as feces. In Hirschsprung disease (congenital megacolon), a section of the large intestine is missing the nerve network that controls the intestine's rhythmic contractions.

Children with Hirschsprung disease can have symptoms that suggest intestinal obstruction—bile-stained vomit, a swollen abdomen, and refusal to eat. If only a small section of the intestine is affected, a child may have milder symptoms and may not be diagnosed until later in childhood. These children may have ribbonlike stools and a swollen abdomen; they often fail to gain weight. In rare cases, constipation is the only symptom. Delayed passage of stool (meconium) by a newborn raises the suspicion of Hirschsprung disease.

Hirschsprung disease can also lead to life-threatening toxic enterocolitis, which produces sudden fever, a swollen abdomen, and explosive and, at times, bloody diarrhea.

A barium enema is often performed. Rectal biopsy and measurement of the pressure inside the rectum (manometry) are the only tests that can reliably be used to diagnose Hirschsprung disease.

Severe Hirschsprung disease must be treated quickly to prevent toxic enterocolitis. Hirschsprung disease is usually treated with surgery to remove the abnormal section of intestine and to connect the normal intestine to the rectum and anus. In some cases, for example, if the child is quite ill, the surgeon connects the lower end of the normal part of the intestine to an opening made in the abdominal wall (colostomy). Stool can thus pass through the opening into a collection bag, restoring normal movement of food through the intestines. The abnormal section of intestine is left disconnected from the rest of the intestine. The normal part of the intestine can be reconnected to the rectum and anus when the child is older.

Bone and Muscle Defects

Birth defects can occur in any bone or muscle, although the bones and muscles of the skull, face, spine, hips, legs, and feet are affected most often. Bones and muscles may develop incompletely. Also, structures that normally align together may be separated or misaligned. Usually bone and muscle defects result in abnormal appearance and function of the affected part of the body. Most of these defects are repaired surgically if symptoms are troublesome. Often, the surgery is complex and involves reconstructing deformed or absent body parts.

FACIAL DEFECTS

- Cleft lip, a separation of the upper lip, prevents infants from closing their lips around a nipple.
- Cleft palate, a split in the roof of the mouth, interferes with eating and speaking.
- The lower jaw may be too small, interfering with eating and breathing.

The most common defects of the skull and face are cleft lip and cleft palate. **Cleft lip** is a separation of the upper lip, usually just below the nose. **Cleft palate** is a split in the roof of the mouth resulting in a passageway into the nose. Cleft lip and cleft palate often occur together.

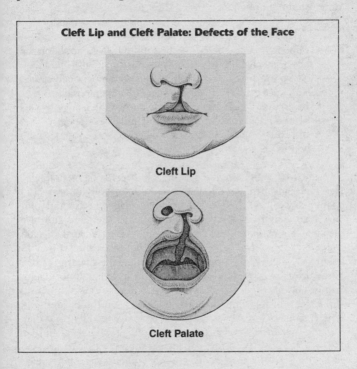

Cleft Lip and Cleft Palate: Defects of the Face

Cleft Lip

Cleft Palate

Cleft lip is disfiguring and prevents the infant from closing his lips around a nipple. A cleft palate interferes with eating and speech. A dental device can temporarily seal the roof of the mouth so the infant can suckle better. Cleft lip and cleft palate can be permanently corrected with surgery. The likelihood of cleft lip and cleft palate can be reduced if a woman takes folic acid before pregnancy and through the 1st trimester of pregnancy.

Another type of facial defect is a small lower jaw (mandible). Pierre Robin and Treacher Collins syndromes, which are characterized by several defects in the head and face, are among the causes of a small lower jaw. If the lower jaw is too small, the infant may have difficulty eating or breathing. Surgery may correct or diminish the problem.

LIMB AND JOINT DEFECTS

- Limb and joint defects may be caused by genetic abnormalities or mechanical forces.
- Newborns may be born with a dislocated hip, usually treated with a harness that holds the legs in a certain position.
- In clubfoot, the foot and ankle are twisted out of shape because the bones or muscles are underdeveloped.
- In arthrogryposis multiplex congenita, some joints cannot bend.

Limbs or joints can be missing, deformed, or incompletely developed at birth. A child with one limb or joint abnormality is more likely to have another related abnormality. Limbs and joints may form abnormally; for example, bones in the hand and forearm may be missing because of a genetic defect. Normal development of a limb can also become disrupted in the womb; for example, a finger can stop growing because the finger gets constricted by fibers. Another cause for limb and joint abnormalities is mechanical force; for example, pressure may cause the hip to dislocate. Chromosomal abnormalities can cause limb and joint abnormalities. Sometimes the cause is unknown. The drug thalidomide, which was taken by some pregnant women in the late 1950s and early 1960s for morning sickness, caused a variety of limb defects—usually short, poorly functioning appendages developed in place of arms and legs.

Abnormalities of the arms and legs may occur in a horizontal fashion (for example, if the arm is shorter than normal) or in a lengthwise fashion (for example, the arm is abnormal on the thumb side [from the elbow to the thumb] but normal on the little finger side). Children often become very adept at using a malformed limb, and an artificial limb (prosthesis) can often be constructed to make the limb easier to use.

Hand defects are common. Sometimes a hand does not form completely; part or all of the hand may be missing. For example, the person may have too few fingers. Sometimes a hand does not develop; for example, the fingers may not separate, producing a weblike hand. Some hand defects involve extra fingers; the little fingers or thumbs are most commonly duplicated. Overgrowth may occur, in which the hands or individual fingers are too large. Surgery is usually carried out to correct the hand defect and provide as much function as possible.

In **congenital dislocation of the hip,** also called developmental dysplasia of the hip, the newborn's hip socket and the thighbone (femoral head), which normally form a joint, become separated, often because the hip has a socket that is not deep enough to hold the head of the femur. Dislocation of the hip is a disorder more common in girls, in newborns born in a breech (buttocks-first) position, and in newborns who have close relatives with the disorder. The right and left legs or hips often look different from each other in newborns with the defect.

The doctor can detect the defect when examining the newborn. In infants younger than 4 months, an ultrasound of the hips can confirm the diagnosis; in infants older than 4 months, an x-ray can be used. The use of triple diapers (an older treatment) is not recommended. The best treatment is use of the Pavlik harness. The Pavlik harness is a soft brace that holds the infant's knees spread outward and up toward the chest. However, if the defect persists past the age of 6 months, surgery to fix the hip in the normal position is usually needed.

Clubfoot (talipes equinovarus) is a defect in which the foot and ankle are twisted out of shape or position. The usual clubfoot is a down and inward turning of the hind foot and ankle, with twisting inward of the forefoot. Sometimes the foot only appears abnormal because it was held in an unusual position in the uterus (positional clubfoot). In contrast, true clubfoot is a structurally abnormal foot. With true clubfoot, the bones of the leg or foot or the muscles of the calf are often underdeveloped.

Positional clubfoot can be corrected by immobilizing the joints in a cast and by using physical therapy to stretch the foot and ankle. Early treatment with immobilization is beneficial for true clubfoot, but surgery, often complex, is also generally needed.

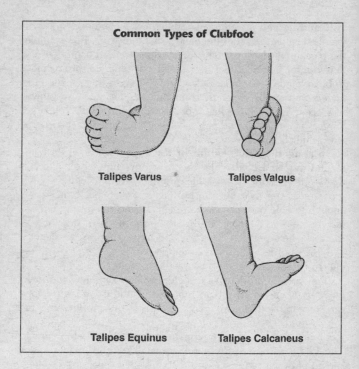

Common Types of Clubfoot

Talipes Varus

Talipes Valgus

Talipes Equinus

Talipes Calcaneus

In **metatarsus adductus,** the foot appears turned inward. Mobility of the joints of the foot and ankle may be limited. Treatment depends on the severity of the deformity and immobility of the foot. Most mild cases resolve spontaneously. Corrective shoes or splints may be needed in more severe cases. Surgery is required only in exceptional instances.

In **arthrogryposis multiplex congenita,** some joints become "frozen" and consequently cannot bend. Many children with this defect have weakened muscles. It is likely that decreased movement of the muscles and joints before birth causes the decreased movement of the joints after birth. The cause is unknown. Sometimes the nerves that would normally move the bones in the affected joints are also impaired. Infants with the defect may also have dislocated hips, knees, or elbows. Placing the limbs in a cast and performing physical therapy, in which the stiff joints are carefully manipulated, may improve joint movements. Surgically freeing the bones from attached tissue sometimes results in more normal joint movement.

Brain and Spinal Cord Defects

- Brain damage may result in mental retardation, seizures, or paralysis.
- Spinal cord damage may result in paralysis, incontinence, or loss of sensation in some parts of the body.
- Computed tomography (CT) and magnetic resonance imaging (MRI) can detect brain and spinal cord defects.
- Some defects can be repaired surgically, but brain or spinal cord damage is usually permanent.

Of the many possible defects in the brain and spinal cord, those known as neural tube defects develop within the first weeks of pregnancy. Others, such as porencephaly and hydranencephaly, develop later in pregnancy. Many brain and spinal cord defects result in visible abnormalities in the head or back.

Symptoms of brain or spinal cord damage may develop if the defect affects brain or spinal cord tissue. Brain damage can be fatal or result in mild or severe disability, which may include mental retardation, seizures, and paralysis. Spinal cord damage can result in paralysis, incontinence, and loss of sensation to areas of the body reached by nerves below the level of the defect. Computed tomography (CT) and magnetic resonance imaging (MRI) can reveal brain and spinal cord defects by showing pictures of the internal structures of those organs.

DID YOU KNOW?

- Many brain and spinal cord defects produce visible abnormalities in the head or back.
- Shunts used to drain fluid in children with hydrocephalus are rarely removed, even if they are no longer needed.

Some defects, such as those that cause visible openings or swellings, can be repaired surgically. However, brain or spinal cord damage from the defect is usually permanent.

NEURAL TUBE DEFECTS

- If the neural tube does not develop normally, the brain, spinal cord, and tissues that surround them may be affected.
- In the most severe and fatal form, brain tissue does not develop.
- In the mildest form, the spine does not close as it normally does, usually causing no symptoms.
- Many defects can be recognized before birth if the doctor tests the mother's blood or the amniotic fluid, which surrounds the fetus.
- Surgery to close neural tube defects is usually done.

The brain and spinal cord develop as a groove that folds over to become a tube (the neural tube). Layers of tissue that come from this tube normally cover the brain and spinal cord (meninges). Sometimes the neural tube does not develop normally, which may affect the brain, spinal cord, and meninges. In the most severe form of neural tube defect, the brain tissue may fail to develop (anencephaly); this defect is fatal. Another type of defect results when the neural tube fails to close completely and remains an open channel. In its mildest form, an open channel defect may affect only bone; for example, in spina bifida occulta (which means hidden spine split in two), the bony spine fails to close, but the spinal cord and meninges are unaffected. This common abnormality usually causes no symptoms. Sometimes, a meningocele develops in which the meninges and other tissue, such as brain tissue (meningoencephalocele) or spinal cord tissue (meningomyelocele), can protrude out of the opening. Sometimes the meninges are not involved when tissue protrudes from the brain (encephalocele) or spinal cord (myelocele). Damage to brain or spinal cord tissue is much more likely when tissue protrudes than when it does not.

In occult spinal dysraphism, newborns are born with visible abnormalities on their lower backs. These include birthmarks, overly pigmented areas (hemangioma and flame nevus), tufts of hair, openings in the skin (dermal sinus), or small lumps (masses). The underlying spinal cord may be connected to the surface, which exposes it to bacteria, greatly increasing the chance for development of meningitis. The nerves of the spinal cord may

Spina Bifida: A Defect of the Spine

In spina bifida, the bones of the spine (vertebrae) do not form normally. Spina bifida can vary in severity. In the least severe, most common type, one or more vertebrae do not form normally, but the spinal cord and the layers of tissues (meninges) surrounding it are not affected. The only symptom may be a tuft of hair, a dimpling, or a pigmented area on the skin over the defect. In a meningocele, a more severe type of spina bifida, the meninges protrude through the incompletely formed vertebrae, resulting in a fluid-filled bulge under the skin. The most severe type is a meningomyelocele, in which the spinal cord protrudes. The affected area appears raw and red, and the infant is likely to be severely disabled.

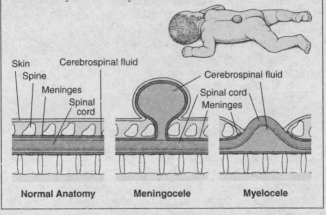

Normal Anatomy   Meningocele   Myelocele

become damaged as the child grows. Or, the spinal cord may have a fatty tumor (lipoma) on it, which also can lead to nerve damage. Therefore, newborns who have these abnormalities should have the underlying soft tissue and spinal cord evaluated using ultrasound or magnetic resonance imaging (MRI).

Genetic factors can make neural tube defects more likely. The defect often develops before the mother knows she is pregnant. Most symptoms from neural tube defects result from brain or spinal cord damage. A defect may be so inconsequential that it is never recognized or so severe that it is fatal. Meningoencephaloceles and meningomyeloceles cause severe disability. These include hydrocephalus, learning disabilities, paralysis with bone and joint abnormalities, decreased sensation of the skin, and bowel and urinary problems.

Many neural tube defects can be detected before birth. A high level of alpha-fetoprotein in the woman's blood or amniotic fluid may indicate a neural tube defect in the fetus. Ultrasound performed late in pregnancy may show the defect or characteristic abnormalities. Folic acid taken just before a woman gets pregnant through the first three months of pregnancy can decrease the risk of neural tube defects by as much as 70%. Neural tube defects are usually closed surgically.

HYDROCEPHALUS

- If the fluid that surrounds the brain cannot drain as it normally does, hydrocephalus develops.
- Affected infants have an abnormally large head and do not develop normally.
- Hydrocephalus may not affect intelligence or may cause mental retardation or learning disabilities.
- Computed tomography (CT), ultrasound, or magnetic resonance imaging (MRI) aids in diagnosis.
- A drain (shunt) is inserted to drain the fluid.

The fluid surrounding the brain (cerebro-spinal fluid) is produced in spaces within the brain called ventricles. The fluid must drain to a different area, where it is absorbed into the blood. When the fluid cannot drain, hydrocephalus (water on the brain) develops. Hydrocephalus often increases the pressure in the ventricles, which compresses the brain. Many conditions, such as a birth defect, bleeding within the brain, or brain tumors can block drainage and cause hydrocephalus.

An abnormally large head may be a symptom of hydrocephalus. The infant usually fails to develop normally. Computed tomography (CT), ultrasound, or magnetic resonance imaging (MRI) of the head reveals the diagnosis as well as the degree of brain compression.

The goal of treatment is to keep pressure normal within the brain. A permanent alternate drainage path (shunt) for cerebrospinal fluid decreases the pressure and volume of the fluid inside the brain. A doctor places the shunt in the ventricles in the brain and runs it under the skin from the head to another site, usually the abdomen (ventriculoperitoneal shunt). The shunt contains a valve that allows fluid to leave the brain if the pressure becomes too high. Although a few children can eventually do without the shunt as they get older, shunts are rarely removed.

If needed, pressure within the brain can often be temporarily reduced with drugs (such as acetazolamide or furosemide) or repeated spinal taps (lumbar punctures) until a shunt is placed.

Some children with hydrocephalus develop normal intelligence. Others are mentally retarded or have learning disabilities.

CHAPTER 5

Chromosomal and Genetic Abnormalities

Chromosomes are structures within cells that contain a person's genes. Abnormalities in chromosomes are always genetic abnormalities. Some genetic abnormalities affect the genes, but do not alter the structure of the chromosomes. Thus, doctors often discuss chromosomal abnormalities separately from the broader category of genetic abnormalities. Some genetic abnormalities, such as sickle cell disease and cystic fibrosis, are very common.

A person normally has 23 pairs of chromosomes, each containing hundreds of genes. The sex chromosomes are one of these pairs of chromosomes. Normal people have 2 sex chromosomes; each is either an X or a Y chromosome. Normal females have two X chromosomes (XX), and normal males have one X and one Y chromosome (XY).

Chromosomal abnormalities can affect any chromosome, including the sex chromosomes. A chromosomal or other genetic abnormality can affect the number of chromosomes, the structure of certain chromosomes, or the composition of chromosomes (for example, genetic material from one chromosome may be attached to another). If the material found in chromosomes is balanced so that the expected amount is found in each cell, no abnormalities occur. If too much (addition) or too little (deletion) genetic material is found within each cell, abnormalities occur. These abnormalities can have profound physical effects.

DID YOU KNOW?

- All chromosomal abnormalities are genetic, but not all genetic abnormalities are chromosomal.
- The older the mother, the greater the chance of a chromosomal abnormality, but the father's age has little effect.
- Some genetic defects (as in Noonan syndrome) can be inherited or can occur spontaneously.
- Some chromosomal and genetic abnormalities result in an abnormal but characteristic physical appearance.
- Many effects of some chromosomal abnormalities (as in Turner and Klinefelter syndromes) begin at puberty.
- Many chromosomal abnormalities can be detected by blood tests in children or by amniocentesis or chorionic villus sampling in fetuses (before birth).
- Some genetic abnormalities can cause learning problems even when intelligence is normal or above normal.

The older a pregnant woman is, the greater the chance that her fetus will have a chromosomal abnormality. The chance of chromosomal abnormalities increases by a barely noticeable degree if the father is older. A marriage between close relatives increases the chance of developing some genetic abnormalities, but usually not chromosomal abnormalities.

Chromosomal abnormalities can cause a wide range of abnormalities or effects, usually birth defects (see page 76) or death of the embryo or fetus before birth. Genetic abnormalities can cause birth defects or diseases (for example, sickle cell disease) or have many different effects.

A person's chromosomes can be analyzed with a sample of blood. A fetus can be tested for chromosomal abnormalities before birth, for example, using amniocentesis or chorionic villus sampling. If the fetus is found to have a chromosomal abnormality, further tests may be performed to detect specific birth defects. Although chromosomal abnormalities cannot be corrected, some of the defects can sometimes be prevented or treated.

WHEN PART OF A CHROMOSOME IS MISSING

A number of syndromes can occur in infants who are missing part of a chromosome. These syndromes are called **chromosome deletion syndromes.**

In the rare **cri du chat syndrome** (cat's cry syndrome, 5p minus syndrome), part of chromosome 5 is missing. An infant with this syndrome is usually underweight at birth; has a small head with many abnormal features, including a round face, small jaw, wide nose, widely separated eyes, and ears set low in the head; and has a high-pitched cry that sounds like a kitten crying. Often the infant seems limp. The high-pitched cry occurs immediately after birth, lasts several weeks, and then disappears. Heart defects are common. Mental and physical development are greatly retarded. Despite these abnormalities, many children with cri du chat syndrome survive to adulthood.

In **Prader-Willi syndrome,** another chromosomal deletion syndrome, mental retardation is common. Many symptoms vary according to the child's age. Newborns with the defect feel limp, feed poorly, and gain weight slowly. Eventually these symptoms resolve. Then, between the ages of 1 and 6, appetite increases, often becoming insatiable. Obsessive-compulsive behaviors are common. Weight gain is excessive, which can lead to other health problems. Obesity can be severe enough to require gastric bypass surgery.

Down Syndrome

- Having an extra chromosome causes Down syndrome, which is characterized by mild to severe mental retardation and certain physical abnormalities.
- Older mothers are more likely than younger ones to contribute the extra chromosome, and fathers sometimes do.
- The average intelligence quotient (IQ) of children with Down syndrome is 50, compared with 100 for normal children.
- Children have a small head, a broad and flat face, slanting eyes, small ears, and often heart defects.
- The diagnosis may be made before birth and is confirmed by chromosome analysis.
- Life expectancy ranges from 45 to 55 years, depending on the severity of mental retardation.

An extra chromosome, making three of a kind, is called trisomy. The most common trisomy in a newborn is trisomy 21 (three copies of chromosome 21). Trisomy 21 causes about 95% of the cases of Down syndrome. Older mothers, especially those older than 35, contribute an extra chromosome more often than do younger mothers. As a result, they more often bear children with Down syndrome. However, the extra chromosome may come from the father.

Symptoms

In Down syndrome, physical and mental development is delayed. Infants with Down syndrome tend to be quiet, passive, and have somewhat limp muscles. The intelligence quotient (IQ) among children with Down syndrome varies but averages about 50, compared with normal children, whose average IQ is 100. Children with Down syndrome have better visual motor skills (such as drawing) than skills that require hearing. Thus, their language skills typically develop slowly. Early intervention with educational and other services improves the functioning of young children with Down syndrome.

DID YOU KNOW?

- Early educational intervention can help children with Down syndrome function better.

Children with Down syndrome tend to have a small head, a face that is broad and flat with slanting eyes and a short nose. The tongue is large. The ears are small and set low in the head. The hands are short and broad, with a single crease across the palm. The fingers are short; the fifth finger, which often has two instead of three sections, curves inward. A space is visible between the first and second toes.

Children with Down syndrome often have heart defects. Many people with Down syndrome develop thyroid disease. They are prone to hearing problems because of recurring ear infections and the associated accumulation of inner ear fluid (serous otitis). They are also prone to vision problems because of problems in their corneas and lenses. They are prone to neck abnormalities, making it important for the doctor to check neck x-rays before allowing older children to participate in vigorous exercise. Many people with Down syndrome develop symptoms of Alzheimer-like dementia in their 30s, such as memory loss, further lowering of intellect, and personality changes.

Diagnosis

The diagnosis of Down syndrome can often be made before birth. An infant with Down syndrome has a physical appearance that suggests the diagnosis. A doctor confirms the diagnosis by testing the infant's chromosomes for trisomy 21 or other disorders of the 21st chromosome. After the diagnosis is made, doctors use tests, such as ultrasound and blood tests, along with examinations by specialists, to detect abnormalities associated with Down syndrome. Treating abnormalities that are detected can often prevent them from impairing health.

Prognosis

Most children with Down syndrome survive to adulthood. Life expectancy for a child with Down syndrome with mild or moderate retardation is 55 years and with profound mental retardation is 45 years. Many have progressively worsening mental functioning. Heart abnormalities are often treatable with drugs or surgery. Heart disease and leukemia account for most deaths among children with Down syndrome.

Fragile X Syndrome

- Abnormalities in an X chromosome causes delayed development, mental retardation (in some children), and prominent ears, chin, and forehead.

The symptoms of fragile X syndrome are caused by abnormalities in DNA on the X chromosome. Usually, affected boys inherit the condition from their mothers.

Many children with the syndrome have normal intelligence. However, the syndrome is the most commonly diagnosed genetic cause of mental retardation besides Down syndrome. The severity of symptoms, including mental retardation, is worse in boys than in girls with the disorder. Symptoms, which are often subtle, include delayed development; large, protuberant ears; a prominent chin and forehead; and, in boys, large testes (most apparent after puberty). The joints may be abnormally flexible, and heart disease (mitral valve prolapse) may occur. Features of autism may develop. Women may experience menopause in their mid 30s.

DID YOU KNOW?

- Fragile X syndrome is the second most commonly diagnosed genetic cause of mental retardation after Down syndrome.
- Early educational intervention can help children with fragile X syndrome function better.

The presence of abnormal DNA on the fragile X chromosome can be detected by tests before or after birth. The greater the number of abnormal repetitions of DNA found, the more likely the child will have symptoms.

Early intervention, including speech and language therapy and occupational therapy, can help children with fragile X syndrome to maximize their abilities. Stimulants, antidepressants, and anti-anxiety drugs may be beneficial for some children.

Turner Syndrome

In Turner syndrome (gonadal dysgenesis), girls are born with one of the two X chromosomes partially or completely missing.

- The neck may have loose folds of skin or webbing, and girls remain short, do not mature sexually, and have some learning difficulties.
- Heart, kidney, and eye defects often develop, as do diabetes mellitus and thyroid disorders.
- Symptoms suggest the diagnosis, which is confirmed by chromosome analysis.
- Girls may be given growth hormone to stimulate growth, followed by estrogen to stimulate sexual maturation.

Many newborns with Turner syndrome have swelling (lymphedema) on the backs of their hands and tops of their feet. Swelling or loose folds of skin are often evident over the back of the neck. Many other abnormalities often develop, including a webbed neck (wide skin attachment between the neck and shoulders), a low hairline at the back of the neck, a broad chest with wide-spaced nipples, and poorly developed nails.

As a girl with Turner syndrome gets older, she has no menstrual periods (amenorrhea), and the breasts, vagina, and labia remain childlike rather than undergoing the changes of puberty. The ovaries usually do not contain developing eggs. A girl or woman with Turner syndrome is virtually always short; obesity is common.

Other disorders often develop. Heart defects include narrowing of part of the aorta (coarctation of the aorta). Kidney and eye

Detecting Abnormalities Before Birth

Chorionic villus sampling and amniocentesis are used to detect abnormalities in a fetus. During both procedures, ultrasonography is used for guidance.

In chorionic villus sampling, a sample of chorionic villi (part of the placenta) is removed by one of two methods. In the transcervical method, a doctor inserts a flexible tube (catheter) through the vagina and cervix into the placenta. In the transabdominal method, a doctor inserts a needle through the abdominal wall into the placenta. In both methods, a sample of the placenta is suctioned out with a syringe and analyzed.

In amniocentesis, a doctor inserts a needle through the abdominal wall into the amniotic fluid. A sample of fluid is withdrawn for analysis.

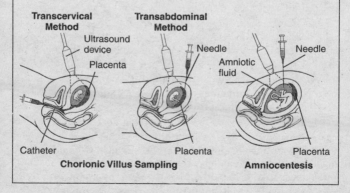

Transcervical Method — Ultrasound device, Placenta, Catheter — **Chorionic Villus Sampling**

Transabdominal Method — Needle, Placenta

Needle, Amniotic fluid, Placenta — **Amniocentesis**

defects, diabetes mellitus, and thyroid diseases are common. Occasionally, abnormal blood vessels in the intestine cause bleeding.

Many girls with Turner syndrome have difficulty in assessing visual and spatial relationships and have problems with planning and attention. They tend to score poorly on certain performance tests and in mathematics, even if they achieve average or above-average scores on verbal intelligence tests. Mental retardation is uncommon.

A doctor may suspect the diagnosis because of the newborn's abnormal appearance. However, suspicion often does not develop until the teenage years, when the girl fails to mature sexually. Analysis of the chromosomes confirms the diagnosis.

Treatment with a hormone normally secreted from the brain (growth hormone) can stimulate growth. Treatment with the female hormone estrogen is usually not started until after satisfactory growth has been achieved. Estrogen treatment may improve planning, attention, and assessment of visual and spatial relationships as well as stimulating sexual maturation.

Noonan Syndrome

- A genetic defect causes short stature, heart defects, and sometimes a webbed neck, droopy eyes, and delayed sexual maturation.

Noonan syndrome is a genetic defect that causes a number of physical abnormalities, usually including short stature, heart defects, and an abnormal appearance.

Noonan syndrome can be inherited or can develop unpredictably in children whose parents have normal genes. Although children with the syndrome have normal chromosomal structure, they have many characteristics typical of Turner syndrome. In the past, Noonan syndrome was called "male Turner syndrome." Boys or girls can be affected. The gene responsible for Noonan syndrome has been localized to chromosome 12.

Symptoms may include webbing of the neck, low-set ears, droopy eyelids, short stature, shortened fourth (ring) fingers, a high-arched palate, and heart and blood vessel abnormalities. Intelligence may be impaired. Most affected people are short. Boys may have underdeveloped or undescended testes. In girls, the ovaries may be underactive or stop working. Puberty may be delayed, and infertility may develop.

Growth may be improved by treatment with growth hormone. After satisfactory growth, testosterone treatment may help boys whose testes are underdeveloped. Testosterone stimulates the development of a more masculine appearance.

Triple X Syndrome

- Female infants are born with three X chromosomes, causing problems with verbal skills and sometimes infertility.

Girls with triple X syndrome tend to have slightly lower intelligence and particular problems with verbal skills. Sometimes the syndrome causes infertility, although some women with triple X syndrome have given birth to physically normal children who had normal chromosomes.

Extremely rare cases of infants with four or even five X chromosomes have been identified. The more X chromosomes the girl has, the greater the chance of mental retardation and physical abnormalities.

Klinefelter Syndrome

- Male infants are born with an extra X chromosome (usually causing problems with language), small testes, sparse facial hair, breast enlargement, and infertility.

Klinefelter syndrome is relatively common. Most boys with Klinefelter syndrome have normal or slightly decreased intelligence. Many have speech and reading disabilities and difficulties with planning. Most have problems with language skills. Early problems with language may lead to problems with social interactions that affect behavior, and these children often get into trouble at school. Although their physical characteristics can vary greatly, most are tall with long arms but otherwise normal in appearance.

Puberty usually occurs at the normal time, but the testes remain small. At puberty, growth of facial hair is often sparse, and the breasts may enlarge somewhat (gynecomastia). Men and boys with the syndrome are usually infertile. Men with Klinefelter syndrome develop diabetes mellitus, chronic lung disease, varicose veins, hypothyroidism, and breast cancer more often than other men.

The syndrome is usually first suspected at puberty, when most of the symptoms develop. Analysis of the chromosomes confirms the diagnosis.

Boys with Klinefelter syndrome usually benefit from speech and language therapy and eventually can do well in school. Some men benefit by taking supplemental male hormones such as testosterone. The hormones improve bone density, making fractures less likely, and stimulate development of a more masculine appearance.

XYY Syndrome

- Male infants are born with an extra Y chromosome, causing a tall stature and problems with language.

Boys with XYY syndrome tend to be tall and have difficulties with language. The IQ tends to be slightly lower than that of other family members. Learning disabilities, attention deficit disorder, and minor behavioral disorders can develop. The XYY syndrome was once thought to cause aggressive or violent criminal behavior, but this theory has been disproved.

Long QT Syndrome

- Children are born with an abnormality of the heart's electrical system, predisposing the heart to beat too fast.
- Children may lose consciousness or die suddenly, and some are born deaf.
- Electrocardiography (ECG) is done in children or young adults who lose consciousness inexplicably.
- Beta-blockers are usually effective, but if not, a pacemaker or pacemaker-internal defibrillator may help.

Long QT syndrome is an abnormality of the heart's electrical system. Long QT syndrome may affect as many as 1 of 7,000 people. In the United States, it may cause sudden death in 3,000 to 4,000 children and young adults each year. In children, this disorder is usually due to a genetic abnormality. A person with the disorder may have family members who died suddenly and inexplicably.

In most adults, long QT syndrome is caused by use of a drug or a disorder.

People who have long QT syndrome are predisposed to developing an unusually fast heart rate, which often occurs during physical activity or emotional excitement. When the heart rate is too fast, the brain may not receive enough blood. The result is loss of consciousness. Some people with long QT syndrome are also born deaf. But about one third of people have no symptoms. Long QT syndrome can cause sudden death at a young age.

DID YOU KNOW?

- In the United States, long QT syndrome may cause sudden death in 3,000 to 4,000 children and young adults each year.

Doctors may recommend electrocardiography (ECG) for children or young adults who have suddenly and inexplicably lost consciousness. The procedure may be performed with the person at rest or after receiving intravenous drugs or the person may be asked to walk on a treadmill or pedal an exercise bicycle in a procedure called exercise stress testing.

Beta-blockers are effective for most children and adults. For children who do not respond to drugs, a pacemaker or a combination pacemaker-internal defibrillator may be tried. An internal defibrillator can shock the heart, reviving the child, whenever the heart develops a lethal rhythm abnormality. Occasionally, as an alternative, a nerve in the neck is cut in a procedure called cervicothoracic sympathectomy. Cutting this nerve can help prevent the fast heart rate that causes sudden death.

CHAPTER 6

Mental Retardation

Mental retardation is significantly subaverage intellectual functioning present from birth or early infancy, causing limitations in the ability to conduct normal activities of daily living.

- Causes can be genetic or as a result of a disorder that interferes with the brain's development.
- Some cases result from problems during the mother's pregnancy or during the birth of the child.
- The child's level of functioning and other associated physical or behavioral problems depend on the level of retardation.
- Evaluation includes formal psychological and perhaps other testing.
- Support from many specialists helps children achieve the highest level of functioning possible.

Mental retardation is not a specific medical disorder like pneumonia or strep throat, and it is not a mental health disorder. A person with mental retardation has significantly below average intellectual functioning that limits his ability to cope with two or more activities of normal daily living (adaptive skills). These activities include the ability to communicate; live at home; take care of oneself, including making decisions; participate in leisure, social, school, and work activities; and be aware of personal health and safety.

People with mental retardation have varying degrees of impairment. While recognizing each person's individuality, doctors find it helpful to classify a person's level of functioning. Intellectual functioning levels can be based on the results of intelligence quotient (IQ) tests or on the level of support a person requires. Support is categorized as intermittent, limited, extensive, or pervasive. Intermittent means occasional support; limited means support such as a day program in a sheltered workshop; extensive means daily, ongoing support; pervasive means a high level of support for all activities of daily living, possibly including full-time nursing care.

Based only on IQ test scores, about 3% of the total population are considered to have mental retardation. However, if classification is based on the need for support, only about 1% of people have significant retardation.

Levels of Mental Retardation

LEVEL	INTELLI-GENCE QUO-TIENT (IQ) RANGE	ABILITY AT PRESCHOOL AGE (BIRTH TO 6 YEARS)	ABILITY AT SCHOOL AGE (6 TO 20 YEARS)	ABILITY AT ADULT AGE (21 YEARS AND OLDER)
Mild	52–68	Can develop social and communication skills; motor coordination is slightly impaired; often not diagnosed until later age	Can learn up to about the 6th-grade level by late teens; can be expected to learn appropriate social skills	Can usually achieve enough social and vocational skills for self-support, but may need guidance and assistance during times of unusual social or economic stress
Moderate	36–51	Can talk or learn to communicate; social awareness is poor; motor coordination is fair; can profit from training in self-help	Can learn some social and occupational skills; can progress to elementary school level in schoolwork; may learn to travel alone in familiar places	May achieve self-support by performing unskilled or semiskilled work under sheltered conditions; needs supervision and guidance when under mild social or economic stress

Levels of Mental Retardation (Continued)

LEVEL	INTELLI-GENCE QUO-TIENT (IQ) RANGE	ABILITY AT PRESCHOOL AGE (BIRTH TO 6 YEARS)	ABILITY AT SCHOOL AGE (6 TO 20 YEARS)	ABILITY AT ADULT AGE (21 YEARS AND OLDER)
Severe	20–35	Can say a few words; able to learn some self-help skills; has limited speech skills; motor coordination is poor	Can talk or learn to communicate; can learn simple health habits; benefits from habit training	May contribute partially to self-care under complete supervision; can develop some useful self-protection skills in controlled environment
Profound	19 or below	Extremely retarded, little motor coordination; may need nursing care	Some motor coordination; limited communication skills	May achieve very limited self-care; usually needs nursing care

Causes

A wide variety of medical and environmental conditions can cause mental retardation. Some are genetic; some are present before or at the time of conception; others occur during pregnancy, during birth, or after birth. The common factor is that something interferes with the growth and development of the brain. However, doctors can identify a specific cause in only about one third of people with mild mental retardation and in two thirds of people with moderate to profound mental retardation.

Symptoms

Some children with mental retardation have abnormalities apparent at birth or shortly thereafter. These abnormalities may be physical as well as neurologic and may include unusual facial features, a head that is too large or too small, deformities of the hands or feet, and various other abnormalities. Sometimes such children have an outwardly normal appearance but have other signs of serious illness, such as seizures, lethargy, vomiting, abnormal urine odor, and failure to feed and grow normally. During their first year,

SOME CAUSES OF MENTAL RETARDATION

Before or At Conception

- Inherited disorders (such as phenylketonuria, hypothyroidism, fragile X syndrome)
- Chromosome abnormalities (for example, Down syndrome)

During Pregnancy

- Severe maternal malnutrition
- Infections with HIV, cytomegalovirus, herpes simplex; toxoplasmosis, rubella
- Toxins (alcohol, lead, methylmercury)
- Drugs (phenytoin, valproate, isotretinoin, cancer chemotherapy)
- Abnormal brain development (spina bifida, myelomeningocele)

During Birth

- Insufficient oxygen (hypoxia)
- Extreme prematurity

After Birth

- Brain infections (meningitis, encephalitis)
- Severe head injury
- Malnutrition of the child
- Severe emotional neglect or abuse
- Toxins (lead, mercury)
- Brain tumors and their treatments

many children with more severe mental retardation have delayed development of motor skills, being slow to roll, sit, and stand.

However, most children with mental retardation do not develop symptoms that are noticeable until the preschool period. Symptoms become apparent at a younger age in those more severely affected. Usually, the first problem parents notice is a delay in language development. Children with mental retardation are slower to use words, put words together, and speak in complete sentences. Their social development is sometimes slow, because of cognitive impairment and language deficiencies. Children with mental retardation may be slow to learn to dress and feed themselves. Some parents may not consider the possibility of retardation until the child is in school or preschool and is unable to keep up with age-appropriate expectations.

Children with mental retardation are somewhat more likely than other children to have behavioral problems, such as explosive outbursts, temper tantrums, and physically aggressive behavior. These behaviors are often related to specific frustrating situations compounded by an impaired ability to communicate and control impulses. Older children may be gullible and easily taken advantage of or led into minor misbehavior.

About 10 to 40% of people with mental retardation also have a mental health disorder (dual diagnosis). In particular, depression is common, especially in children who are aware that they are different from their peers or who are maligned and mistreated because of their disability.

Diagnosis

Many children are evaluated by teams of professionals, including a pediatric neurologist or developmental pediatrician, a psychologist, speech pathologist, occupational or physical therapist, special educator, social worker, or nurse.

Doctors evaluate a child suspected of having mental retardation by testing intellectual functioning and looking for a cause. Even though mental retardation is usually irreversible, identifying a disorder that caused the retardation may allow doctors to predict the child's future course, plan any interventions that can increase the child's level of functioning, and counsel parents on the risk of having another child with that disorder.

Newborns with physical abnormalities or other symptoms suggestive of a condition associated with mental retardation often need laboratory tests to help detect metabolic and genetic disorders. Imaging tests, such as computed tomography (CT) or magnetic resonance imaging (MRI), may be performed to look for structural problems within the brain.

Some children who are delayed in learning language and mastering social skills have conditions other than mental retardation. Because hearing problems interfere with language and social development, a hearing evaluation is typically performed. Emotional problems and learning disorders also can be mistaken for mental retardation. Children who have been severely deprived of normal love and attention (see page 550) for long periods of time may appear retarded. A child with delays in sitting or walking (gross motor skills) or in manipulating objects (fine motor skills) may have a neurologic disorder not associated with mental retardation.

Because mild developmental problems are not always noticed by parents, doctors routinely perform developmental screening tests during well-child visits. Doctors use simple tests, such as the Denver Developmental Screening Test, to quickly evaluate the child's cognitive, verbal, and motor skills. Questions can be asked of the parents to help the doctor determine the child's level of functioning. Children who perform significantly below their age level on these screening tests are referred for formal testing.

Formal testing has three components: interviews with parents, observations of the child, and norm-referenced tests. Some tests, such as the Wechsler Intelligence Scale for Children-III (WISC-III), measure intellectual ability. Other tests, such as the Vineland Adaptive Behavior Scales, assess areas such as communication, daily living skills, social abilities, and motor skills. Generally, these formal tests accurately compare a child's intellectual and social abilities with those of others his age. However, children of different cultural backgrounds, non-English speaking families, and very low socioeconomic status are more likely to perform poorly on these tests. Because of this, a diagnosis of mental retardation requires that the doctor integrate the test data with information obtained

DID YOU KNOW?

- Doctors can identify a specific cause in only about one third of children with mild mental retardation.
- Mental retardation can occasionally be a complication of severe abuse.
- The Federal Individuals with Disabilities Educational Act requires public schools to provide free and appropriate education to children and adolescents with mental retardation or other developmental disorders.

from parents and direct observations of the child. A diagnosis of mental retardation is appropriate only when both intellectual and adaptive skills are significantly below average.

Prevention and Prognosis

Prevention mainly applies to genetic and infectious disorders and to accidental injuries. Doctors may recommend genetic testing for people with a family member or other child with a known inherited disorder, particularly ones related to mental retardation, such as phenylketonuria, Tay-Sachs disease, or fragile X syndrome. Identification of a gene for an inherited disorder allows genetic counselors to help parents evaluate the risk of having an affected child. Women who plan to get pregnant should receive necessary vaccinations, particularly against rubella. Women who are at risk for infectious disorders that may be harmful to a fetus, such as rubella and HIV, should be tested for these before getting pregnant.

Proper prenatal care lowers the risk of having a child with mental retardation. Folic acid, a vitamin supplement, taken before conception and early in pregnancy can help prevent certain kinds of brain abnormalities. Advances in the practices of labor and delivery and in the care of premature infants have helped to reduce the rate of mental retardation related to prematurity.

Certain tests, such as ultrasound, amniocentesis, chorionic villus sampling, and various blood tests, can be performed during pregnancy to identify conditions that often result in mental retardation. Amniocentesis or chorionic villus sampling is often used for women at high risk of having a baby with Down syndrome. A few conditions, such as hydrocephalus and severe Rh incompatibility, may be treated during pregnancy. Most conditions, however, cannot be treated, and early recognition can serve only to prepare the parents and allow them to consider the option of abortion.

Because mental retardation sometimes coexists with serious physical problems, the life expectancy of children with mental retardation may be shortened, depending on the specific condition. In general, the more severe the retardation and the more physical problems the child has, the shorter the life expectancy. However, a child with mild mental retardation has a relatively normal life expectancy.

Treatment

The child with mental retardation is best cared for by a multidisciplinary team consisting of the primary care doctor, social workers, speech and physical therapists, psychologists, educators, and others. Together with the family, these people develop a comprehensive, individualized program for the child, which is begun as soon as the diagnosis of mental retardation is suspected. The parents and siblings of the child also need emotional support, and the whole family should be an integral part of the program.

The full array of a child's strengths and weaknesses must be considered in determining what kind of support is needed. Factors such as physical disabilities, personality problems, mental illness, and interpersonal skills all help determine how much support is needed.

All children with mental retardation benefit from education. The Federal Individuals with Disabilities Education Act requires public schools to provide free and appropriate education to children and adolescents with mental retardation or other developmental disorders. Education must be provided in the least restrictive, most inclusive setting possible—where the children have every opportunity to interact with nondisabled peers as well as equal access to community resources.

A child with mental retardation usually does best living at home. However, some families cannot provide care at home, especially for children with severe, complex disabilities. This decision is difficult and requires extensive discussion between the family and their entire support team. Having a child with severe disabilities at home can be disruptive and requires dedicated care that many parents may not be able to provide. The family may need psychologic support. A social worker can organize services to assist the family. Help can be provided by day care centers, housekeepers, child caregivers, and respite care facilities. Most adults with mental retardation live in community-based residences that provide services appropriate to the person's needs, with work and recreational opportunities.

CHAPTER 7

Cerebral Palsy

Cerebral palsy is poor muscle control, spasticity, paralysis, and other neurologic problems resulting from brain injury before, during, or shortly after birth.

- Most often, the cause of the brain injury cannot be determined.
- Symptoms range from barely noticeable clumsiness to severe spasticity.
- Cerebral palsy is difficult to recognize in young infants.
- As infants mature, poor development, spasticity, and muscle weakness become more noticeable.
- Many children with cerebral palsy have other disabilities such as mental retardation, behavioral problems, or seizures.
- Cerebral palsy cannot be cured, but therapy can help children achieve their highest potential.

Cerebral palsy affects 2 to 4 of every 1,000 infants, but it is 10 times more common in premature infants. It is particularly common in infants of very low birth weight.

Cerebral palsy is not a disease; it is a constellation of symptoms that result from damage to the parts of the brain that control muscle movements (motor areas). Sometimes children with cerebral palsy have damage to other parts of the brain as well. The brain damage that results in cerebral palsy may occur during pregnancy, during birth, after birth, or in early childhood. Once the brain damage has occurred, it does not get worse even though the child's symptoms may change with growth and maturation. Brain damage occurring after age 5 is not considered cerebral palsy.

Causes

Many different types of injury to the brain can cause cerebral palsy, and most often a specific cause cannot be identified. Birth injuries and poor oxygen supply to the brain before, during, and immediately after birth cause 10 to 15% of cases. Prenatal infections, such as rubella, toxoplasmosis, or cytomegalovirus infection, sometimes result in cerebral palsy. Premature infants are particularly vulnerable, possibly in part because the blood vessels of the brain are poorly developed and bleed easily. High levels of bilirubin in the blood can lead to a form of brain damage called kernicterus. During the first years of life, severe illness, such as inflammation of the tissues covering the brain (meningitis), sepsis, trauma, and severe dehydration, can cause brain injury and result in cerebral palsy.

DID YOU KNOW?

- Cerebral palsy is not a disease but a collection of symptoms that result from damage to the brain.
- Cerebral palsy is more common in infants who are premature or have a very low birth weight.
- Brain damage that occurs after age 5 is not considered cerebral palsy.
- Life expectancy is usually normal.

Symptoms

The symptoms of cerebral palsy can range from barely noticeable clumsiness to severe spasticity that contorts the child's arms and legs, requiring mobility aids, such as braces, crutches, and wheelchairs.

There are four main types of cerebral palsy: spastic, choreoathetoid, ataxic, and mixed. In all forms of cerebral palsy, speech may be hard to understand because the child has difficulty controlling the muscles involved in speech. Because nonmotor parts of the brain also may be affected, many children with cerebral palsy have other disabilities, such as mental retardation, behavioral problems, difficulty seeing or hearing properly, and seizure disorders.

In the spastic type, which occurs in about 70% of children with cerebral palsy, the muscles are stiff and weak. The stiffness may affect both arms and both legs (quadriplegia), mainly the legs (diplegia), or only the arm and leg on one side (hemiplegia). The affected arms and legs are poorly developed, stiff, and weak. Children with spastic quadriplegia are the most severely affected. They commonly have mental retardation (sometimes severe) along with seizures and trouble swallowing. Trouble with swallowing makes these children prone to choking on secretions from the mouth and stomach (aspiration). Aspiration injures the lungs, causing difficulty breathing. Repeated aspiration can permanently damage the lungs. Children with spastic diplegia usually have normal mental development and rarely have seizures. About one fourth of children with spastic hemiplegia have below-normal intelligence, and one third have seizures.

In the choreoathetoid type, which occurs in about 20% of children with cerebral palsy, the muscles spontaneously move slowly and without normal control. Movements of the arms, legs, and body may be writhing, abrupt, and jerky. Strong emotion makes the movements worse; sleep makes them disappear. These children usually have normal intelligence and rarely have seizures.

In the ataxic type, which occurs in about 10% of children with cerebral palsy, coordination is poor and movements are shaky. These children also have muscle weakness and trembling. Children with this disorder have difficulty making rapid or fine movements and walk unsteadily, with their legs widely spaced.

In the mixed type, two of the above types, most often spastic and choreoathetoid, are combined. This type occurs in many children with cerebral palsy.

Diagnosis

Cerebral palsy is difficult to diagnose during early infancy. As the baby matures, poor development, weakness, spasticity, or lack of coordination becomes noticeable. Although laboratory tests cannot identify cerebral palsy, a doctor may perform blood tests, electrical studies of muscle (electromyography), a muscle biopsy, and computed tomography (CT) or magnetic resonance imaging (MRI) of the brain to clarify the nature of the brain damage and to look for other disorders. The doctor might recommend additional testing if the child's symptoms appear to be evolving in a way not typical of cerebral palsy. The specific type of cerebral palsy often cannot be distinguished before the child is 18 months old.

Prognosis and Treatment

The prognosis usually depends on the type of cerebral palsy and on its severity. More than 90% of children with cerebral palsy survive into adulthood. Only the most severely affected—those incapable of any self-care—have a substantially shortened life expectancy.

Cerebral palsy cannot be cured; its problems are lifelong. However, much can be done to improve a child's mobility and independence. Physical therapy, occupational therapy, and braces may improve muscle control and walking, particularly when rehabilitation is started as early as possible. Surgery may be performed to cut or lengthen tendons of the stiff muscles that limit motion. Sometimes cutting certain nerve roots coming from the spinal cord improves the spasticity. Speech therapy may make speech much clearer and help with swallowing problems. Seizures can be treated with anticonvulsant drugs. Drugs taken by mouth, such as dantrolene and baclofen, are sometimes used to help spasticity, but their benefits are limited by side effects. Some treatments deliver drugs directly to the nerves and muscles that are affected. Botulinum toxin can be injected into spastic muscles.

Children with cerebral palsy grow normally and attend regular schools if they do not have severe intellectual and physical disabilities. Other children require extensive physical therapy, need special education, and are severely limited in activities of daily living, requiring some type of lifelong care and assistance. However, even severely affected children can benefit from education and training.

Information and counseling are available to parents to help them understand their child's condition and potential, and to assist with problems as they arise. Loving parental care combined with assistance from public and private agencies, such as community health agencies and vocational rehabilitation organizations, can help a child reach his highest potential.

CHAPTER 8

Common Problems in Infants and Very Young Children

Few children make it through their first years without minor problems. Crying, problems with feeding, and an occasional fever are common. These problems become health concerns only when they are extreme—for example, when children cry too much, when they are not growing well, or when a high fever is due to a serious infection. Fortunately, most childhood problems are not severe. Many children experience rashes. Very rarely, families face the tragedy of sudden infant death syndrome (SIDS).

Fussiness, Excessive Crying, and Colic

Fussiness *is the inability of an infant to settle down or be soothed.* **Excessive crying** *is crying over long hours by a healthy infant whose basic needs are met.* **Colic** *is a pattern of excessive crying over weeks that is loud, piercing, constant, and that occurs at intervals, between which the infant acts normally.*

- Doctors check for possible causes.
- If no cause for crying is found, there is no specific treatment.
- Holding, rocking, or patting the infant may help, as may white noise or vibration from a fan or car ride.

Fussiness, excessive crying, and colic occur most commonly between the second week and third month of life. Their cause is usually unknown, but excessive crying is sometimes associated with excess air in the digestive tract (for example, from not burping after eating or from swallowing air while crying). Excessive crying can be due to an infection, such as an ear or urinary tract infection or meningitis. Other causes of crying are gastroesophageal reflux (see page 382), milk allergy, eruption of a tooth, a hair caught around a finger or toe (hair tourniquet), or a corneal abrasion.

Parents of children with excessive crying or colic should consult a doctor if there is nothing they can do to stop the child's crying or if the child has other symptoms, such as fever or poor feeding. Doctors try to diagnose and treat known causes of fussiness and crying. Infections may or may not require antibiotics. Gastroesophageal reflux can be treated by a number of strategies (see page 383). Air in the digestive tract can be diminished by adequately burping the child. A change of formula may treat symptoms of milk allergy; however, parents should consult with their doctor before changing the formula. Crying from teething improves with time. A hair tourniquet needs to be removed. Corneal abrasions are treated with an antibiotic ointment or drops to prevent infection.

DID YOU KNOW?

- Excessive crying and colic usually stop by the time infants are 3 or 4 months old.

If there is no medical reason for an infant's crying, the doctor may diagnose excessive crying or colic. Parents of infants with colic typically note that their child does not seem ill, even though he is crying vigorously during certain hours of the day. There is no specific treatment. If mothers who are breastfeeding notice that certain foods lead to increased crying in their infants, they should avoid eating these foods. Many infants get some relief from being held, rocked, or patted or from the "white noise" and vibration of a fan, washing machine, or car ride. A pacifier or swaddling clothes may also be comforting. Feeding sometimes soothes the child, but parents should avoid overfeeding in an attempt to stop the crying. If left alone, some children will cry themselves to sleep.

Excessive crying and colic can be exhausting and stressful for parents. Parents should take advantage of nighttime crying interludes to lay the infant on his back in his crib to encourage self-soothing and sleep. Emotional support from friends, family, neighbors, and doctors is key to coping. Parents should ask for whatever help they need (with siblings, errands, or child care) and share their feelings and fears. Overwhelmed parents can take comfort in the fact that, despite the extreme distress the crying or colicky infant appears to be in, excessive crying and colic usually disappear by 3 to 4 months of age and cause no long-term harm.

Teething

- When teeth are coming in, children may cry, be irritable, drool, and constantly chew on food and objects.
- Chewing on hard, cold objects may relieve discomfort; acetaminophen or ibuprofen may also help.

A child's first tooth usually appears by 6 months of age, and a complete set of 20 primary or first teeth usually develops by age 3. Before a tooth appears, the child may cry, be irritable, and sleep and eat poorly. The child may drool, have red and tender gums, and constantly chew on food and objects during tooth eruption. During teething, the child may have a mildly elevated temperature (below 100°F). Children with higher temperatures and those who are especially fussy should be evaluated by a doctor because these symptoms are not due to teething.

DID YOU KNOW?

- Teething does not normally cause high fevers or excessive crying.

Teething infants get some relief from chewing on hard, cold objects, such as a frozen bagel or banana. Parents should prevent the infant from biting off large pieces, which can choke the child. Firm rubber teething rings and teething biscuits are also useful. Massaging the child's gums with or without ice may help. Teething gels may provide relief for a few minutes. If a child is extremely uncomfortable, acetaminophen or ibuprofen is usually effective for pain.

Feeding Problems

- Simple measures solve some feeding problems—for example, burping infants who spit up.
- Vomiting usually stops on its own but sometimes requires medical attention.
- Dehydration may result from vomiting, diarrhea, or inadequate fluid intake.
- Dehydrated infants and children are treated with fluids and electrolytes, usually given by mouth.

Feeding problems in infants and young children are usually minor but sometimes have serious consequences.

Spitting up (burping up) is the effortless return of swallowed formula or breast milk through the mouth or nose after feeding. Almost all infants spit up, because infants cannot sit upright during and after feedings. Also, the valve (sphincter) that separates the esophagus and stomach is immature and does not keep all of the stomach's contents in place. Spitting up gets worse when an infant eats too fast or swallows air. Spitting up usually stops between the ages of 7 and 12 months.

Spitting up can be reduced by feeding an infant before he gets very hungry, burping him every 4 to 5 minutes, placing him in an upright position during and after feeding, and making certain the bottle nipple lets out only a few drops with pressure or when the bottle is upside down. Spitting up that seems to cause an infant discomfort, interferes with feeding and growth, or persists into early childhood is called gastroesophageal reflux and may require medical attention (see page 382). If the material that is spit up is green (indicating bile), bloody, or causes any coughing or choking, medical attention is needed.

Vomiting is the uncomfortable, forced throwing up of feedings. It is never normal. Vomiting in infants is most often the result of viral gastroenteritis. It can also be caused by infections elsewhere in the body. Less commonly, vomiting occurs because of a serious medical disorder. Infants between the ages of 2 weeks and

4 months may rarely have forceful (projectile) vomiting after feedings because of a blockage at the stomach outlet (hypertrophic pyloric stenosis). Vomiting can also be caused by life-threatening disorders, such as meningitis, intestinal blockage, and appendicitis. These disorders usually cause severe pain, lethargy, and continuous vomiting that does not get better with time.

Most vomiting caused by gastroenteritis stops on its own. Giving the child fluid and electrolytes (such as sodium and chloride) from solutions available in stores or pharmacies prevents or treats dehydration. Older children can be given popsicles or gelatin, although red versions of these foods can be confused with blood if the child vomits again. A doctor should see any child who has severe abdominal pain, is unable to drink and retain fluids, is lethargic or acting extremely ill, vomits for more than 12 hours, vomits blood or green material (bile), or is unable to urinate. These symptoms may signal dehydration or a more severe condition.

DID YOU KNOW?

- Spitting up usually stops by the time infants are 7 to 12 months old.
- Spitting up requires medical attention if the material is green or bloody, if it causes coughing or choking, or if the infant is not gaining weight.
- Vomiting requires medical attention if the child has severe abdominal pain, cannot drink and retain fluids, is lethargic or acting extremely ill, vomits for more than 12 hours, vomits blood or green material, or cannot urinate.
- Infants should not be fed automatically every time they cry and should not be allowed to always have a bottle with them.
- Plain water, juice, and colas are not good for treating dehydration because water does not contain enough salt and because juice and colas contain too much sugar.

Overfeeding is the provision of more nutrition than a child needs for healthy growth. Overfeeding occurs when children are automatically fed as a response to crying, when they are given a bottle as a distraction or activity, or when they are allowed to keep a bottle with them at all times. Overfeeding also occurs when parents reward good behavior with food or expect a child to finish his food even if he is not hungry. In the short term, overfeeding causes spitting up and diarrhea. In the long term, overfed children can become obese (see page 206).

Underfeeding is the provision of less nutrition than a child needs for healthy growth. It is one of many causes of failure to thrive (see page 153) and may be related to the child or the caregiver. Underfeeding may result when a fussy or distracted infant does not sit well for feedings or has difficulty sucking or swallowing. Underfeeding can also result from improper feeding techniques and errors in formula preparation (see page 22). Poverty and poor access to nutritious food are major reasons for underfeeding. Occasionally, abusive parents and parents with mental health disorders purposely withhold food from their children.

Community social agencies (such as the Women, Infants and Children [WIC] program) can help parents purchase formula and can teach them proper techniques for formula preparation and feeding. If an infant is so far below expected weight that he needs supervised feedings, then the doctor may admit the child to a hospital for evaluation. If the parents are abusive or neglectful, child protective services may be called.

Dehydration is caused by excess fluid loss, such as from vomiting and diarrhea, or by inadequate fluid intake, such as when an infant does not take in enough milk through breastfeeding. Children who are moderately dehydrated are less interactive or playful, cry without tears, have a dry mouth, and urinate fewer than 2 or 3 times a day. Children who are severely dehydrated become sleepy or lethargic. Sometimes dehydration causes the concentration of salt in the blood to fall or rise abnormally. Changes in salt concentration make the symptoms of dehydration worse and can worsen lethargy. In severe cases, the child can have seizures or suffer brain damage and die.

Dehydration is treated with fluids and electrolytes, such as sodium and chloride. In severe cases, intravenous fluids are needed.

TREATING DEHYDRATION

Minor illnesses that cause vomiting and diarrhea can lead to dehydration in children. In infants, dehydration is treated by encouraging an infant to drink fluids that contain electrolytes. Breast milk contains all the fluids and electrolytes an infant needs and is the best treatment. If an infant is not breastfeeding, oral electrolyte solutions should be given. These can be bought as powders or liquids at drug or grocery stores without a prescription. The amount of solution to give a child depends on the child's age, but generally should be about $1^{1}/_{2}$ to $2^{1}/_{2}$ ounces of solution in a 24-hour period for each pound the child weighs.

Children older than 1 year may try small sips of juices or clear soups, clear sodas diluted to half-strength with water, or popsicles. Plain water, juice, and colas are not good for treating dehydration at any age because the salt content of water is too low and because juice and colas have a high sugar content and ingredients that irritate the digestive tract.

Treatment of dehydration at any age is more effective if children are first given small, frequent sips of fluids about every 10 minutes. The amount of fluid can slowly be increased and given at less frequent intervals if the child can keep the fluid down without vomiting or getting severe diarrhea. Infants who digest fluids over 12 to 24 hours can then resume drinking formula from a bottle. Older children can try broths or soups and bland foods (for example, bananas, toast, rice). Infants and young children who are unable to digest any fluids, or who develop listlessness and other serious signs of dehydration, may require more intensive treatment with intravenous fluids or electrolyte solutions given through a nasogastric tube

Bowel Problems

- Diarrhea is usually due to viral gastroenteritis but can be caused by many other disorders.
- The most common problem caused by acute diarrhea is dehydration.
- Constipation may be hard to identify because, for some infants, having infrequent bowel movements is normal.
- Constipation usually results from dehydration, inadequate dietary fiber, or a change in feeding habits.

- Constipation is usually treated with diet.
- Parents should consult a doctor before they give their child a laxative, suppository, or enema.

The number and consistency of stools for a healthy child vary with age and diet. For example, infants who are breastfed normally have mustard-colored stools that are soft and seedy. However, repeated watery bowel movements for a time lasting longer than 12 hours are never normal.

Diarrhea is frequent, watery bowel movements. Acute diarrhea starts suddenly and improves in one to several days. Acute diarrhea is most often caused by viral gastroenteritis, which is especially likely when vomiting accompanies the diarrhea. Typically, vomiting occurs at the beginning of the illness and then tapers off, while diarrhea continues. Acute diarrhea can also be caused by a bacterial or parasitic infection; an infection elsewhere in the body, such as an ear or respiratory tract infection; and as a side effect from the use of antibiotics. Acute diarrhea is a concern mainly because it can cause dehydration. Therefore, the main treatment is administering fluids and electrolytes. Bacterial infections are treated with antibiotics. Antibiotics that cause diarrhea may be discontinued, but only after consultation with a doctor.

Chronic diarrhea lasts for weeks or months. The most common causes of chronic diarrhea in infants and young children are cystic fibrosis, celiac disease, giardiasis, sugar malabsorption, and food allergy. In less developed countries, malnutrition is the most common cause of chronic diarrhea.

DID YOU KNOW?

- Some infants and young children have bowel movements only once every 3 to 4 days.

Constipation is the infrequent passing of hard, dry stools (see page 391). Constipation may be difficult to recognize because some infants and young children have bowel movements only once every 3 to 4 days. In general, children are constipated when they have not had a bowel movement in 5 or more days, when the stools are hard or cause pain, or when drops of blood are seen in the diaper or stool.

Constipation in infants is usually caused by dehydration, insufficient fiber in the diet, or a change in feeding patterns. Rarely, medical disorders, such as inadequate nerve supply to the large intestine (Hirschsprung disease), low thyroid hormone levels, or calcium or potassium abnormalities cause constipation. The use of certain drugs (such as antihistamines, anticholinergic drugs, and opioids) is another rare cause.

Treatment of constipation varies with the age of the child. Infants younger than 2 months of age who consume adequate amounts of formula or breast milk can be given a teaspoon of light corn syrup in their morning and evening bottles. Apple or prune juice is good for infants between 2 and 4 months of age. Infants between 4 months and 1 year can get relief from high-fiber cereals or from strained apricots, prunes, or plums. Children older than 1 year should be given high-fiber foods, such as fruits, peas, cereals, graham crackers, beans, and spinach. Parents should not give their child a laxative, suppository, or enema without first consulting a doctor. For older children with significant constipation, doctors may use various drugs. Treatment of rare disorders includes surgery for Hirschsprung disease, thyroid hormone replacement for low thyroid hormone levels, and calcium supplements for abnormal calcium levels.

Separation Anxiety

Separation anxiety is the fear young children have that their parents will leave them.

- At about age 8 months, infants normally begin to feel some anxiety when they are separated from their parents.
- Parents should not limit or stop separations because doing so may interfere with normal development.
- If separation anxiety repeatedly interferes with going to childcare or preschool or playing with peers, medical attention may be needed.

Children with separation anxiety panic and cry when a parent leaves them, even if only to go into an adjacent room. Separation anxiety is normal for infants at about 8 months of age, is most intense between 10 and 18 months of age, and generally resolves by 2 years of age. The intensity and duration of a child's separation anxiety vary and depend partly on the child-parent relationship. For example, separation anxiety in a child with a strong and healthy attachment to a parent resolves sooner than in a child whose connection is less strong.

Separation anxiety occurs at a time when infants start to become aware that their parents are unique individuals. Because they have incomplete memory and no sense of time, these young children fear the departure of their parents may be permanent. Separation anxiety resolves as a young child develops a sense of memory and keeps an image of the parents in mind when they are gone. The child recollects that in the past the parents returned.

Parents should not limit or forgo separations in response to separation anxiety; this could compromise the child's maturation and development. When parents leave the home (or leave the child at a childcare center), they should encourage the person with whom they are leaving the child to create distractions. The parent should then leave without responding at length to a child's crying. If the parents are staying at home but in a different room, they should not return immediately in response to crying, but instead call to the child from the other room. This teaches the child that parents are still present even though the child cannot see them. Separation anxiety may be worse when a child is hungry or tired, so feeding the child and letting him nap before leaving may also help.

Separation anxiety at the normal age causes no long-term harm to the child. Separation anxiety that lasts beyond age 2 may or may not be a problem depending on the extent to which it interferes with the child's development. It is normal for children to feel some fear upon leaving for preschool or kindergarten. This feeling should diminish with time. Rarely, excessive fear of separations inhibits a child from attending childcare or preschool or keeps him from playing normally with peers. This anxiety is probably abnormal (separation anxiety disorder—see page 532). In this case, the parents should seek medical attention for the child.

Skin Rashes

- Diaper rash is usually caused by irritation and relieved by frequently changing diapers and sometimes by using an ointment.
- Eczema is a red, scaly, dry patchy rash, treated, if necessary, with moisturizers, corticosteroid creams, and anti-itch drugs.
- Cradle cap is a red and yellow crusty rash, treated by shampooing regularly and massaging mineral oil into the scalp.
- Other rashes may be caused by fungal or viral infections.

Skin rashes in infants and young children are not usually serious and can have various causes.

Diaper rash (diaper dermatitis) is a bright red rash caused by irritation from prolonged skin contact with urine or stool anywhere beneath a child's diaper. Typically, the areas of the skin that touch the diaper are most affected. Diaper rash can also be caused by infection with the fungus *Candida*, typically causing a bright red rash in the creases of the skin and small red spots. Less often, diaper rash is caused by bacteria. Diaper rash does not always bother the child. It can be prevented or minimized by using diapers with absorbent gel, by avoiding restrictive plastic diapers or pants that trap moisture, and by frequent changing of diapers when they are soiled. Breastfed babies tend to have fewer diaper rashes because their stools contain fewer enzymes and other substances that can irritate the skin.

The main treatment for diaper rash is frequent removal or change of a child's diapers. The child's skin should be washed gently with mild soap and water. Often the rash improves with these measures alone. Use of a skin moisturizer and barrier ointment, such as zinc, petroleum jelly, or vitamin A & D cream, may help. Antifungal cream may be necessary if the doctor diagnoses a *Candida* infection. Antibiotic cream can be used if the rash is caused by bacteria.

Eczema (atopic dermatitis) is a red, scaly, dry rash that tends to appear in patches, and comes and goes. Although the cause is unknown, eczema tends to run in families and in many cases is present in children who have allergies. Most children outgrow eczema, but for others eczema is a lifelong condition. Children with severe cases may develop infections intermittently of some particularly affected areas. Treatment includes use of skin moisturizers, gentle soaps, humidified air, corticosteroid creams, and anti-itch drugs. Efforts to control dust mites and other triggers of a child's allergies may occasionally improve the condition.

Cradle cap (seborrheic dermatitis) is a red and yellow scaling, crusty rash that occurs on an infant's head and occasionally in the skin folds. The cause is not known. Cradle cap is harmless and disappears in most children by 6 months of age. Cradle cap can be treated by regularly shampooing and massaging mineral oil into the scalp. The scales may be worked off with a fine comb. Cradle cap that does not improve with these measures may need further treatment, such as selenium shampoo or corticosteroid creams.

Tinea is a fungal infection of the skin. In children, infections of the scalp (tinea capitis) and body (tinea corporis, or "ringworm") are most common. Diagnosis is based on the appearance of the skin or scalp and by analyzing scrapings of the skin with a microscope. Sometimes shining a special light (Wood's light) on the scalp can help diagnose tinea capitis. Treatment of tinea capitis is with griseofulvin taken by mouth and application to the scalp of an antifungal cream such as ciclopirox, clotrimazole, econazole, ketoconazole, miconazole, oxiconazole, or sulconazole. Treatment of tinea corporis is usually by application to the skin of an antifungal, such as one of those used for tinea capitis or naftifine or terbinafine as a cream, lotion, or gel. Some children have an inflammatory reaction to the fungal infection that leads to a scalp mass (kerion), which may require additional treatment.

Molluscum contagiosum is a cluster of flesh-colored pearly pimples or bumps caused by a viral skin infection that usually disappears without treatment.

Milia are small pearly cysts on the face of newborns caused by the first secretions of the child's oil glands. Like newborn acne (see page 38), milia require no treatment and disappear soon after birth.

Other skin rashes in young children are often caused by viral infections. Rashes caused by roseola and erythema infectiosum (fifth disease) are usually harmless and generally improve without treatment (see page 301). Rashes caused by measles, rubella, and chickenpox are becoming less common or rare because children are receiving vaccines.

Undescended and Retractile Testes

- One or both testes may not move from the abdomen into the scrotum just before birth as they normally do.
- In some boys, the testes easily move back and forth between the scrotum and the abdomen but usually become stationary by puberty.
- Surgery to bring the testes down into the scrotum is done if testes have not descended by age 1 year.

Undescended testes (cryptorchidism) are testes that remain in the abdomen instead of descending into the scrotum just before birth. About 3 of every 100 boys have undescended testes at birth. Most testes descend on their own within 6 months. Boys born prematurely are much more likely to have the condition; so are boys whose family members had undescended testes. Half of the boys with the condition have an undescended testis only on the right, and one fourth are affected on both sides.

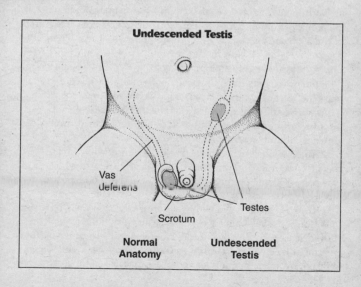

Undescended Testis

Vas Deferens

Scrotum

Testes

Normal Anatomy

Undescended Testis

Undescended testes cause no symptoms. However, undescended testes can become twisted in the abdomen (testicular torsion), impair sperm production later in life, and increase the risk of hernia and testicular cancer. Surgery is generally performed to bring the testes down into the scrotum if the testes remain undescended at 1 year of age.

DID YOU KNOW?

- In most infants with undescended testes, the testes descend by age 6 months.

Retractile (hypermobile) testes are descended testes that easily move back and forth between the scrotum and the abdomen. Retractile testes do not lead to cancer or other complications. The testes usually stop retracting by puberty and do not require surgery or other treatment.

Fever

Fever is a rise in body temperature in response to infection, injury, or inflammation.

- Fever results usually from common infections and rarely from serious infections.
- Infants and children are usually irritable, do not sleep or feed well, and may lose interest in activities.
- Doctors try to determine the cause of the fever.
- Acetaminophen or ibuprofen can relieve the fever.

Body temperatures vary, and temperature elevations up to 100.3°F (about 38°C) can be normal in healthy children. Therefore, minor temperature elevations that do not distress a child do not require medical attention. Temperatures of 100.4°F (38°C) and higher are considered abnormal and generally deserve attention, particularly in infants younger than 3 months.

Causes and Symptoms

Fever is usually the result of common infections, such as colds and "stomach flu" (gastroenteritis). These infections are usually viral and get better without treatment. Less commonly, fever develops because of infection in the ear, lung, bladder, or kidney; these are usually bacterial infections that require antibiotics. In infants on rare occasions, fever may be the only sign of a bloodstream infection (occult bacteremia) (see page 274), which can lead to meningitis and overwhelming infection (sepsis), two life-threatening conditions. Persistent fever in infants with no other symptoms may also signal a urinary tract infection. These children usually appear ill. Many conditions besides infection cause fever in children, but all are rare. Unlike fevers that occur with common infections, these fevers persist for more than a few days.

Fevers can occur after routine vaccinations and are not a reason to avoid recommended vaccines. Giving the infant acetaminophen or ibuprofen at the time of vaccination and afterward minimizes the risk of getting a fever or lowers the fever itself.

Infants with fever are usually irritable and may not sleep or feed well. Older children lose their interest in play, although sometimes children with high fevers appear surprisingly well. The irritability and disinterest that fever usually causes worsen the higher the fever gets. Occasionally, a rapidly rising fever can cause seizures (febrile seizures), and even more rarely, a fever gets so high that children become lethargic and unresponsive.

DID YOU KNOW?

- Infants younger than 3 months who have temperatures of 100.4°F (38°C) or higher should be seen by a doctor.
- Fevers can occur after routine vaccinations and are not a reason to avoid subsequent vaccinations.

Diagnosis and Treatment

Detecting fever is not a challenge, but determining its cause can be. If the fever is low grade (100.3°F or below) and of short duration, no testing or treatment may be needed. In other cases, knowledge of the child's symptoms and a thorough examination help doctors find the cause. In general, any infant with a temperature of 100.4°F or higher should be seen by a doctor, as should older children with higher or recurring fevers.

In infants younger than 2 months of age who have a fever, doctors may order blood and urine tests and perform a spinal tap (lumbar puncture) to look for occult bacteremia and meningitis. The reason for these tests is that in infants, the source of fever is difficult to determine. They are also at risk of serious infection compared with older children because of their immature immune system. Doctors may also order an x-ray if the infant's breathing is abnormal. After 2 months of age, testing may not be needed, but many doctors order blood and urine tests and perform a spinal tap if the source of the fever is not obvious and the child appears ill. For children 3 months of age and older, doctors rely more on the child's behavior and physical examination to determine which

---

HOW TO TAKE A CHILD'S TEMPERATURE

A child's temperature can be taken from the rectum, the ear, the mouth, or the armpit. Rectal temperatures can be taken with a glass or digital thermometer.

Rectal temperatures are most accurate; that is, they come closest to the child's true internal body temperature. To take a rectal temperature, a thermometer with a coat of petroleum jelly around the bulb should be gently inserted about ½ to 1 inch into the child's rectum while the child is lying face down. The child should be kept from moving. The thermometer should be kept in place for 2 to 3 minutes before removing it and taking a reading.

Ear temperatures are taken with a digital device that measures infrared radiation from the eardrum. Ear thermometers are unreliable in infants younger than 3 months of age. To take an ear temperature, the person should form a seal around the opening of the ear with the thermometer probe and press the start button. A digital readout provides the temperature.

Oral temperatures are taken by placing a glass or digital thermometer under the child's tongue for 2 to 3 minutes. Oral temperatures provide reliable readings but are difficult to take in young children, who usually cannot keep their mouth gently closed around the thermometer to get an accurate reading.

Armpit temperatures are taken by placing a glass or digital thermometer in the child's armpit for 4 to 5 minutes. Armpit temperatures are least accurate because the armpit is cooler than the rectum, ear, or mouth.

tests to order. Doctors may order blood and urine tests for children younger than 3 years old with high fevers if they cannot determine the source of fever after examining the child.

Most fevers do not require treatment except to make the child feel better. Acetaminophen and ibuprofen are used. Aspirin is not safe for lowering fever because it can interact with certain viral infections and cause a serious condition called Reye's syndrome (see page 299). A warm (not cold) bath can sometimes make an older child feel better by reducing the fever. Rubbing the child down with alcohol or witch hazel is not recommended. The fumes can be harmful; in addition, it may come into contact with the eyes or the child might accidentally ingest it.

Additional treatment depends on the child's age and cause of the fever. Rarely, fevers persist and doctors are unable to determine their source even after extensive testing; this is called fever of unknown origin.

Febrile Seizures

- Febrile seizures are triggered by a fever, causing the entire body to shake.
- Children with febrile seizures should be taken to the emergency department.
- Phenobarbital or another anticonvulsant may be used to prevent subsequent seizures.

Seizure disorders involve periodic disturbances of the brain's electrical activity, resulting in some degree of temporary brain dysfunction.

Febrile seizures (convulsive seizures) are seizures that are triggered by a fever. They occur in about 4% of children aged 6 months to 5 years but most often occur in children aged 9 to 20 months. Febrile seizures tend to run in families. Most children who have a febrile seizure have only one, and most seizures last for less than 15 minutes. Febrile seizures may be simple or complex. In simple febrile seizures, the entire body shakes (in a generalized seizure) for less than 15 minutes. In complex febrile seizures, the entire body shakes for more than 15 minutes, only one side of the body shakes—a partial seizure—for more than 15 minutes, or seizures occur at least twice within 24 hours. Children who have complex febrile seizures are slightly more likely to develop a seizure disorder later in life.

Children with febrile seizures should be taken to the emergency department for evaluation. Whether a child has meningitis or encephalitis may not be clear, and these disorders must be ruled out. Usually, no treatment is given for a simple febrile seizure other than drugs to reduce the fever. For simple febrile seizures that recur or for complex febrile seizures, phenobarbital may be given to prevent seizures. However, phenobarbital can markedly interfere with the ability of the child to learn. Other anticonvulsants may be used instead.

Failure to Thrive

Failure to thrive is a delay in physical growth and weight gain that can lead to delays in development and maturation.

- Many environmental and social factors can prevent children from getting enough nutrition, as can some medical disorders.
- Doctors compare the child's weight and rate of growth with standard height-weight charts.
- Treatment depends on the cause but usually includes nutritious, high-calorie feedings given on a regular schedule.

Failure to thrive is a diagnosis given to children who are consistently underweight or who do not gain weight for unclear reasons. There are many causes. Failure to thrive may be the result of environmental, emotional, physical, and medical factors that prevent a child from growing normally.

Many environmental and social factors can interact to keep the child from getting the nutrition he needs. Parental neglect or abuse, parental mental health disorders, and chaotic family situations in which routine, nutritious meals are insufficiently provided, may all blunt a child's growth, appetite, and intake of food. The amount of money a family has to spend on food and the nutritional value of the food they buy also affect growth. Inadequate intake of food may reflect inadequate parenting and environmental stimulation.

Sometimes failure to thrive is caused by a medical disorder in the child; sometimes the disorder is as minor as difficulty chewing or swallowing. Medical disorders, such as gastroesophageal reflux, narrowing of the esophagus, or intestinal malabsorption, may also affect a child's ability to retain, absorb, or process food. Infection, tumor, hormonal or metabolic disorders, heart disease, kidney disease, genetic disorders, and human immunodeficiency virus (HIV) infection are other physical reasons for failure to thrive.

Diagnosis

Doctors diagnose failure to thrive when a child's weight or rate of growth is well below what it should be when compared with past measurements or standard height-weight charts (see page 159). If the rate of growth is adequate, the child may be small for his or her age but still growing normally.

To determine why a child may be failing to thrive, doctors ask parents specific questions about feeding; bowel habits; social and financial stability of the family, which might affect the child's access to food; and illnesses that the child has had or that run in the family. The doctor examines the child, looking for signs of conditions that could explain the child's growth delay. The doctor makes decisions about blood and urine tests and x-rays based on this evaluation. More extensive testing is performed only if the doctor suspects an underlying disease.

DID YOU KNOW?

- If children are undernourished during their first year, mental development may remain below normal even if physical growth improves.

Treatment and Prognosis

Treatment depends on the underlying cause. If a physical cause is found, specific treatment is given. Otherwise, treatment depends on how far below normal the child's weight is. Mild to moderate failure to thrive is treated with nutritious, high-calorie feedings given on a regular schedule. Parents may be counseled about family interactions that are damaging to the child and about financial and social resources available to them. Severe failure to thrive is treated in the hospital where social workers, nutritionists, feeding specialists, psychiatrists, and other specialists work together to determine the most likely causes of the child's failure to thrive and the best approach to feeding.

Because the first year of life is important for brain development, children who become undernourished during this time may fall permanently behind their peers, even if their physical growth improves. In about half of these children, mental development, especially verbal skills, remains below normal, and these children often have social and emotional problems in adulthood.

Sudden Infant Death Syndrome

Sudden infant death syndrome (SIDS) is the sudden, unexpected death of a seemingly healthy infant during sleep.

- The cause is unknown but may involve an abnormality in breathing control.
- Placing infants on their back to sleep, removing extra bedding and toys from the bed, and protecting infants from exposure to cigarette smoke are recommended for all infants and reduce the likelihood of SIDS.
- Parents of an infant who had SIDS can benefit from counseling and support from people who have had experience with the disorder.

Although SIDS (also called crib death) is very rare, it is the most common cause of death in infants between the ages of 2 weeks and 1 year. It most often affects children between the second and fourth month of life. The syndrome occurs worldwide. SIDS is more common in premature infants, those who were small at birth, those that previously needed resuscitation, and those with upper respiratory tract infections. For unknown reasons, black and American Indian infants are at a higher risk. It is more common among infants in families with low incomes, whose mothers are single or who used cigarettes or illicit drugs during pregnancy, and who had brothers or sisters who also died of SIDS.

The cause of SIDS is unknown. It may be due to an abnormality in the control of breathing. Some infants with SIDS show signs of having had low levels of oxygen in their blood and having had periods when they stopped breathing. Laying infants down to sleep on their stomach has been linked to SIDS.

DID YOU KNOW?

- Sudden infant death syndrome is most common among infants 2 to 4 months old.
- Sudden infant death syndrome, though rare, is the most common cause of death in infants 2 weeks to 1 year old.

Despite the known risk factors for SIDS, there is no certain way to prevent it. However, putting an infant to sleep on his back on a firm mattress prevents many but not all cases. The number of SIDS deaths has decreased as more parents have put their infants to sleep on their back. Parents should also remove pillows, bumper guards, and toys that could block an infant's breathing. Protecting the infant from overheating may also help but is not proven. Preventing infants from breathing second-hand cigarette smoke may help and clearly has other health benefits.

Most parents who have lost an infant to SIDS are grief-stricken and unprepared for the tragedy. They usually feel guilty. They may be further traumatized by investigations conducted by police, social workers, or others. Counseling and support from specially trained doctors and nurses and other parents who have lost an infant to SIDS are critical to helping parents cope with the tragedy. Specialists can recommend reading materials, web sites, and support groups to assist parents.

CHAPTER 9

Normal Preschool and School-Aged Children

Between the ages of 1 and 13, children's physical, intellectual, and emotional capabilities expand tremendously. Children progress from barely tottering to running, jumping, and playing organized sports. At age 1, most children can utter only a few recognizable words; by age 10, most can write book reports and use computers. Physical, intellectual, and social development, however, proceed at an individual pace.

Milestones From Ages 18 Months to 6 Years

AGE	GROSS MOTOR SKILLS	FINE MOTOR SKILLS
18 months	Walks well	Draws vertical stroke Makes a tower of 4 cubes
2 years	Runs with coordination Climbs on furniture	Handles a spoon well Makes a tower of 7 cubes
2½ years	Jumps Walks upstairs	Scribbles in a circular pattern Opens doors

(Continued)

157

Milestones From Ages 18 Months to 6 Years (Continued)

AGE	GROSS MOTOR SKILLS	FINE MOTOR SKILLS
3 years	Mature gait in walking Rides tricycle	Favors using one hand over the other Copies a circle
4 years	Walks downstairs, alternating feet Hops	Copies a cross Dresses self
5 years	Skips	Copies a square Draws a person in 6 parts
6 years	Walks along a straight line from heel to toe	Writes name

Physical Development

- Physical growth slows around age 1 and progresses steadily and predictably through adolescence.
- Most children can physically control their bowels and bladder at about age 3.

Physical growth begins to slow around age 1. At the same time, parents may notice a decrease in appetite. Some children seem to eat virtually nothing yet continue to grow and thrive. Children who are beginning to walk have an endearing physique, with the belly sticking forward and the back curved. They may also appear to be quite bow-legged. By 3 years of age, muscle tone increases and the proportion of body fat decreases, so the body begins to look leaner and more muscular. Most children are physically able to control their bowels and bladder at this time.

DID YOU KNOW?

- Doubling a child's height at age 24 months fairly accurately predicts adult height.
- Encouragement and praise teach toileting skills more effectively than does punishment.

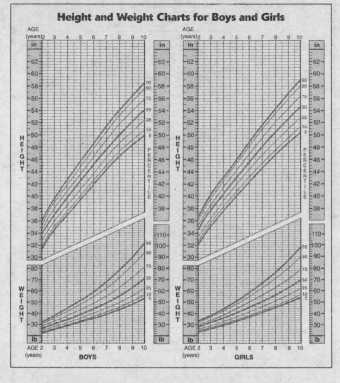

Height and Weight Charts for Boys and Girls

BOYS

GIRLS

Source: The National Center for Health Statistics in collaboration with the National Center for Chronic Disease Prevention and Health Promotion (2000). www.cdc.gov/growthcharts

During the preschool and school years, growth in height and weight is steady. The next major growth spurt occurs in early adolescence. During the years of steady growth, most children follow a predictable pattern. The doctor reports how the child is growing in relation to other children his age and monitors the child's weight gain compared to his height. Some children can become obese at an early age. Doubling the child's height at age 24 months fairly accurately predicts his adult height.

TOILET TEACHING

Most children can be taught to use the toilet when they are between 2 and 3 years of age. Using the toilet to defecate is usually accomplished first. By age 5, the average child can go to the toilet alone, managing all aspects of dressing, undressing, wiping, and hand-washing. However, about 30% of healthy 4-year-olds and 10% of 6-year-olds have not yet achieved regular nighttime bladder control.

Recognizing signs of the child's readiness is the key to toilet teaching. Readiness is signaled when the child:

- Has dry periods lasting several hours
- Wants to be changed when wet
- Shows an interest in sitting on a potty chair or toilet
- Is able to follow simple commands

Children are usually ready to start training between the ages of 18 and 24 months. Despite physical readiness to use the toilet, some children may not be emotionally ready. To avoid a lengthy struggle over toileting, it is best to wait until the child indicates emotional readiness. When he is ready, he will ask for help in the bathroom or make his way to his potty chair on his own.

The timing method is the most commonly used method of toilet teaching. A child who seems ready is introduced to the potty chair and gradually asked to sit on it briefly while fully clothed. The child is then encouraged to practice taking his pants down, sitting on the potty chair for no more than 5 or 10 minutes, and redressing. Simple explanations are given repeatedly and are reinforced by placing wet or dirty diapers in the potty bowl. Praise or a reward is given for successful behavior. Anger or punishment for accidents or for lack of success may be counterproductive. The timing method works well for children with predictable bowel and urine schedules. Teaching children with unpredictable schedules is better delayed until they can anticipate the need to visit the bathroom on their own.

A child who resists sitting on the toilet may be allowed to get up and try again after a meal. If resistance continues for days, postponing the teaching for several weeks is the best strategy. Giving praise or a reward for sitting on the toilet and producing results is effective. Once the pattern is established, rewards can be given for every other success and then gradually withdrawn. Power struggles are unproductive and may strain the parent-child relationship.

Intellectual Development

- By age 4, most children have a complex understanding of time, can tell simple stories, and can have conversations with adults or children.
- By age 7, children can focus on several things at the same time, make connections, and understand different points of view.

At the age of 2, most children understand the concept of time in broad terms. Many 2- and 3-year-olds believe that anything that happened in the past happened "yesterday," and anything that will happen in the future will happen "tomorrow." A child at this age has a vivid imagination but has difficulty distinguishing fantasy from reality. By age 4, most children have a more complicated understanding of time. They realize that the day is divided into morning, afternoon, and night. They can even appreciate the change in seasons.

From 18 months to 5 years of age, a child's vocabulary quickly expands from about 50 words to several thousand words. Children can begin to name and to actively ask about objects and events. By age 2, they begin to put two words together in short phrases, progressing to simple sentences by age 3. Pronunciation improves, with speech being half-understandable to a stranger by age 2 and fully understandable by age 4. A 4-year-old child can tell simple stories and can engage in conversation with adults or other children.

DID YOU KNOW?

- Many 2- and 3-year-olds believe that anything that happened in the past happened yesterday, and anything that will happen in the future will happen tomorrow.

Even before 18 months of age, children can listen to and understand a story being read to them. By age 5, children are able to recite the alphabet and to recognize simple words in print. These skills are all fundamental to learning how to read simple words, phrases, and sentences. Depending on exposure to books and natural abilities, most children begin to read by age 7.

By age 7, a child's intellectual capabilities have become more complex. By this time, a child becomes increasingly able to focus on more than one aspect of an event or situation at the same time. For example, a school-aged child can appreciate that a tall, slender container can hold the same amount of water as a short, broad one. He can appreciate that medicine can taste bad but can make him feel better, or that his mother can be mad at him but can still love him. The child is increasingly able to understand another person's perspective and so learns the essentials of taking turns in games or conversations. In addition, a school-aged child is able to follow agreed-upon rules of games. The child is also increasingly able to reason using the powers of observation and multiple points of view.

Social and Emotional Development

- Temperaments, which vary from child to child, affect emotion and behavior.
- At about age 9 months, children become anxious about separation from their parents.
- By age 2 or 3, they start testing their limits in their quest for more independence, sometimes resulting in temper tantrums.
- Between age 18 months and 2 years, children begin establishing gender identity.
- At age 3 to 5, fantasy play and imaginary friends are common.
- At age 7 to 12 years, children progress in developing a concept of relationships with peers and family members.

Emotion and behavior are based on the child's developmental stage and on his temperament. Every child has an individual temperament, or mood. Some children may be cheerful and adaptable and easily develop regular routines of sleeping, waking, eating, and other daily activities; these children tend to respond positively to new situations. Other children are not very adaptable and may have great irregularities in their routine; these children tend to respond negatively to new situations. Still other children are in between.

At about 9 months of age, infants normally become more anxious about being separated from their parents. Separations at bedtime and at childcare may be difficult and can be marked by temper tantrums; this behavior can last for many months. For many older children, a special blanket or stuffed animal serves at this time as a "transitional object" that acts as a symbol for the absent parent.

At 2 to 3 years of age, a child begins to test his limits and do what he has been forbidden to do, simply to see what will happen. The frequent "no's" that children hear from parents reflect the struggle for independence at this age. Although distressing to both the parent and child, tantrums are normal because they help children express their frustration during a time when they cannot verbalize their feelings well. Parents can help decrease the number of tantrums by not letting the child become overtired or unduly frustrated, and by predicting the child's behavior and avoiding situations that are likely to induce tantrums. Rarely, temper tantrums need to be evaluated by a doctor (see page 180). Some young children have particular difficulty controlling their impulses and need their parents to set stricter limits around which there can be some safety and regularity in their world.

DID YOU KNOW?

- Tantrums are normal and help children express their frustrations at a time when they are not yet able to talk about them.
- Fantasy play helps children learn to resolve conflicts with parents or other children.

At age 18 months to 2 years, children typically begin to establish gender identity. During the preschool years, children also acquire a notion of gender role, of what boys and girls typically do. Exploration of the genitals is expected at this age and signals that children are beginning to make a connection between gender and body image.

Between 2 and 3 years of age, children begin to play more interactively with other children. Although they may still be possessive about toys, they may begin to share and even take turns in play. Asserting ownership of toys by saying, "That is mine!" helps establish the sense of self. Although children of this age strive for independence, they still need their parents nearby for security and support; for example, they may walk away from their parents when they feel curious only to later hide behind their parents when they are fearful.

At 3 to 5 years of age, many children become interested in fantasy play and imaginary friends. Fantasy play allows children to safely act out different roles and strong feelings in acceptable ways. Fantasy play also helps children grow socially; they learn to resolve conflicts with parents or other children in ways that will help them vent frustrations and maintain self-esteem. Also at this time, typical childhood fears like that of "the monster in the closet" emerge. These fears are normal.

At 7 to 12 years of age, children work through numerous issues: self-concept, the foundation for which is laid by competency in the classroom; relationships with peers, which are determined by the ability to socialize and fit in well; and family relationships, which are determined in part by the approval the child gains from his parents and siblings. Although many children seem to place a high value on the peer group, they still look primarily to parents for support and guidance. Siblings can serve as role models and as valuable supports and critics in what can and cannot be done. This period of time is very active for children, who engage in many activities and are eager to explore new activities. At this age, children are eager learners and often respond well to advice about safety, healthy lifestyles, and avoidance of high-risk behaviors.

Promoting Optimal Health and Development

- Establishing healthy eating habits is important.
- Parents can encourage curiosity and learning by providing books and music, reading with the child, limiting use of television and electronic games, and, when the child is in school, showing interest in homework.
- By observing the child's response to a childcare setting, parents can better choose a good environment for their child.

There are a number of ways parents can help their children achieve the best possible health. For example, obesity can be prevented with healthy eating patterns and regular exercise.

The child should consume a variety of healthy foods, including fruits and vegetables along with protein. Regular meals and small nutritious snacks encourage healthy eating in even a picky preschooler. Although the child may avoid some healthy foods, such as broccoli or beans, for a period of time, it is important to continue to offer healthy foods. In addition, parents should limit intake of fruit juices. Some children lose their appetite for food at mealtime if they drink too much fruit juice. A child who drinks from a bottle should be weaned by about 1 year of age to prevent excess juice and milk intake and to avoid tooth decay.

Promoting optimal development in a child works best if approached with flexibility, keeping the individual child's age, temperament, developmental stage, and learning style in mind. A coordinated approach involving parents, teachers, and the child usually works best. Throughout these years, children need an environment that promotes lifelong curiosity and learning. The child should be provided with books and music. Reading to a child and other activities that promote early language skills are important because a young brain is able to learn these skills well. The same is true of music. A routine of daily interactive reading, with parents asking as well as answering questions, helps children pay attention, read with comprehension, and encourages their interest in learning activities. Limiting television and electronic games encourages more interactive play.

DID YOU KNOW?

- Whether child care is provided in or out of the child's home, a young child can do well.
- At preschool, children can learn important social skills as well as learn to recognize letters, numbers, and colors.

Playgroups and preschool have benefits for many young children. Children can learn important social skills, such as sharing. In addition, they may begin to recognize letters, numbers, and colors; learning these skills makes the transition to school smoother. Importantly, in a structured preschool setting, potential developmental problems can be identified and addressed early.

Parents who are in need of childcare may wonder what the best environment is and whether care by others may actually harm their child. Available information suggests that young children can do well both in their own home and in care out of the home, as long as the environment is loving and nurturing. By closely watching the child's response to a given childcare setting, parents are better able to choose the best environment. Some children thrive in a childcare environment where there are many children; others may fare better in their own home or in a smaller group.

When the child begins to receive homework assignments, parents can help by showing interest in the child's work, by being available to sort through questions but not finishing the work themselves, by providing a quiet work environment at home for the child, and by communicating with the teacher about any concerns. As the school years progress, parents need to consider their child's needs when selecting extracurricular activities. Many children thrive when offered the opportunity to participate in team sports or learn a musical instrument. These activities may also provide a venue for improving social skills. On the other hand, some children become stressed if they are "over-scheduled" and expected to participate in too many activities. Children need to be encouraged and supported in their extracurricular activities without having unrealistic expectations placed on them.

Preventive Health Care Visits

- Preventive health care visits should be scheduled at intervals suggested by the doctor.
- Doctors monitor children's physical growth and development.
- Doctors do various screening tests, give routine vaccinations, and perform a general physical examination.
- Safety can be discussed with the parents and with children when they are old enough.

Scheduled visits to the doctor provide parents with information about their child's growth and development. Such visits also give parents an opportunity to ask questions and seek advice. The American Academy of Pediatrics recommends that after the first year of life children see their doctor for preventive health care visits at 12, 15, 18, and 24 months of age and then yearly until age 21 years. Visits can be made more often based on the advice of the doctor or the needs of the family.

A variety of measurements, screening procedures, and vaccinations are performed (see page 32) at each visit. Height and weight are checked. Good growth is one indicator that the child is generally healthy. Head circumference is not routinely measured after the age of 18 months. Beginning at age 3, blood pressure is measured at each visit.

Preventive visits may include a check of vision and hearing. Some children may need to have their blood checked for anemia or an increased level of lead (see page 240). The age of the child and various other factors determine which tests are performed. Some doctors also recommend that the child's urine be checked, although the value of such testing has not been established.

The doctor also asks questions to see how the child has progressed intellectually since the last visit. For example, the doctor may want to know if an 18-month-old has begun to speak or if a 7-year-old has begun to read. In the same way, doctors often ask age-appropriate questions about the child's behavior. Does the 18-month-old child have tantrums? Does the 2-year-old sleep through the night? Does the 6-year-old wet the bed at night? Parents and doctors can discuss these types of behavioral and developmental issues during the preventive health care visits and together design approaches to any behavioral or developmental problems.

Child safety is discussed during preventive visits. Specific safety concerns are based on the age of the child. For a 6-month-old, the doctor may wish to talk about childproofing the house to prevent unintentional poisonings or injury. For a 5-year-old, the discussion might be focused on the potential hazards of guns in the home and gun safety. Parents should take the opportunity to bring up topics that are most relevant to their unique family situation. As the child gets older, he can be an active participant in these discussions.

Keeping Children Safe

SAFETY ISSUE	TIPS
Age 1 Year and Older	
Burns	Keep children out of the kitchen during cooking and away from hot objects, such as stoves, grills, or space heaters.
	Turn the water heater temperature down to 120°F (49°C).
	Keep pot handles turned inward and use back burners as much as possible.
	Do not carry a child and hot liquids or food at the same time.
	Keep electrical appliances and cords out of reach.
	Put plastic safety plugs in all electrical outlets.
	Keep matches and lighters out of reach.
	Always test the bathwater before putting children in.
Cars	Install child safety or booster seats according to the instructions.
	Always use approved child safety seats appropriate for the child's size and weight.
	Seat children in the backseat.
	Do not leave children alone in a car.
	Keep cars and their trunks locked.
Falls	Use gates on stairways and window guards on windows.
	Keep doors to dangerous areas (such as those to the outside or basement) locked.
	Remove sharp-edged furniture from rooms the child sleeps or plays in.
Fire	Test smoke alarms monthly, and replace batteries once a year.
	Do not smoke in the home.
	Use flame-retardant sleepwear for children.
	Buy a fire extinguisher for the home.
Firearms	Do not keep guns in the house if possible.
	Store guns unloaded and in a locked place. Store ammunition in a separate locked place.
	Ask about guns and their storage at homes where children play or spend time.

Keeping Children Safe (Continued)

SAFETY ISSUE	TIPS
Age 1 Year and Older	
Home	Keep emergency telephone numbers by the telephone.
	Have heating systems and fireplaces cleaned and inspected regularly.
Poisoning	Use safety caps on all drugs (including vitamins) and toxic household products.
	Keep them in their original containers.
	Store them out of sight and out of reach in a locked cabinet.
	Do not keep lye drain cleaners in the home.
	Use safety latches on cabinets and drawers.
	Never call drugs candy.
	Discard old or outdated drugs and household products.
	Keep poisonous plants out of children's reach.
	Install carbon monoxide detectors.
	In older homes, remove leaded paint.
Toys	Give children age-appropriate toys.
	Check toys for small or easy-to-pull-off parts that children could put in their mouth and choke on.
Water	Do not leave a child alone in or near a bathtub, containers of water, swimming pools, or any other water, even for a moment.
	Empty containers of water when finished with them.
	Keep bathroom doors closed.
	If there is a swimming pool, fence it and install a self-latching gate.
Age 2 Years and Older	
Burns	Teach children not to play with matches and lighters.
Falls	Make sure children play only on playground equipment with a soft surface (such as sand or wood chips) under it.
	Teach children how to use playground equipment safely.

(Continued)

Keeping Children Safe (Continued)

SAFETY ISSUE	TIPS
Age 2 Years and Older	
Street	Do not let children play or ride a tricycle in the street.
Age 5 Years and Older	
Bicycles, roller blades, and skateboards	Make sure children wear a helmet when they bike or skate.
	Do not let children bike or skate in the street or after dark.
Emergencies	Teach children to alert an adult if an emergency occurs.
	Teach children to call 911 or other emergency telephone numbers.
	Make sure children know their name, address, and telephone number.
Fire	Teach children what to do if the smoke alarm goes off.
	Have an escape plan and practice it.
	Teach children to stop, drop, and roll if their clothes catch on fire.
Poisoning	Teach children about poisons, including dangerous household products, lawn chemicals, and poisonous plants (particularly mushrooms).
Street	Teach children to stop at the curb or edge of the street.
	Teach children never to cross a street without an adult.
Water	Teach children to swim.
	Do not let children swim without adult supervision.
	Encourage the buddy system.
	Do not let children swim in fast-moving water or canals.
	Teach children to check the depth of water before jumping or diving in.
	Make sure children wear life jackets in boats.

Keeping Children Safe (Continued)

SAFETY ISSUE	TIPS
Age 8 Years and Older	
Bicycles	Teach children the rules of riding on the street.
	Watch children ride to make sure they can ride with control, follow the rules, and use good judgment.
	Make sure children come home by dark.
Firearms	Teach children that guns are not toys and are not to be played with.
Sports	Make sure children wear the necessary protective equipment for their sport.
	Talk to the coach about what equipment is needed.

Finally, the doctor performs a complete physical examination. In addition to examining the child from head to toe, including the heart, lungs, abdomen, genitals, and head and neck, the doctor may ask the child to perform some age-appropriate tasks. To check gross motor skills (such as walking and running), the doctor may ask a 4-year-old to hop on one foot. To check fine motor skills (manipulating small objects with the hands), the child may be asked to draw a picture or copy some shapes.

CHAPTER 10

Behavioral and Developmental Problems in Young Children

Children acquire many skills as they grow. Some skills, such as controlling urine and stool, depend mainly on the level of maturity of the child's nerves and brain. Others, such as behaving appropriately at home and in school, are the result of a complicated interaction between the child's physical and intellectual (cognitive) development, health, temperament, and relationship with parents, teachers, and caregivers.

DID YOU KNOW?

- Behavioral problems may develop from normal, easily acquired bad habits.
- The best results occur when children want to change their behavior.
- Praising children and spending time with them each day are usually more effective than punishing them.
- Sometimes bad behavior, if it does not hurt other people, is best ignored.

Behavioral and developmental problems can become so troublesome that they threaten normal relationships between the child and others. Some behavioral problems, such as bed-wetting, can be mild and resolve quickly. Other behavioral problems, such as those that arise in children with attention deficit/hyperactivity disorder (ADHD), can require ongoing treatment. Most of the problems described in this chapter arise out of developmentally normal bad habits that children easily acquire. The goal of treatment is to change the bad habits by getting the child to want to change his behavior. This goal often takes persistent changes in actions by the parents, which in turn result in improved behaviors by the child.

BEHAVIORAL PROBLEMS DUE TO SUBOPTIMAL PARENTING

A number of relatively minor problems of behavior may be due to suboptimal parenting. Note that all of these behaviors occur during the normal course of childhood. They become behavioral problems when they affect the family relationship.

Child-parent interactional problems are difficulties in the relationship between a child and his parents, which may begin during the first few months of life. The relationship may be strained because of a difficult pregnancy or delivery or due to the mother suffering from depression after delivery or receiving inadequate support from the father, relatives, or friends. Contributing to the strain are a baby's unpredictable feeding and sleeping schedules. Most babies do not sleep through the night until 3 to 4 months of age. Poor relationships may slow the child's development of mental and social skills and cause failure to thrive.

A doctor or nurse can discuss the temperament of an individual baby and offer the parents information on the development of infants and helpful tips for coping. The parents may then be able to develop more realistic expectations, accept their feelings of guilt and conflict as normal, and try to rebuild a healthy relationship. If the relationship is not repaired, the child may continue to have problems later.

A vicious circle pattern is a cycle of negative (naughty) behavior by the child that causes a negative (angry) response from the parent or caregiver, followed by further negative behavior by the child, leading to a further negative response from the parent. Vicious circles usually begin when a child is aggressive and resistant. The parents or caregivers respond by scolding, yelling, and spanking. Vicious

(Continued)

BEHAVIORAL PROBLEMS DUE TO SUBOPTIMAL PARENTING
(Continued)

circles may also result when parents react to a fearful, clinging, or manipulative child with overprotection and overpermissiveness.

The vicious circle pattern may be broken if parents learn to ignore bad behavior that does not affect the rights of others, such as temper tantrums or refusals to eat. For behavior that cannot be ignored, distraction or a time-out procedure can be tried. Parents should also praise the child for good behavior.

Discipline problems are inappropriate behaviors that develop when discipline is ineffective. Efforts to control a child's behavior through scolding or physical punishments such as spanking may work briefly if used sparingly. However, these approaches generally tend not to alter the bad behavior sufficiently and may reduce the child's sense of security and self-esteem. Moreover, spanking can get out of hand when the parent is angry. Therefore, spanking is not recommended. A time-out procedure can be helpful. However, punishments become ineffective when overused. Furthermore, threats that the parents will leave or send the child away can be psychologically damaging.

Praise and reward can reinforce good behavior. Because most children prefer attention for inappropriate behavior to no attention at all, the parents should create special times each day for pleasant interactions with the child.

Eating Problems

- When children are about 1 year old, they eat less because growth slows down.
- Children should be offered meals and snacks at regular times and not be forced to eat.
- Overeating during childhood increases the number of fat cells formed, and that number does not change, making weight loss more difficult.

Some eating problems can be behavioral in nature.

Undereating: A decrease in appetite, caused by a slowing growth rate, is common in children around 1 year of age. However, an eating problem may develop if a parent or caregiver tries to coerce the child to eat or shows too much concern about the child's appetite or eating habits. When parents coax and threaten, children with eating problems may refuse to eat the food in their mouths. Some children may respond to parental attempts at force-feeding by vomiting.

Decreasing the tension and negative emotions surrounding mealtimes may be helpful. Emotional scenes can be avoided by putting food in front of the child and removing it in 20 to 30 minutes without comment. The child should be allowed to eat whatever he chooses from offered food at mealtimes and scheduled snacks in the morning and afternoon. Food and fluids other than water should be restricted at all other times. Young children should be offered 3 meals and 2 to 3 snacks each day. Mealtimes should be scheduled at a time when other family members are eating; distractions, such as television, should be avoided. Sitting at a table is encouraged. Using these techniques balances the child's appetite, amount of food eaten, and nutritional needs.

Overeating: Overeating is another problem. Overeating can lead to childhood obesity (see page 206). Once fat cells form, they do not go away. Thus, obese children are more likely than children of normal weight to be obese as adults. Because childhood obesity can lead to adult obesity, it should be prevented or treated.

Bed-Wetting

- Bed-wetting is very common, can be corrected, and is nothing to feel guilty about.
- Usually, bed-wetting occurs because the nerves that supply the bladder are slow to mature.
- Limiting fluids after dinner, encouraging children to urinate before going to bed, using alarms that detect urine, and giving age-appropriate rewards for dry nights can help.
- If these measures are ineffective, older children may be given imipramine or desmopressin.

About 30% of children still wet the bed at age 4, 10% at age 6, 3% at age 12, and 1% at age 18. Bed-wetting is more common in boys than in girls and seems to run in families.

Bed-wetting is usually caused by slow maturation of the nerves that supply the bladder, so that the child fails to awaken appropriately when the bladder fills and needs emptying. Bed-wetting can accompany such sleep disorders as sleepwalking and night terrors (see page 178). A physical disorder—usually a urinary tract infection—is found in only 1 to 2% of children who wet the bed. Other disorders, such as diabetes, rarely cause bed-wetting. Bed-wetting occasionally is caused by psychologic problems, either in the child or in another family member, and is occasionally part of a constellation of symptoms that suggests the possibility of sexual abuse.

Sometimes bed-wetting stops and then begins again. The relapse usually follows a psychologically stressful event or condition, but a physical cause, especially a urinary tract infection, may be responsible.

Treatment

Parents and the child need to know that bed-wetting is quite common, that it can be corrected, and that nobody should feel guilty about it. An older child who has bed-wetting can take responsibility by limiting fluids after dinner (especially caffeinated beverages), urinating before going to bed, recording wet and dry nights, and changing clothing and bedding when wet. Parents may choose to give the child age-appropriate rewards (positive reinforcement) for dry nights.

DID YOU KNOW?

- Bed-wetting usually has a physical, not a psychologic cause.
- Alarms that detect urine cure bed-wetting in about 70% of children.

For children younger than 6, parents can avoid giving the child fluids 2 to 3 hours before bedtime and encourage the child to urinate just before going to bed. In most children of this age, time and physical maturation solve the problem.

For children older than 6 to 7 years, some form of treatment is often indicated. Bed-wetting alarms, which awaken a child when a few drops of urine are detected, are the most effective treatment available. They cure bed-wetting in about 70% of the children, and only about 10 to 15% of children start wetting the bed again after the alarms are discontinued. Alarms are relatively inexpensive and are easy to set up. In the first few weeks of use, the child awakens only after fully urinating. In the next few weeks, the child awakens after urinating a small amount and may wet the bed less often. Eventually, the need to urinate wakes the child before the bed is wet. Most parents find that the alarm can be removed after a 3-week dry period.

If bed-wetting persists in an older child after alarms and age-appropriate rewards have been tried, the doctor may prescribe imipramine, or, more commonly, desmopressin. Imipramine is an antidepressant drug but has been used to treat bed-wetting because it relaxes the bladder and tightens the sphincter that blocks urine flow. If imipramine is going to work, it usually does so in the first week of treatment. This rapid response is the only real advantage of the drug, particularly if the parents and child feel they need to cure the problem quickly. After 1 month without bed-wetting, the drug dose is decreased over 2 to 4 weeks, then discontinued. However, about 75% of children eventually start wetting the bed again. If this happens, a 3-month course of the drug may be tried.

An increasingly popular drug for bed-wetting is desmopressin tablets or nasal spray. This drug reduces the output of urine, which reduces bed-wetting. This drug is used for a 1- to 3-month period and then discontinued as soon as possible. It can be used intermittently, such as when the child goes to camp.

Encopresis

Encopresis is the accidental passing of bowel movements that is not caused by illness or physical abnormality.

- The most common causes are resistance to toilet teaching (in toddlers) and constipation (in older children).

About 17% of 3-year-olds and 1% of 4-year-olds have encopresis, most often from resistance to toilet teaching. However, chronic constipation, which stretches the bowel wall and reduces the child's awareness of a full bowel, impairing muscle control, sometimes causes encopresis. Often a vicious cycle develops in which the child is constipated, so he withholds stool because it is painful to have a bowel movement. Withholding stool only exacerbates the constipation, and so on. The constipation becomes so severe that stool leaks around the impaction.

A doctor first tries to determine the cause. If the cause is constipation, a laxative or other medication is prescribed and other measures are instituted to ensure regular bowel movements. Once regular bowel movements are achieved, the leakage often stops. If these measures fail, diagnostic tests may be performed, such as abdominal x-rays and rarely a biopsy of the rectal wall, in which a tissue sample is taken and examined under a microscope. If a physical cause is found, it often can be treated. In the most severe cases, psychologic counseling may be needed for children whose encopresis is the result of resistance to toilet teaching or other behavioral problems.

Sleep Problems

- Nightmares are cause for concern only when they occur very often.
- Children who have night terrors are very frightened and inconsolable at the time but usually go back to sleep and do not remember the episode.
- Night terrors and sleepwalking usually stop on their own.
- Children aged 1 to 2 years often resist going to bed because of separation anxiety or a desire for control.
- Children who awaken during the night may benefit from following a bedtime routine (including a brief story), sleeping with a favorite doll or blanket, and having a night-light.

For most children, sleep problems are intermittent or temporary and often do not need treatment.

Nightmares: Nightmares are frightening dreams that occur during rapid eye movement (REM) sleep. A child having a nightmare can awaken fully and can vividly recall the details of the dream. Nightmares are not a cause for alarm, unless they occur very often. They can occur more often during times of stress, or even when the child has seen a video containing aggressive content. If nightmares occur often, parents can keep a diary to see if they can identify the cause.

Night Terrors and Sleepwalking: Night terrors, episodes of incomplete awakening with extreme anxiety shortly after falling asleep, are most common between the ages of 3 and 8. The child screams and appears frightened, with a rapid heart rate and rapid breathing. The child does not seem to be aware of the parents' presence and does not talk. He may thrash around violently and does not respond to comforting. After a few minutes, he goes fully back to sleep. Unlike with nightmares, the child is not able to recall these episodes. Night terrors are dramatic because the child screams and is inconsolable during the episode. About one third of children with night terrors also experience sleepwalking (rising from bed and walking around while apparently asleep, also called somnambulism. About 15% of children between the ages of 5 and 12 have at least one episode of sleepwalking.

Night terrors and sleepwalking almost always stop on their own, although occasional episodes may occur for years; usually, no treatment is needed. If a disorder persists into adolescence or adulthood and is severe, treatment may be necessary. In children who need treatment, night terrors may sometimes respond to a sedative or certain antidepressants; however, these drugs are potent and can have side effects and should be used only in extreme cases. Installing a lock on the outside of the bedroom door keeps a child from wandering but may frighten the child.

DID YOU KNOW?

- Most sleep problems are temporary and do not require treatment.
- Providing children with an attachment object (such as a teddy bear) often helps them go to bed.

Resistance to Going to Bed: Children, particularly between the ages of 1 and 2, often resist going to bed. Young children often cry when left alone in their cribs, or they climb out and seek their parents. This behavior is related to separation anxiety (see page 532) and, in older children, to the child's attempts to control more aspects of his environment.

Resistance to going to bed is not helped if parents stay in the room at length to provide comfort or let the child get up. To control the problem, a parent may have to sit quietly in the hallway in sight of the child and make sure the child stays in bed. The child then learns that getting out of bed is not allowed. The child also learns that the parents cannot be enticed into the room for more stories or play. Eventually, the child settles down and goes to sleep. Providing the child with an attachment object (like a teddy bear) is often helpful.

Awakening During the Night: Children often awaken during the night, but they usually fall back to sleep on their own. Repeated night awakening often follows a move, an illness, or another stressful event. Sleeping problems may be worsened when the child takes long naps late in the afternoon or is overstimulated by playing before bedtime.

Allowing the child to sleep with the parents because of the night awakening is likely only to prolong the problem. Also counterproductive are playing with or feeding the child during the night, spanking, and scolding. Returning the child to bed with simple reassurance is usually more effective. A bedtime routine that includes reading a brief story, offering a favorite doll or blanket, and using a small night-light (in children who are older than 3) is often helpful. Parents and other caregivers should also try to keep to a routine each night, so that the child learns what is expected. If the child is physically healthy, allowing him to cry for 20 to 30 minutes often teaches him that he needs to settle himself down, which will diminish the night awakening.

Temper Tantrums

- Temper tantrums often result from a combination of the child's personality, immediate circumstances, and normal behavior for the child's stage of development.
- Parents should ask the child to stop, and if the child does not, they should remove the child from the situation (for example by using a time-out).

Temper tantrums are common in childhood. They usually appear toward the end of the first year, are most common between the ages of 2 and 4, and are typically infrequent after age 5. If tantrums are frequent after age 5, they may persist throughout childhood.

Causes include frustration, tiredness, or hunger. Children may also have temper tantrums to seek attention or to manipulate parents to obtain something, or to avoid doing something. Parents often place the blame on themselves (because of imagined poor parenting) when the real cause is often a combination of the child's personality, immediate circumstances, and developmentally normal behavior. An underlying psychologic, medical, or social problem may rarely be the cause and is more likely if a tantrum lasts for more than 15 minutes or if tantrums occur multiple times each day.

A child who is having a temper tantrum may shout, scream, cry, thrash about, roll on the floor, stamp with his feet, and throw things. Some of the behavior may be ragelike and potentially harmful; he may become red in the face and hit or kick.

To stop a tantrum, parents should first ask the child simply and firmly to do so. If that fails and if the behavior is sufficiently disruptive, the child may have to be removed physically from the situation. At this point, a time-out procedure can be very effective. A time-out procedure is a discipline technique used by parents to interrupt the child's disruptive behavior. A time-out is most effective in children 2 and older. After repeatedly misbehaving, the child is calmly sent or taken to a chair for a set period—1 minute for each year of age, up to a maximum of 5 minutes. If the child gets up early or does not quiet down within the set period, the timer is reset.

Breath-Holding Spells

A breath-holding spell is an episode in which the child stops breathing and loses consciousness for a short period immediately after a frightening or emotionally upsetting event.

- Breath-holding usually occurs subconsciously as part of a tantrum or after a scolding.
- Breath-holding may occur when something triggers a nerve response that slows the heart.

Breath-holding spells occur in 5% of otherwise healthy children. They usually begin in the second year of life. They disappear by age 4 in 50% of children and by age 8 in about 83% of children. The 17% of children who continue to have spells as adults lose consciousness as a reaction to emotional stress. Breath-holding spells can take one of two forms.

The **cyanotic form** of breath-holding, which is most common, is initiated subconsciously by young children often as a component of a temper tantrum or in response to a scolding or other upsetting event. Episodes peak at about 2 years and are rare after 5 years. During the episode, a child holds his breath (without necessarily being aware he is doing so) until he loses consciousness. Typically, the child cries out, breathes out, then stops breathing. Shortly afterward, the child's skin begins to turn blue and he becomes unconscious. A seizure may occur. After the loss of consciousness (which generally lasts for seconds only), breathing resumes and normal skin color and consciousness return. It may be possible to interrupt the episode by placing a cold rag on the child's face when the spell begins. Despite the frightening nature of the episode, the parents must try to avoid reinforcing the initiating behavior in the cyanotic form. As the child recovers, parents should put the child safely in bed. Parents should enforce household rules; the child cannot have "free rein" of the house just because these spells follow temper tantrums. Distracting the child and avoiding situations that will likely lead to tantrums are good strategies.

The **pallid form** typically follows a painful experience, such as falling and banging the head or being suddenly startled. The brain sends out a signal (via the vagus nerve) that severely slows the heart rate, producing loss of consciousness. Thus, in this form, the loss of consciousness and stoppage of breathing (which are both temporary) result from a nerve response to being startled that leads to slowing of the heart.

The child stops breathing, rapidly loses consciousness, and becomes pale and limp. A seizure may occur. The heart typically beats very slowly during an attack. After the attack, the heart speeds up again, breathing restarts, and consciousness returns without any treatment. Because this type is rare, if the attacks occur often, further diagnostic evaluation and treatment may be needed.

School Avoidance

- Some children avoid school by making excuses (such as a faked illness) or by directly refusing to go.
- Reasons for avoiding school vary from anxiety to school-related social issues.
- The best approach is to reassure the child and continue sending the child to school.
- If the problem persists, therapy with a psychologist or psychiatrist may be needed.

Avoiding school occurs in about 5% of all school-aged children and affects girls and boys equally. It is most likely to occur between ages 5 and 6 and between ages 10 and 11.

The cause is often unclear, but psychologic factors (such as anxiety and depression) and social factors (such as having no friends, feeling rejected by peers, or being bullied) may contribute. A sensitive child may be overreacting with fear to a teacher's strictness or rebukes. Younger children tend to fake illness or make other excuses to avoid school. The child may complain of a stomachache, nausea, or other symptoms that justify staying home. Some children directly refuse to go to school. Alternatively, the child may go to school without difficulty but become anxious or develop various symptoms during the school day, often going regularly to the nurse's office. This behavior is unlike that of adolescents, who may decide not to attend school (truancy, playing "hooky"—see page 214).

School avoidance tends to result in poor academic performance, family difficulties, and difficulties with the child's peers. Most children recover from school avoidance, although some develop it again after a real illness or a vacation.

Home tutoring is generally not a solution. A child with school avoidance should return to school immediately, so that he does not fall behind in his schoolwork. If school avoidance is so intense that it interferes with the child's activity and if the child does not respond to simple reassurance by parents or teachers, referral to a psychologist or psychiatrist may be warranted.

Treatment should include communication between parents and school personnel, regular attendance at school, and sometimes therapy involving the family and child with a psychologist.

Therapy includes treatment of underlying causes as well as behavioral techniques to cope with the stresses at school.

WHAT ARE STRESS-RELATED BEHAVIORS?

Each child handles stress differently. Certain behaviors that help children deal with stress include thumb sucking, nail biting, and, sometimes, head banging.

Thumb sucking (or sucking a pacifier) is a normal part of early childhood, and most children stop by the time they are 1 or 2 years old, but some continue into their school-age years. Occasional thumb sucking is normal at times of stress, but habitual sucking past the age of about 5 can alter the shape of the roof of the mouth, cause misalignment of teeth, and lead to teasing from other children. Occasionally, persistent thumb sucking can be the sign of an underlying emotional disorder.

All children eventually stop thumb sucking. Parents should intervene only if their child's dentist advises them to, or if they feel their child's thumb sucking is socially unhealthy. Parents need to gently encourage the child to understand why it would be good to stop. Once the child signals a willingness to stop, gentle verbal reminders are a good start. These can be followed by symbolic rewards put directly on the thumb, such as a colored bandage, fingernail polish, or a star drawn with a nontoxic colored marker. If necessary, additional measures, such as a plastic guard over the thumb, overnight elbow splinting to prevent a child from bending it, or "painting" the thumbnail with a bitter substance can be used. However, none of these measures should be used against the child's will.

Nail biting is a common problem in young children. The habit typically disappears as the child gets older, but is typically related to stress and anxiety. Children who are motivated to stop can be taught to substitute other habits (for example, twirling a pencil).

Head banging and **rhythmic rocking** are common among healthy toddlers. While alarming to parents, the children do not seem to be in distress and actually appear to derive comfort from the activity.

Children usually outgrow rocking, rolling, and head banging between 18 months and 2 years of age, but repetitive actions sometimes still occur in older children and adolescents.

Children with autism and certain other developmental problems also may bang their heads. However, these conditions have additional symptoms that make their diagnosis apparent.

Although children almost never damage themselves by these behaviors, this possibility (and the noise) can be reduced by pulling the crib away from the wall, taking off the wheels or placing carpet protectors under them, and applying a padded crib bumper to the inside of the crib.

Attention Deficit/Hyperactivity Disorder

Attention deficit/hyperactivity disorder (ADHD) is poor or short attention span and impulsiveness inappropriate for the child's age; some children also manifest hyperactivity.

- Attention deficit/hyperactivity disorder may cause more problems at school because of the rules and constraints.
- Children cannot pay attention or concentrate long enough to finish a task.
- Routines, a school intervention plan, modified parenting techniques, behavior therapy, and psychostimulant drugs (such as methylphenidate) may help.
- Most children do not outgrow their inattentiveness, but by adolescence or adulthood, they have learned to adapt.

Although there is considerable controversy about incidence, it is estimated that ADHD affects 5 to 10% of school-aged children and is diagnosed 10 times more often in boys than in girls. Many features of ADHD are often noticed before age 4 and invariably before age 7, but they may not interfere significantly with academic performance and social functioning until the middle school years. ADHD was previously just called "attention deficit disorder"; however, the common occurrence of hyperactivity in affected children—which is really a physical extension of attention deficit—led to a change in the current terminology.

ADHD can be inherited. Recent research indicates that the disorder is caused by abnormalities in neurotransmitters (substances that transmit nerve impulses within the brain). The symptoms of ADHD range from mild to severe and can become exaggerated or become a problem in certain environments, such as in the child's home or at school. The constraints of school and organized lifestyles make ADHD a problem, whereas in prior generations, the symptoms may not have interfered significantly with children's functioning because such restraints were often much fewer. Although some of the symptoms of ADHD also occur in children without ADHD, they are more frequent and severe in children with ADHD.

DID YOU KNOW?

- Most children with attention deficit/hyperactivity disorder become productive adults, adjusting to work better than to school.

Symptoms

ADHD is primarily a problem with sustained attention, concentration, and task persistence (ability to finish a task). The child may also be overactive and impulsive. Many preschool children are anxious, have problems communicating and interacting, and behave poorly. They seem inattentive. They may fidget and squirm. They may be impatient and answer out of turn. During later childhood, such children may move their legs restlessly, move and fidget their hands, talk impulsively, forget easily, and they may be disorganized. They are generally not aggressive.

About 20% of children with ADHD have learning disabilities and about 80% have academic problems. Work may be messy, with careless mistakes and an absence of considered thought. Affected children often behave as if their mind is elsewhere and they are not listening. They often do not follow through on requests or complete schoolwork, chores, or other duties. There may be frequent shifts from one incomplete task to another.

About 40% of affected children may have issues with self-esteem, depression, anxiety, or opposition to authority by the time they reach adolescence. About 60% of young children have such problems as temper tantrums, and most older children have a low tolerance for frustration.

SIGNS OF ADHD

All signs do not have to be present for a diagnosis of attention deficit/hyperactivity disorder (ADHD). However, signs of inattention must always be present for a diagnosis. Signs must be present in two or more situations (for example, home and school) and must interfere with social or academic functioning.

Signs of inattention

- Often fails to pay close attention to details
- Has difficulty sustaining attention in work and play
- Does not seem to listen when spoken to directly
- Often does not follow through on instructions and fails to finish tasks
- Often has difficulty organizing tasks and activities
- Often avoids, dislikes, or is reluctant to engage in tasks that require sustained mental effort
- Often loses things
- Is easily distracted by extraneous stimuli
- Is often forgetful

Signs of hyperactivity

- Often fidgets with hands or feet or squirms
- Often leaves seat in classroom and elsewhere
- Often runs about or climbs excessively
- Has difficulty playing or engaging in leisure activities quietly
- Is often on the go or acts as if "driven by a motor"
- Often talks excessively

Signs of impulsivity

- Often blurts out answers before questions have been completed
- Often has difficulty awaiting his turn
- Often interrupts or intrudes on others

Diagnosis

The diagnosis is based on the number, frequency, and severity of symptoms. Symptoms must be present in at least two separate environments (typically, home and school)—occurrence of symptoms just at home or just at school and nowhere else does not qualify as ADHD. Often, diagnosis is difficult because it depends on the judgment of the observer. There is no laboratory test for ADHD. Questionnaires about various aspects of behavior can help the doctor make the diagnosis. Because learning disabilities are common, many children receive psychologic testing both to help determine if ADHD exists and to detect the presence of specific learning disabilities.

ADHD: EPIDEMIC OR OVERDIAGNOSIS?

An increasing number of children are diagnosed with attention deficit/hyperactivity disorder (ADHD). However, there is a growing concern among doctors and parents that many children are misdiagnosed. A high activity level may be completely normal and be simply an exaggeration of normal childhood temperament. Alternatively, it may have a variety of causes, including emotional disorders or abnormalities of brain function, such as ADHD.

Generally, 2-year-olds are active and seldom stay still. A high activity and noise level is common up until age 4. In these age groups, such behavior is normal. Active behavior can cause conflicts between parents and child and may worry parents. It also can create problems for others who supervise such children, including teachers.

Determining whether a child's activity level is abnormally high should not simply depend on how tolerant the annoyed person is. However, some children are clearly more active than average. If the high activity level is combined with short attention span and impulsivity, it may be defined as hyperactivity and considered part of ADHD.

Scolding and punishing children whose high activity level is within normal limits usually backfires, increasing the child's activity level. Avoiding situations in which the child has to sit still for a long time or finding a teacher skilled in coping with such children may help. If simple measures do not help, a medical or psychologic evaluation may be useful to rule out an underlying disorder such as ADHD.

Treatment and Prognosis

To minimize the effects of ADHD, structures, routines, a school intervention plan, and modified parenting techniques are often needed. Some children who are not aggressive and who come from a stable and supportive home environment may benefit from drug treatment alone. Behavior therapy conducted by a child psychologist is sometimes combined with drug treatment. Psychostimulant drugs are the most effective drug treatment.

Methylphenidate is the psychostimulant drug most often prescribed. It is as effective as other psychostimulants (such as dextroamphetamine) and is probably safer. A number of slow-release (longer-acting) forms of methylphenidate are available in addition to the regular form and allow for one time per day dosing. Side effects of methylphenidate include sleep disturbances, such as insomnia, appetite suppression, depression or sadness, headaches, stomachaches, and high blood pressure. All of these side effects disappear if the drug is discontinued; however, most children have no side effects except perhaps a decreased appetite. However, if taken in large doses for a long time, methylphenidate can occasionally slow the child's growth; therefore, doctors monitor weight gain.

A number of other drugs can be used to treat inattentiveness and behavioral symptoms. These include clonidine, amphetamine-based drugs, antidepressants, antianxiety drugs, and a new drug called atomoxetine. Sometimes, combinations of drugs are used.

Children with ADHD generally do not outgrow their inattentiveness, although those with hyperactivity tend to become somewhat less impulsive and hyperactive with age. However, most adolescents and adults learn to adapt to their inattentiveness. Other problems that emerge or persist in adolescence and adulthood include poor academic achievement, low self-esteem, anxiety, depression, and difficulty in learning appropriate social behaviors. Importantly, the vast majority of children with ADHD become productive adults, and people who have ADHD seem to adjust better to work than to school situations. Some adults are prescribed medications for continuing ADHD. If the disorder is untreated in childhood, the risk of alcohol or substance abuse or suicide may increase.

Learning Disorders

Learning disorders involve an inability to acquire, retain, or broadly use specific skills or information, resulting from deficiencies in attention, memory, or reasoning and affecting academic performance.

- Learning disorders affect only certain functions, usually reading, writing, or mathematics.
- Children may be slow learning to name colors, count, read, and write or may have trouble communicating.
- Children are evaluated for physical disorders that could interfere with learning and are given intelligence and academic tests.
- The best approach is carefully tailoring education to each child.

Learning disorders are quite different from mental retardation and occur in children with normal or even high intellectual function. Learning disorders affect only certain functions, whereas in a child with mental retardation, difficulties affect cognitive functions broadly. There are three main types of learning disorders: reading disorders, disorders of written expression, and mathematics disorders. Thus, a child with a learning disorder may have significant difficulty understanding and learning math, but have no difficulty reading, writing, and performing well in other subjects. Dyslexia is the best known of the learning disorders. Learning disorders do not include learning problems that are due primarily to problems of vision, hearing, coordination, or emotional disturbance.

Although the causes of learning disorders are not fully understood, they include abnormalities in the basic processes involved in understanding or in using spoken or written language or numerical and spatial reasoning.

An estimated 3 to 15% of school children in the United States may need special educational services to compensate for learning disorders. Boys with learning disorders may outnumber girls five to one, although girls are often not recognized or diagnosed as having learning disorders.

Many children with behavioral problems perform poorly in school and are tested by educational psychologists for learning disorders. However, some children with certain types of learning disorders hide their deficits well, avoiding diagnosis, and therefore treatment, for a long time.

DID YOU KNOW?

- Boys with learning disorders may outnumber girls five to one, although the number of girls may be underestimated.

Symptoms

A young child may be slow to learn the names of colors or letters, to assign words to familiar objects, to count, and to progress in other early learning skills. Learning to read and write may be delayed. Other symptoms may be a short attention span and distractibility, halting speech, and a short memory span. The child may have difficulty with activities that require fine motor coordination, such as printing and copying.

A child with a learning disorder may have difficulty communicating. Some children initially become frustrated and later develop behavioral problems, such as being easily distracted, hyperactive, withdrawn, shy, or aggressive.

Diagnosis and Treatment

Children who are not reading or learning at the grade level expected for their verbal or intellectual abilities should be evaluated. Testing of hearing and eyesight should be carried out, because problems with these senses can also interfere with reading and writing skills.

A doctor examines the child for any physical disorders. The child takes a series of intelligence tests, both verbal and nonverbal, and academic tests of reading, writing, and arithmetic skills.

The most useful treatment for a learning disorder is education that is carefully tailored to the individual child. Measures such as eliminating food additives, taking large doses of vitamins, and analyzing the child's system for trace minerals are often tried but unproven. No drug treatment has much effect on academic achievement, intelligence, and general learning ability. Because some children with a learning disorder also have ADHD, certain drugs, such as methylphenidate, may improve attention and concentration, enhancing the child's ability to learn.

Dyslexia

Dyslexia is a specific reading disorder involving difficulty separating single words from groups of words and parts of words (phonemes) within each word. It occurs because the brain has difficulty connecting sounds with symbols (letters).

- Children with dyslexia have difficulty articulating words, remembering the names of letters and numbers, and putting sounds and letters in the correct order.
- Children who are not progressing in word-learning skills by the middle or end of first grade should be tested.
- Affected children are taught techniques for recognizing and pronouncing words, including phonics using multisensory cues.

Dyslexia is a particular type of learning disorder that affects an estimated 3 to 5% of children. It is identified in more boys than girls; however, it may simply go unrecognized more often in girls. Dyslexia tends to run in families.

Dyslexia occurs when the brain has difficulty making the connection between sounds and symbols (letters). This difficulty is caused by poorly understood problems with certain connections in the brain. The problems are present from birth and may cause spelling and writing errors and reduced speed and accuracy when reading aloud. People with dyslexia do not have problems understanding spoken language.

Symptoms and Diagnosis

Preschool children with dyslexia may be late in speaking, have speech articulation problems, and have difficulty remembering the names of letters, numbers, and colors. Dyslexic children often have difficulty blending sounds, rhyming words, identifying the positions of sounds in words, segmenting words into sounds, and identifying the number of sounds in words. Delays or hesitations in choosing words, making word substitutions, and naming letters and pictures are early indicators of dyslexia. Problems with short-term memory for sounds and for putting sounds in the correct order are common.

Many children with dyslexia confuse letters and words with similar ones. Reversing the letters while writing—for instance, *on* instead of *no,* and *saw* instead of *was*—or confusing letters—for instance, *b* instead of *d, w* instead of *m, n* instead of *h*—is common. However, many children without dyslexia will reverse letters in kindergarten or first grade.

Children who are not progressing in word-learning skills by the middle or end of first grade should be tested for dyslexia.

Treatment

The best treatment for word recognition is direct instruction that incorporates multisensory approaches. This type of treatment consists of teaching phonics with a variety of cues, usually separately and, when possible, as part of a reading program.

Indirect instruction for word recognition is also helpful. This instruction usually consists of training to improve word pronunciation or reading comprehension. Children are taught how to process sounds.

Component-skills instruction for word recognition is also helpful. It consists of training to blend sounds to form words, to segment words into word parts, and to identify the positions of sounds in words.

Indirect treatments, other than those for word recognition, may be used but are not recommended. Indirect treatments can include using tinted lenses that allow words and letters to be read more easily, eye movement exercises, or visual perceptual training. Drugs such as piracetam have also been tried. The benefits of most indirect treatments have not been proved and may provide unrealistic expectations and delay the teaching that is needed.

CHAPTER 11

Normal Adolescents

During adolescence (usually encompassing ages 10 to 21), children become young adults. They mature socially and physically. Notably, they become sexually mature and socially independent. During this time, the adolescent develops a sense of who he or she is and learns to form intimate relationships with people who are not members of the family.

Physical Development

- Most boys and girls reach adult height and weight during adolescence.
- In boys, the genitals usually enlarge first, then pubic hair appears, followed by facial and underarm hair.
- In most girls, breasts begin to develop first, then pubic and underarm hair appears, followed by menstruation about 2 years after breasts begin to develop.

Normal growth during adolescence includes sexual maturation and an increase in body size. The timing and speed with which these changes occur vary and are affected by both heredity and environment. Physical maturity begins at an earlier age today than it did a century ago. For example, girls have their first menstrual period at a considerably younger age than their counterparts did 100 years ago. The reason is probably improvements in nutrition, general health, and living conditions.

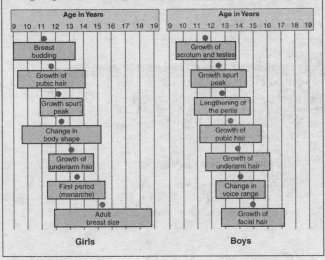

Milestones in Sexual Development

During puberty, sexual development usually occurs in a set sequence. The tempo of change varies from person to person but occurs within a range of ages, indicated by a box in the diagram. The average age at which a change begins is indicated by a dot.

During adolescence, most boys and girls reach adult height and weight, although there is considerable variation in when this occurs. The growth spurt in boys occurs between the ages of 13 and 15½ years; a gain of 4 inches can be expected in the year of maximum growth. The growth spurt in girls occurs between the ages of 11 and 13½ years; a gain of 3½ inches can be expected in the year of maximum growth. In general, boys become heavier and taller than girls. By age 18, boys have about ¾ inch of growth remaining and girls have slightly less.

DID YOU KNOW?

- Adolescent boys can grow up to 4 inches during a year.
- Girls today start menstruating at a much younger age than in years past.
- In girls, height increases most before menstruation starts.

In boys, the first changes in sexual characteristics are enlargement of the scrotum and testes, followed by lengthening of the penis. Internally, the seminal vesicles and prostate gland enlarge. Next, pubic hair appears. Hair grows on the face and in the underarms about 2 years after it appears in the pubic area. The first ejaculation usually occurs between the ages of 12½ and 14, about 1 year after the penis begins to lengthen. Breast enlargement on one side or both is common in young adolescent boys and usually disappears within a year.

In the majority of girls, the first visible sign of sexual maturation is breast budding, closely followed by the growth spurt. Soon afterward, pubic and underarm hair appears. The first menstrual period generally starts about 2 years after the breasts begin to enlarge. Height increases most before menstruation begins.

Intellectual and Behavioral Development

- Thinking becomes more abstract and logical.
- These new reflective capabilities may lead to self-consciousness and questioning of values and behavior standards.

In early adolescence, a child begins to develop the capacity for abstract, logical thought. This increased sophistication leads to an enhanced awareness of self and the ability to reflect on one's own being. Because of the many noticeable physical changes of adolescence, this self-awareness often turns into self-consciousness, with an accompanying feeling of awkwardness. The adolescent also has a preoccupation with physical appearance and attractiveness and a heightened sensitivity to differences from peers.

The adolescent also applies his new reflective capabilities to moral issues. Preadolescents understand right and wrong as fixed and absolute. The adolescent questions standards of behavior and frequently rejects tradition—often to the consternation of parents. Ideally, this reflection culminates in the development and internalization of the adolescent's own moral code.

Many adolescents begin to engage in risk-taking behaviors, such as fast driving, substance abuse, sexual experimentation, and sometimes, theft and other illegal activities. Some experts think this behavior occurs in part because adolescents may feel a sense of power and immortality.

Social Development

- Peer groups often replace the family as the primary social focus.

During childhood, the family is the center of the child's life. During adolescence, the peer group often begins to replace the family as the child's primary social focus. Peer groups are often established because of distinctions in dress, appearance, attitudes, hobbies, interests, and other characteristics that may appear profound or trivial to outsiders. Initially, peer groups are usually same-sex but typically become mixed later in adolescence. These groups assume an importance to adolescents because they provide validation for the adolescent's tentative choices and support in stressful situations.

DID YOU KNOW?

- Being without a peer group may make adolescents feel different and alienated and act in dysfunctional or antisocial ways.

Those adolescents who, for various reasons, find themselves without a peer group often develop intense feelings of being different and alienated. Although these feelings often have little permanent effect, they may worsen any potential for dysfunctional or antisocial behavior. At the other extreme, the peer group assumes too much importance for some adolescents. Gang membership and behavior are more common when the home and social environments are unable to counterbalance the often dysfunctional demands of the peer group (see page 216).

Development of Sexuality

- As adolescents mature sexually, they may engage in sexual behaviors.

- Providing information and advice about safe-sex practices is important.
- Some adolescents develop homosexual feelings, which may cause stress and fears of abandonment and may even trigger physical threats at school.

During early adolescence, an increasing interest in sexual anatomy and pubertal changes develops. These changes (or lack thereof) often are a source of anxiety. As adolescents mature emotionally and sexually, they may begin to engage in sexual behaviors. Masturbation among boys is nearly universal and is common among girls. Sexual behavior with others often begins as extended petting, but sometimes progresses to oral sex, vaginal intercourse, and anal sex. By late adolescence, sexuality has shifted from being exploratory to being an expression of intimacy and sharing. Appropriate advice on safe-sex practices is essential.

Some adolescents explore homosexual activities but ultimately do not continue to be interested in same-sex relationships. Other adolescents never have any interest in opposite-sex relationships. Doctors do not understand exactly why homosexual feelings develop, but it is not something adolescents "learn" from their peers or the media.

DID YOU KNOW?

- Masturbation among boys is nearly universal and is common among girls.
- Some adolescents explore and eventually lose interest in homosexual activities.

Homosexual adolescents face an emotional burden as their sexuality develops. Many teenagers are made to feel unwanted if they express homosexual desires. Such pressure (especially during a time when social acceptance is critically important) can cause severe stress. Problems can be made worse by comments and even physical threats made at school. A fear of abandonment by parents, sometimes real, may lead to dishonest or at least incomplete communication between adolescents and their parents. Threats of physical violence should be taken seriously and reported to school officials.

The emotional development of homosexual adolescents is best helped by supportive friends and family members. Family and friends should express the same interest and involvement as they would for heterosexual adolescents.

Preventive Health Care Visits

- At annual visits, doctors monitor physical, emotional, and intellectual maturation, perform a detailed physical examination, screen for sexually transmitted diseases in sexually active adolescents, and provide advice about healthy lifestyles and injury prevention.
- Doctors and adolescents also discuss developmental, psychosocial, and behavioral issues.
- Parents can talk to doctors about how to handle the changes that occur during adolescence.

Annual health care visits allow a doctor to continue monitoring the adolescent's physical growth and sexual maturation. In most cases for older adolescents, the parent is not present during the examination. Examination of the skin (checking for acne), evaluation of the degree of sexual maturation, and examination of the back for scoliosis are particularly important in adolescence. Screening for sexually transmitted diseases should be performed for adolescents who are sexually active.

Other appropriate screening tests might include a blood cholesterol level for adolescents whose families have a history of high cholesterol or heart disease and tuberculosis testing for adolescents with a history of exposure to tuberculosis. The doctor also makes sure the adolescent has had all appropriate vaccinations, particularly hepatitis B, which may not have been given in childhood, and tetanus, which requires a booster. Newly recommended vaccinations for adolescents include meningococcal conjugate vaccination, pertussis vaccination, and, for girls, vaccine against human papillomavirus.

The bulk of the doctor's visit with the adolescent encompasses discussions and questions about developmental, psychosocial, and behavioral issues. Typically, the doctor asks questions about an adolescent's home environment, academic achievement and goals, activities and hobbies, engagement in risk-taking behaviors, and emotional health. Equally important is counseling about physical and psychosocial development, healthy lifestyles, and injury prevention. Other discussions include the importance of wearing seatbelts, the dangers of drinking and driving, peer pressure, potential for becoming dependent on drugs or alcohol, readiness for parenthood, responsible sexual behavior, and avoiding violence. The doctor may provide a list of resources (for example, books, phone numbers, web sites) for the adolescent. For older adolescents, the doctor often discusses issues of confidentiality within the doctor-patient relationship, and it is developmentally appropriate for older adolescents to be alone with the doctor during at least part of the preventive health care visit.

The doctor should also ask the parents about how they are handling the changes that come with adolescence. Specific questions about limit-setting, spending quality time with the adolescent, and discussion of expectations for behavior are typically included in the interview with the parents. Typically, the adolescent is not present for the interview with the parents.

CHAPTER 12

Problems in Adolescents

The most common problems adolescents face relate to growth and development, childhood illnesses that continue into adolescence, and experimentation with risky or illegal behavior. As adolescents try new behaviors, they become vulnerable to injury, legal consequences, and sexually transmitted diseases. Heterosexually active girls are at risk of becoming pregnant. Traumatic injuries, particularly from car and motorcycle accidents, are the leading cause of death and disability among adolescents. Interpersonal violence has become a particular problem among adolescents.

DID YOU KNOW?

- Puberty may occur too early or too late, causing distress in the child or adolescent.

Adolescence is a time when mental health disorders (see page 513), such as depression and schizophrenia, can become apparent, leading to a risk of suicide. Eating disorders, such as anorexia nervosa (see page 527), are particularly common in adolescent girls. Obesity has become an epidemic in the adolescent population.

WHEN PUBERTY STARTS TOO EARLY

Precocious puberty and pseudoprecocious puberty are sexual maturation that begins before age 7 in a girl or before age 9 in a boy. True precocious puberty is caused by the early release of certain sex hormones (gonadotropins) from the pituitary gland. These hormones cause the ovaries or testes to develop and begin secreting other sex hormones, such as estrogen or testosterone. The estrogen or testosterone causes the development of puberty and the appearance of adult physical characteristics. This early hormone release may be caused by a tumor or other abnormality in the pituitary gland or the hypothalamus (the region of the brain that controls the pituitary gland).

In pseudoprecocious puberty, high levels of testosterone or estrogen are produced by a tumor or other abnormality in the adrenal gland or in a testis or ovary. These hormones do not cause the testes or ovaries themselves to mature but do cause a child to look more like an adult.

In both conditions, pubic and underarm hair grows, adult body odor develops, and the child's body shape changes. Acne may appear. A boy develops facial hair, his penis lengthens, and his appearance becomes more masculine. A girl develops breasts and may start to have menstrual periods, especially if she has true precocious puberty. Height increases rapidly but stops at an early age. Therefore, the final height is shorter than would be expected. In true precocious puberty, the sex glands (ovaries or testes) also mature and enlarge, whereas in pseudoprecocious puberty, the sex glands remain immature. True precocious puberty is 2 to 5 times more common in girls.

Testotoxicosis is a rare hereditary form of pseudoprecocious puberty that affects boys; it results directly from maturation of the testes, independent of the hypothalamus or pituitary gland. Similarly, McCune-Albright syndrome is a genetic (but not hereditary) disorder that results in pseudoprecocious puberty; this disorder is more common in girls.

Doctors measure blood hormone levels and take x-rays of the hand and wrist to estimate bone maturity. They perform an ultrasound of the pelvis and adrenal glands and computed tomography (CT) or magnetic resonance imaging (MRI) of the head to check for tumors in the adrenal glands, hypothalamus, or pituitary gland. A test to measure the effect of gonadotropin-releasing hormone on pituitary hormone levels can help doctors diagnose the cause.

In true precocious puberty, taking a drug such as long-acting injections of leuprolide (synthetic gonadotropin-releasing hormone) or daily injections of deslorelin or histrelin stops the pituitary gland from producing sex hormones by desensitizing it to the effects of the body's own gonadotropin-releasing hormone. In pseudoprecocious puberty, a doctor may try to inhibit the action of the sex hormones with various drugs. The antifungal drug ketoconazole reduces the levels of testosterone circulating in the blood in boys who have testotoxicosis. A drug called testolactone reduces the levels of estrogen in adolescents who have McCune-Albright syndrome. In both of these conditions, spironolactone or cyproterone may also be useful.

When a tumor is responsible for true precocious or pseudoprecocious puberty, removing it may cure the condition.

Delayed Sexual Maturation

Delayed sexual maturation is a delay in the onset of puberty and the development of the sexual organs.

- Sexual maturation may be delayed by various disorders, cancer treatment, and, less commonly, genetic disorders and brain tumors.
- Pubic hair does not appear, testes do not enlarge in boys, and breasts do not grow and menstruation does not occur in girls.
- Bone x-rays may be taken to see whether bones are maturing on schedule, and blood and imaging tests may be done to check for various disorders.

The onset of sexual maturation (puberty) takes place when one part of the brain, the hypothalamus, sends a chemical signal to another part of the brain, the pituitary gland. This signal tells the pituitary gland to begin releasing hormones called gonadotropins, which stimulate the growth of the sex organs (the testicles in boys and the ovaries in girls). The growing organs secrete sex hormones, such as testosterone (in boys) and estrogen (in girls). These hormones cause the development of sexual characteristics, including pubic and axillary hair in both sexes, facial hair and muscle mass in boys, and breast growth in girls, and of sexual desire (libido).

Some adolescents do not start their sexual development at the usual age. A delay may be perfectly normal, and in some families sexual maturation tends to occur later. In such adolescents, the growth rate before puberty is usually normal, and they otherwise appear healthy. Although the growth spurt and sexual maturation are delayed, they eventually proceed normally.

Various chronic diseases, such as diabetes mellitus, inflammatory bowel disease, kidney disease, cystic fibrosis, and anemia, can delay or prevent sexual development. Development may be delayed in adolescents receiving radiation therapy or cancer chemotherapy. Adolescents, particularly girls, who become very thin because of excessive exercise or dieting often have delayed sexual maturation, including an absence of menstruation.

There are many uncommon causes of delayed sexual maturation. Chromosomal abnormalities (such as Turner syndrome in girls (see page 117) and Klinefelter syndrome in boys (see page 120) and other genetic disorders can affect production of hormones. A tumor that damages the pituitary gland or the hypothalamus can lower the levels of gonadotropins or stop production of the hormones altogether. A mumps infection can damage the testicles and prevent puberty.

Symptoms and Diagnosis

In boys, the symptoms of delayed sexual maturation are lack of testicular enlargement by age $13^{1}/2$, lack of pubic hair by age 15, or a time lapse of more than 5 years from the start to the completion of genital enlargement. In girls, the symptoms are lack of breast development by age 13, more than 5 years from the beginning of breast growth to the first menstrual period, lack of pubic hair by age 14, or failure to menstruate by age 16. A short height (short stature) may indicate delayed maturation in both boys and girls.

Although adolescents are typically uncomfortable about being different from their peers, boys in particular are likely to feel psychologic stress and embarrassment from delayed puberty. Girls who remain smaller and less sexually mature than their peers are not stigmatized as quickly.

If an adolescent appears healthy and has no signs of any disorder—particularly if other family members were slow to mature—the doctor may elect to wait 6 to 12 months before conducting extensive testing. After this time, x-rays are often used to evaluate bone maturity. Adolescents whose bone maturity is delayed are probably just slow overall developers. Those with age-appropriate bone maturity are more likely to have delayed sexual maturation. They require blood tests to measure various hormone levels, as well as tests for diabetes, anemia, and other disorders that can delay sexual development. Sometimes a chromosomal analysis may be performed. Computed tomography (CT) or magnetic resonance imaging (MRI) may be performed to ensure that there is no brain tumor.

Treatment

The treatment for delayed sexual maturation depends on its cause. Once a chronic underlying disorder has been treated, maturation usually proceeds. An adolescent who is naturally late in developing needs no treatment, although if the adolescent is severely stressed by the lack of development or development is extremely delayed, some doctors may give supplemental sex hormones to begin the process sooner. A genetic disorder cannot be cured, although replacing hormones may help sexual characteristics develop. Surgery may be needed for adolescents with tumors.

Short Stature

Short stature is height below normal for the child's age (according to standard charts for age and height).

- Sometimes short stature is caused by a disorder.

The pituitary gland regulates the amount of growth hormone produced, which is an important factor in determining stature. If the pituitary gland produces too little growth hormone, abnormally slow growth and short stature with normal proportions (pituitary dwarfism) can result. Most short children, however, have normally functioning pituitary glands and are short because their growth spurt is late or their parents are relatively short. Chronic illnesses that affect the heart, lungs, kidneys, or intestine can also result in short stature. Abnormalities in the bone can also lead to very short stature.

Pituitary dwarfism is treated with growth hormone. Growth hormone is also used sometimes to increase height in children who have short stature but normally functioning pituitary glands, but this use is controversial. Some parents feel that short stature is a disorder, but most doctors do not approve of the use of growth hormone in these children. Regardless of the cause of short stature, pituitary hormone is effective only if given before the growth plates in the long bones become inactive. X-rays can help determine whether the growth plates are inactive.

Obesity

Obesity is the accumulation of excessive body fat.

- Obesity increases the risk of high blood pressure and type 2 diabetes.
- Usually, the cause is eating too much and exercising too little.
- The best approach is to encourage permanent changes in eating habits and increased physical activity.

Obesity is twice as common in adolescents as it was 30 years ago. Although most of the complications of obesity occur in adulthood, obese adolescents are more likely than other adolescents to have high blood pressure and type 2 diabetes. Although fewer than one third of obese adults were obese as adolescents, most obese adolescents remain obese in adulthood.

The factors that influence obesity among adolescents are the same as those among adults. Parents often are concerned that obesity is the result of some type of endocrine disease, such as hypothyroidism, but such disorders are rarely the cause. Adolescents with weight gain caused by endocrine disorders are usually of small stature and have other signs of the underlying condition. Most obese adolescents simply eat too much and exercise too little. They also tend to be tall for their age. Because of society's stigma against obesity, many obese adolescents have a poor self-image and become increasingly sedentary and socially isolated.

DID YOU KNOW?

- Most obese adolescents remain obese as adults.
- Obesity is rarely caused by an endocrine disorder.

Intervention for obese adolescents should be focused on developing healthy eating and exercise habits rather than on losing a specific amount of weight. Caloric intake is reduced by establishing a well-balanced diet of ordinary foods, making permanent changes in eating habits, and increasing physical activity. Summer camps for obese adolescents usually help them lose a significant amount of weight, but without continuing effort, the weight is usually regained. Counseling to help adolescents cope with their problems, including poor self-esteem, may be helpful.

Drugs that help reduce weight are generally not used during adolescence because of concerns about safety and possible abuse. One exception is for obese adolescents with a strong family history of type 2 diabetes; they are at high risk for developing diabetes. The drug metformin, which is used to treat diabetes, may help them lose weight and also lower their risk of becoming diabetic.

Acne

Acne is a common skin condition producing pimples on the face and upper torso.

- Hair follicles become clogged with sebum (the oily substance produced by glands in the skin), dead skin cells, and bacteria.
- Skin pores may have a tiny dark or white center or become pimples, which sometimes become large, red, painful, pus-filled lumps.
- Squeezing or otherwise opening pimples increases the risk of scarring.
- Gently washing the affected areas once or twice a day with a mild soap can help, but antibacterials and other drugs may be needed.

Acne is caused by an interaction between hormones, skin oils, and bacteria that results in inflammation of hair follicles. Acne occurs mostly on the face, upper chest, shoulders, and back and is characterized by pimples, cysts, and sometimes abscesses. Both cysts and abscesses are pus-filled pockets, but abscesses are somewhat larger and deeper.

Sebaceous glands, which secrete an oily substance (sebum), lie in the dermis, the middle layer of skin. These glands are attached to the hair follicles. The sebum, along with dead skin cells, passes up from the sebaceous gland and hair follicle and out to the surface of the skin through the pores.

Acne results when a collection of dried sebum, dead skin cells, and bacteria clog the hair follicles, blocking the sebum from leaving through the pores. If the blockage is incomplete, a blackhead (open comedo) develops; if the blockage is complete, a whitehead (closed comedo) develops. The blocked sebum-filled hair follicle promotes overgrowth of the bacteria *Propionibacterium acnes*, which are normally present in the hair follicle. These bacteria break down the sebum into substances that irritate the skin. The resulting inflammation and infection produce the skin eruptions that are commonly known as acne pimples. If the infection worsens, an abscess may form, which may rupture into the skin, creating even more inflammation.

DID YOU KNOW?

- Antibacterial or abrasive soaps, alcohol pads, and heavy frequent scrubbing are not recommended for acne.
- People with acne can eat any food (for example, pizza and chocolate) but should follow a balanced diet.
- Severe scarring due to acne can be treated surgically or with chemical peels, laser resurfacing, or injections of substances to raise the scarred area.

Acne occurs mainly during puberty, when the sebaceous glands are stimulated by increased hormone levels, especially the androgens (such as testosterone), resulting in excessive sebum production. By a person's early to mid 20s, hormone production stabilizes and acne usually disappears. Other conditions that involve hormonal changes can affect the occurrence of acne as well. For example, acne may occur with each menstrual period in young women and may clear up or substantially worsen during pregnancy. The use of certain drugs, particularly corticosteroids and anabolic steroids, can cause acne by stimulating the sebaceous glands. Certain cosmetics may worsen acne by clogging the pores.

Because acne naturally varies in severity for most people— sometimes worsening, sometimes improving—pinpointing the factors that may produce an outbreak is difficult. Acne is often worse in the winter and better in the summer, for unknown reasons. There is no relationship, however, between acne and specific foods or sexual activity.

Symptoms

Acne ranges from mild to very severe. Yet, even mild acne can be vexing, especially to teenagers, who see each pimple as a major cosmetic challenge.

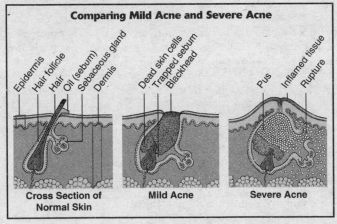

Comparing Mild Acne and Severe Acne

Epidermis · Hair follicle · Hair · Oil (sebum) · Sebaceous gland · Dermis

Dead skin cells · Trapped sebum · Blackhead

Pus · Inflamed tissue · Rupture

Cross Section of Normal Skin   **Mild Acne**   **Severe Acne**

People with mild (superficial) acne develop only a few noninflamed blackheads or a moderate number of small, mildly irritated pimples. Most acne occurs on the face but is also common on the shoulders, back, and upper chest. Anabolic steroid use typically causes acne on the shoulders and upper back. Blackheads appear as tiny, dark dots at the center of a small swelling of normal-colored skin. Pimples are mildly uncomfortable and have a white center surrounded by a small area of reddened skin. People with severe (deep, or cystic) acne have numerous large, red, painful pus-filled lumps (nodules) that sometimes even join together under the skin into giant, oozing abscesses.

Mild acne usually does not leave scars. However, squeezing pimples or trying to open them in other ways increases inflammation and the depth of injury to the skin, making scarring more likely. The nodules and abscesses of severe acne often rupture and, after healing, typically leave scars. Scars may be tiny, deep holes (ice pick scars); wider pits of varying depth; or large, irregular indentations. Acne scars last a lifetime and, for some people, are cosmetically significant and a source of psychologic stress.

Treatment

General care of acne is very simple. Affected areas should be gently washed once or twice a day with a mild soap. Antibacterial or abrasive soaps, alcohol pads, and heavy frequent scrubbing provide no added benefit and may further irritate the skin. Cosmetics should be water-based; very greasy products can worsen acne. Although there are no restrictions on specific foods (for example, pizza or chocolate), a healthy, balanced diet should be followed.

Beyond these routine measures, acne treatment depends on the severity of the condition. Mild acne requires the simplest treatment, which poses the fewest risks of side effects. More severe acne or acne that does not respond to preliminary treatment requires additional treatment.

Mild Acne Drugs used to treat mild acne are applied to the skin (topical drugs). They work by either killing bacteria (antibacterials) or drying up or unclogging the pores.

The two most commonly prescribed antibacterials are the antibiotics clindamycin and erythromycin. Benzoyl peroxide, another effective antibacterial, is available with or without a prescription.

Older nonprescription creams that contain salicylic acid, resorcinol, or sulfur work by drying out the pimples and causing slight scaling. These drugs, however, are less effective than antibiotics or benzoyl peroxide.

If topical antibacterials fail, doctors use other topical prescription drugs that help unclog the pores. The most common such drug is tretinoin. Tretinoin is very effective but is irritating to the skin and makes it more sensitive to sunlight. Doctors therefore use this drug cautiously, starting with low concentrations and infrequent applications, which can be gradually increased. Benzoyl peroxide inactivates tretinoin, so the two must not be applied together. Other drugs with effects similar to tretinoin include adapalene, azelaic acid, and tazarotene.

Blackheads and whiteheads can be removed by a doctor. A large pimple may be opened with a sterile needle. Other instruments, such as a loop extractor, can also be used to drain plugged pores and pimples.

Severe Acne: Antibiotics given by mouth, including tetracycline, doxycycline, minocycline, and erythromycin, are reserved for the treatment of severe acne. People may need to take one of these drugs for weeks, months, or even years to prevent a recurrence. Some of these drugs have potentially serious side effects, so close monitoring by a doctor is necessary. Girls who take antibiotics for a long time sometimes develop vaginal yeast infections that may require treatment with other drugs. If controlling the yeast infection proves difficult, oral antibiotic therapy for acne may not be practical.

For the most severe acne, when antibiotics do not work, oral isotretinoin is the best treatment. Isotretinoin, which is related to the topical drug tretinoin, is the only drug that can potentially cure acne. However, isotretinoin can have very serious side effects. *Isotretinoin can harm a developing fetus, and sexually active girls taking it must use strict contraceptive measures so they do not become pregnant.* Other, less serious side effects may occur as well. Therapy generally continues for 20 weeks. If more therapy is needed, it should not be restarted for at least 4 months.

Other acne treatments are useful for specific people. For example, a girl with severe acne that worsens with her menstrual period may be helped by taking oral contraceptives. This treatment takes 2 to 4 months to produce results.

Doctors sometimes treat large, inflamed nodules or abscesses by injecting corticosteroids into them. Occasionally, a doctor cuts open a nodule or abscess to drain it.

Treatment of severe acne scars depends on their shape, depth, and location. Individual scars of any depth may be cut out and the skin sewn back together. Wide indented scars can be improved cosmetically in a procedure called subcision, in which small cuts are made under the skin to release the scar tissue. This procedure often allows the skin to resume its normal contours. Multiple shallow scars may be treated with chemical peels or laser resurfacing. Dermabrasion, a procedure in which the skin surface is rubbed with an abrasive metal instrument to remove the top layer, also may help remove small scars. Sometimes scars are injected with various substances such as collagen, fat, or a variety of synthetic materials. These substances may raise the scarred area to make it level with the rest of the skin.

Drugs Used to Treat Acne

ACTION	DRUG	SELECTED SIDE EFFECTS	COMMENTS
Kills bacteria (applied topically)			
	Clindamycin	Diarrhea (rarely)	—
	Erythromycin	—	Well tolerated
	Benzoyl peroxide	Dries the skin May discolor clothing and hair	Especially effective when combined with erythromycin
Unclogs pores (applied topically)			
	Tretinoin	Irritates skin; sensitizes skin to sunlight	Acne appears to worsen when tretinoin is started; may take 3 to 4 weeks to notice any improvement; protective clothing and sunscreen should be worn during sun exposure

Drugs Used to Treat Acne (Continued)

ACTION	DRUG	SELECTED SIDE EFFECTS	COMMENTS
Unclogs pores (applied topically)			
	Tazarotene	Irritates skin; sensitizes skin to sunlight	Acne appears to worsen when tazarotene is started; may take 3 to 4 weeks to notice any improvement; protective clothing and sunscreen should be worn during sun exposure
	Adapalene	Some redness, burning, and increased sun sensitivity	As effective as tretinoin but less irritating; protective clothing and sunscreen should be worn during sun exposure
	Azelaic acid	May lighten skin	Minimally irritating; may be used by itself or with tretinoin; should be used cautiously in people with darker skin because of skin-lightening effects
Kills bacteria (taken by mouth)			
	Tetracycline	Sensitizes skin to sunlight	Inexpensive and safe, but must be taken on an empty stomach; protective clothing and sunscreen should be worn during sun exposure
	Doxycycline	Sensitizes skin to sunlight	Protective clothing and sunscreen should be worn during sun exposure
	Minocycline	Headache, dizziness, and skin discoloration	Most effective antibiotic
	Erythromycin	Stomach upset	Bacteria frequently become resistant to erythromycin

(Continued)

Drugs Used to Treat Acne (Continued)

ACTION	DRUG	SELECTED SIDE EFFECTS	COMMENTS
Unclogs pores (taken by mouth)			
	Isotretinoin	Can harm a developing fetus; can affect blood cells, liver, and fat levels; dry eyes, chapped lips, drying of the mucous membranes; pain or stiffness of large joints and lower back with high dosages; has been associated with depression, suicidal thoughts, attempted suicide, and (in rare cases) completed suicide	A sexually active woman should have a pregnancy test before she starts taking isotretinoin and at monthly intervals while she is taking it; contraception or sexual abstinence should begin 1 month before she starts taking the drug and should continue while she takes it and for 1 month after she discontinues it. Blood tests are necessary to make sure the drug is not affecting blood cells, the liver, or fat (triglyceride and cholesterol) levels

School Problems

- Adolescents may have problems in school because they are rebelling and want to be independent.
- Adolescents may fear going to school, choose to skip school periodically, drop out, or do poorly academically.
- If problems are severe, educational testing and a mental health evaluation may help identify the cause.
- Parents and school personnel should try to identify the reason for problems and encourage adolescents to attend school or to consider alternative programs.

School constitutes a large part of an adolescent's existence. Difficulties in almost any area of life often manifest as school problems.

School problems during the adolescent years may be the result of rebellion and a need for independence. Less commonly, they may be caused by mental health disorders, such as anxiety or depression. Substance use, abuse, and family conflict also are common contributors to school problems. Sometimes, inappropriate academic placement—particularly in adolescents with a learning disability or mild mental retardation that was not recognized early in life—causes school problems. In general, adolescents with significant school problems should undergo educational testing and a mental health evaluation. Specific problems are treated as needed, and general support and encouragement are provided.

Particular school problems include fear of going to school, truancy, dropping out, and academic underachievement. Problems that developed earlier in childhood, such as attention deficit/hyperactivity disorder (ADHD) and learning disorders (see page 185 and page 190), may continue to cause school problems for adolescents.

Between 1% and 5% of adolescents develop fear of going to school. This fear may be generalized or related to a particular person (a teacher or another student) or event at school (such as physical education class). The adolescent may develop physical symptoms, such as abdominal pain, or may simply refuse to go to school. School personnel and family members should identify the reason, if any, for the fear and encourage the adolescent to attend school.

Adolescents who are repeatedly truant or drop out of school have made a conscious decision to miss school. These adolescents generally have poor academic achievement and have had little success or satisfaction from school-related activities. They often have engaged in high-risk behaviors, such as having unprotected sex, taking drugs, and engaging in violence. Adolescents at risk for dropping out should be made aware of other educational options, such as vocational training and alternative programs.

Behavioral Problems

- The adolescent's quest for independence may lead to breaking rules, risky behaviors, and even physical confrontations.
- Parents can help adolescents by providing clear guidance and support, by setting consistent limits and monitoring the limits, and by gradually increasing privileges as adolescents show more responsibility.
- Occasionally, professional help is needed.

Adolescence is a time for developing independence. Typically, adolescents exercise their independence by questioning their parents' rules, which at times leads to rule breaking. Parents and doctors must distinguish occasional errors of judgment from a degree of misbehavior that requires professional intervention. The severity and frequency of infractions are guides. For example, drinking habitually, fighting often, frequent truancy and theft are much more significant than isolated episodes of the same activities. Other warning signs include deterioration of performance at school and running away from home.

Children occasionally engage in physical confrontation. However, during adolescence, the frequency and severity of violent interactions increase. Although episodes of violence at school are highly publicized, adolescents are much more likely to be involved with violence (or more often the threat of violence) at home and outside of school. Many factors, including developmental issues, gang membership, access to firearms, substance use, and poverty, contribute to an increased risk of violence for adolescents. Of particular concern are adolescents who, in an altercation, cause serious injury or use a weapon.

Because adolescents are much more independent and mobile than they were as children, they are often out of the direct physical control of adults. In these circumstances, adolescents' behavior is determined by their own moral and behavioral code. The parents guide rather than directly control the adolescents' actions. Adolescents who feel warmth and support from their parents are less likely to engage in risky behaviors. Also, parents who convey clear expectations regarding their adolescents' behavior and who demonstrate consistent limit setting and monitoring are less likely to have adolescents who engage in risky behaviors. Authoritative parenting, as opposed to harsh or permissive parenting, is most likely to promote mature behaviors.

Authoritative parents typically use a system of graduated privileges, in which the adolescent is initially given small bits of responsibility and freedom (such as caring for a pet, doing household chores, picking out clothing, or decorating his room). If the adolescent handles this responsibility appropriately over a period of time, freedom is increased. Abuses of freedom are dealt with by taking away privileges. Each increase in freedom requires close attention by parents to make sure the adolescent is where and with whom he is supposed to be, returns at the proper time, and so forth.

Some parents and their adolescents clash over almost everything. In these situations, the core issue is really control—adolescents want to feel in control of their lives and parents want adolescents to know they still make the rules. In these situations, everyone may benefit from the parents focusing their efforts on the adolescents' actions (attending school, complying with household responsibilities) rather than on expressions (dress, hairstyle, preferred entertainment).

Adolescents whose behavior is still dangerous or otherwise unacceptable despite their parents' best efforts may need professional intervention. Substance abuse is a common trigger of behavioral problems and often requires specific therapy. Behavioral problems may be the first sign of depression or other mental health disorders. Such disorders typically require treatment with drugs as well as counseling. In extreme cases, some adolescents may also need legal intervention in the form of probation.

Drug and Substance Use and Abuse

- Many adolescents experiment with drugs, but drug dependence is uncommon.
- Alcohol is the substance of concern most commonly used by adolescents.

- Parents can discourage smoking by adolescents by not smoking themselves and by openly discussing the hazards of smoking.
- Erratic behavior, mood swings, a change in friends, and declining school performance may be signs of substance abuse.

Substance use among adolescents occurs on a spectrum from experimentation to dependence. The consequences range from none to life threatening, depending on the substance, the circumstances, and the frequency of use. However, even occasional use can produce significant harm, such as overdose, motor vehicle collision, and unwanted pregnancy. Although experimentation and occasional usage are common, actual drug dependence is not.

Alcohol is the substance most often used among adolescents. About 80% of high school seniors reported trying alcohol; some engage in binge drinking, which is defined as having more than 5 drinks in a row. There are risk factors for whether an adolescent will try alcohol. Genetics may be a factor; adolescents who have a family member who is an alcoholic should be made aware of the risk. Adolescents whose friends and siblings drink excessively may think this behavior is acceptable. Society and the media often model drinking as being acceptable. Despite these influences, parents can make a difference by conveying clear expectations to their adolescent regarding drinking, setting limits consistently, and monitoring the adolescent.

The majority of adults who smoke cigarettes begin smoking during adolescence. Nearly one fifth of 9th graders report smoking regularly. If an adolescent reaches the age of 18 to 19 years without becoming a smoker, it is highly unlikely that he will become a smoker as an adult. Factors that increase the likelihood of an adolescent smoking are having parents who smoke (the single most predictive factor), peers who smoke, and poor self-esteem. Using other illegal substances is also a factor. Parents can prevent their adolescent from smoking by not smoking themselves (or quitting), by openly discussing the hazards of tobacco, and by convincing adolescents who already smoke to quit and to seek medical assistance in quitting if necessary.

DID YOU KNOW?

- About 8 in 10 high school seniors report trying alcohol, and more than 6 in 10 report having been drunk.
- Adolescents with a family member who is an alcoholic should be told that a genetic predisposition toward alcoholism is possible.
- Adolescents who do not become smokers by age 18 or 19 years are unlikely to become smokers as adults.
- Using anabolic steroids during adolescence can stunt growth.
- Demanding that a doctor test an adolescent for drug use is not recommended.

Use of illegal substances in adolescents, although decreasing overall in the last few years, remains high. In the year 2000, about 54% of 12th graders had used illegal drugs at some time in their life. About 62% of 12th graders reported having been drunk; 49% reported use of marijuana; 16%, amphetamines; 13%, hallucinogens; 9%, barbiturates; 9%, cocaine; and 2%, heroin. Use of methylenedioxymethamphetamine (Ecstasy), unlike the other drugs mentioned, increased dramatically in the last few years, with 11% of 12th graders reporting use at some time.

Up to 6% of boys in high school, including a number of nonathletes, have used anabolic steroids at least once. A particular problem with anabolic steroid use in adolescents is early closure of the growth plates at the ends of bones, resulting in permanent short stature. Other side effects are common, including behavioral disturbances, liver damage, increased body hair, and acne.

Adolescents as young as 12 to 14 years of age may be involved in substance use. Although there are risk factors for adolescents engaging in substance use, it is difficult to predict which adolescents will engage in the most serious forms of abuse. Parents should look for erratic behavior in their adolescent, mood swings, a change in friends, and declining school performance. If parents notice any of these behaviors, they should discuss their concerns with the adolescent and his doctor (see also page 538).

The doctor can help assess whether an adolescent has a problem with substance use. Some parents simply bring the adolescent into a doctor demanding that he perform a urine drug test. There are a few points for a parent to keep in mind: The doctor cannot force the adolescent to take a drug test if he refuses. Results of a urine test may be falsely negative; factors influencing results are the metabolism of the drug and the time it was last used. Most important, in an atmosphere of accusation and confrontation, it will be difficult for the doctor to obtain a history from the adolescent, which is key to making the diagnosis.

If the doctor thinks the adolescent does have a problem, he can refer the adolescent to a professional with expertise in substance abuse; this person can make the diagnosis and determine the treatment needed. Treatment for adolescents is similar to that of adults but is typically conducted in a setting with other adolescents.

Contraception and Adolescent Pregnancy

- Sexually active adolescents are less apt to use birth control and barrier protection regularly.
- Pregnancy during adolescence causes substantial emotional stress and often interrupts school or job training.
- Pregnant adolescents need help sorting through the difficult choices of abortion, adoption, and parenthood.

Although adolescents may engage in sexual activity, many sexually active adolescents are not fully informed about contraception, pregnancy, and sexually transmitted diseases, including human immunodeficiency virus (HIV) infection. Impulsivity, lack of planning, and concurrent drug and alcohol use decrease the likelihood that adolescents will use birth control and barrier protection.

Any of the adult contraceptive methods may be used by adolescents. Problems with adolescents and contraception revolve around adherence. For example, many adolescent girls who are taking oral contraceptives forget to take them regularly or stop using them for various reasons—often not substituting another form of birth control. Some girls do not feel empowered to ask their male partners to use condoms during sex. Boys generally prefer not to use condoms.

Because adolescence is a transitional stage in life, pregnancy can add significant emotional stress. Pregnant adolescents and their partners tend to drop out of school or job training, thus worsening their economic status, lowering their self-esteem, and straining personal relationships.

Pregnant adolescents, particularly the very young and those who are not receiving prenatal care, are more likely than women in their 20s to have medical problems such as anemia and toxemia. Infants of young mothers (especially mothers younger than 15 years) are more likely to be born prematurely and to have a low birth weight. However, with proper prenatal care, older adolescents have no higher risk of pregnancy problems than adults from similar backgrounds.

DID YOU KNOW?

- Adolescent girls are more likely to have health problems during pregnancy, and their babies are more likely to be premature and have a low birth weight.

Having an abortion does not remove the psychologic problems of an unwanted pregnancy—either for the adolescent girl or her partner. Emotional crises may occur when the pregnancy is diagnosed, when the decision to have an abortion is made, immediately after the abortion is performed, when the baby would have been born, and on the anniversaries of that date. Family counseling and education about contraceptive methods, for both the girl and her partner, can be very helpful.

Parents may have different reactions when their daughter says she is pregnant or their son says his girlfriend is pregnant. Emotions may range from apathy to disappointment and anger. It is important for parents to express their support and willingness to help the adolescent sort through his or her choices. Parents and adolescents need to communicate openly about abortion, adoption, and parenthood—all tough options for the adolescent to struggle with alone.

Emergencies

CHAPTER 13

Poisoning

Poisoning is the harmful effect that occurs when a toxic substance is swallowed, is inhaled, or comes in contact with the skin, eyes, or mucous membranes, such as those of the mouth or nose.

Poisoning is the most common cause of nonfatal accidents in the home. Drugs—prescription, nonprescription, and illegal—are the most common source of serious poisonings and poisoning-related deaths. Other common poisons include gases, household products, agricultural products, plants, industrial chemicals, vitamins, and foods (particularly certain species of mushrooms and fish). However, almost any substance ingested in sufficiently large quantities can be toxic. Young children are particularly vulnerable

---

DID YOU KNOW?

- Most poisonings in children can be prevented.
- In the United States, the local poison center can be reached by dialing 800-222-1222.
- Containers of the poisons or drugs taken should be saved and given to the doctor.
- Every home should have activated charcoal on hand in case of poisoning.
- Most children who are poisoned recover fully if they can be kept alive until the body eliminates the poison.

---

to accidental poisoning in the home. Adolescents and, rarely, younger children may attempt suicide by poisoning themselves.

The damage caused by poisoning depends on the poison, the amount taken, and the age and underlying health of the child who takes it. Some poisons are not very potent and cause problems only with prolonged exposure or repeated ingestion of large amounts. Other poisons are so potent that just a drop on the skin can cause severe damage.

Some poisons produce symptoms within seconds, whereas others produce symptoms only after hours or even days. Some poisons produce few obvious symptoms until they have damaged vital organs—such as the kidneys or liver—sometimes permanently.

First Aid and Prevention

Anyone exposed to a toxic gas should be removed from the source quickly, preferably out into fresh air.

In chemical spills, all contaminated clothing should be removed immediately. The skin should be thoroughly washed with soap and water. If the eyes have been exposed, they should be thoroughly flushed with water. Rescuers must be careful to avoid contaminating themselves.

If the child appears very sick, emergency medical assistance (911 in most areas of the United States) should be called. Bystanders should perform cardiopulmonary resuscitation (CPR) if needed (see page 266). If the child does not appear very sick, a family member or another adult can contact the nearest poison center for advice. In the United States, the local poison center can be reached at 800-222-1222, or through 911. If the caller knows the identity of the poison and the amount ingested, treatment can often be managed at home.

Containers of the poisons or the drugs taken should be saved and given to the doctor. If the poisoning could be serious, the child must be treated as soon as possible. The poison center may recommend giving activated charcoal (see page 228) at home. Drugs should be kept in their original child-resistant containers to prevent accidental poisoning. Expired drugs should be flushed down the toilet. In addition, drugs and poisonous substances should be kept out of sight and beyond a child's reach, preferably in a locked cabinet. All labels should be read before taking or giving any drugs.

NONTOXIC HOUSEHOLD PRODUCTS*

Adhesives
Antacids
Bath oil
Bleach (less than 5% sodium hypochlorite)
Body conditioners
Bubble bath soaps (detergents)
Chalk (calcium carbonate)
Colognes
Cosmetics
Deodorants
Deodorizers, spray and refrigerant
Fabric softeners
Hand lotions and creams
3% hydrogen peroxide, medicinal
Incense
Indelible markers
Ink (black, blue)
"Lead" pencils (which are really made of graphite)
Magic markers
Matches
Mineral oil
Modeling clay
Newspaper
Perfumes
Petroleum jelly
Sachets (essential oils, powders)
Shaving creams and lotions
Soap and soap products
Suntan preparations
Sweetening agents (saccharin, aspartame)
Toothpaste with or without fluoride
Water colors
Wax or paraffin
Zinc oxide
Zirconium oxide

*Almost any substance can be toxic if ingested in sufficient amounts.

Diagnosis and Treatment

Identifying the poison is crucial to successful treatment. Labels on bottles and other information from the child, family members, or other people present best enables the doctor or the poison center to identify poisons. Urine and blood tests may help in identification as well. Sometimes, blood tests can reveal how serious the poisoning is.

Many children who have been poisoned must be hospitalized. The principles for the treatment of all poisoning are the same:

- Prevent additional absorption of the poison
- Increase elimination of the poison
- Give specific antidotes (substances that eliminate, inactivate, or counteract the effects of the poison), if available
- Prevent reexposure

With prompt medical care, most children recover fully. The usual goal of hospital treatment is to keep the child alive until the poison disappears or is inactivated. Eventually, most poisons are inactivated by the liver or are passed into the urine.

Stomach emptying may be attempted if an unusually dangerous poison is involved or if the child appears very sick. In this procedure, a tube is inserted through the mouth or nose into the stomach. Water is poured into the stomach through the tube and is then drained out (gastric lavage) several times.

For many swallowed poisons, hospital emergency departments usually give activated charcoal. Activated charcoal binds to the poison that is still in the digestive tract, preventing its absorption into the blood. Charcoal is usually taken by mouth but may have to be given through a tube that is inserted through the nose into the stomach. Sometimes doctors give charcoal every several hours to help cleanse the body of the poison.

If a poisoning remains life threatening despite the use of charcoal and antidotes, more complicated treatments may be needed. The most common involve filtering poisons directly from the bloodstream—hemodialysis, which uses an artificial kidney (dialyzer) to filter the poisons, or charcoal hemoperfusion, which uses charcoal to help eliminate the poisons. For either of these methods, two small tubes (catheters) are inserted into blood vessels. One is used to drain blood from an artery, and the other to return blood to a vein. The blood is passed through special filters that remove the toxic substance before the blood is returned to the body.

Poisoning often requires additional treatment. For example, a child who becomes very drowsy or comatose may need a breathing tube inserted into the windpipe. The tube is then attached to a ventilator, which mechanically supports the child's breathing. The tube prevents vomit from entering the lungs, and the ventilator ensures adequate breathing. Treatment also may be needed to control seizures, abnormal heart rhythms, low blood pressure, high blood pressure, fever, or vomiting.

If the kidneys stop working, hemodialysis is necessary. If liver damage is extensive, treatment for liver failure may be necessary. If the liver or kidneys sustain permanent, severe damage, organ transplantation may be needed.

Adolescents or children who attempt suicide by poisoning need mental health evaluation and appropriate treatment.

Acetaminophen Poisoning

- Acetaminophen, taken in very high doses, can damage the liver.
- Symptoms may take hours to develop.
- Children are given acetylcysteine to reduce the toxicity of acetaminophen.

More than 100 products contain acetaminophen, a common over-the-counter pain reliever. If several similar products are used at a time, a child may inadvertently be given too much acetaminophen. Many preparations intended for use in children are available in liquid, tablet, and capsule form, and a parent may try several preparations simultaneously or within several hours, not realizing they all contain acetaminophen.

Acetaminophen usually is a very safe drug, but it is not harmless. For poisoning to occur, several times the recommended dose of acetaminophen must be taken. For example, a child who weighs 75 pounds generally needs to take at least 10 325-mg tablets at one time before toxic effects are possible. Death is extremely unlikely unless the child takes more than 20 325-mg tablets. Thus, serious acetaminophen poisoning is unlikely unless a child or adolescent deliberately take an overdose. In very high doses, acetaminophen can damage the liver. Liver failure can follow.

DID YOU KNOW?

• Accidentally giving children too much acetaminophen, although common, is unlikely to cause serious poisoning.

Symptoms and Diagnosis

Most overdoses produce no immediate symptoms. The level of acetaminophen in the blood, measured 2 to 4 hours after ingestion, predicts the severity of the liver damage accurately. If the overdose is very large, symptoms develop in four stages.

- **Stage 1** (after several hours): The child may vomit but does not seem ill.
- **Stage 2** (after 24 hours): Many children have no symptoms until stage 2 when nausea, vomiting, and abdominal pain may develop. At this stage, blood tests show that the liver is functioning abnormally.
- **Stage 3** (after 2 to 5 days): Vomiting becomes worse. Tests show that the liver is functioning poorly, and jaundice and bleeding develop.
- **Stage 4** (after 5 days): The child either recovers quickly or experiences liver failure, which may prove fatal.

Treatment

If acetaminophen was taken within the previous several hours, activated charcoal is usually given.

If the level of acetaminophen in the blood is high, acetylcysteine is generally given by mouth or intravenously to reduce the toxicity of the acetaminophen. Acetylcysteine is given repeatedly for one to several days. Treatment for liver failure may also be necessary.

Aspirin Poisoning

- Aspirin poisoning can occur rapidly after taking a high dose or develop gradually after taking low doses repeatedly.
- Children are given activated charcoal to reduce aspirin absorption.

Ingestion of a high dose of aspirin and similar drugs (salicylates) can lead to rapid poisoning. A child weighing about 75 pounds would have to consume more than 15 325-mg tablets to develop even mild poisoning. An aspirin overdose, therefore, is seldom accidental.

Gradual aspirin poisoning can develop unintentionally by taking aspirin repeatedly at much lower doses. Children with fever who are given only slightly higher than the prescribed dose of aspirin for several days may develop poisoning.

The most toxic form of salicylate is oil of wintergreen (methyl salicylate). Methyl salicylate is a component of products such as liniments and solutions used in hot vaporizers. A young child can die from swallowing less than 1 teaspoonful of pure methyl salicylate. Far less toxic are over-the-counter products containing bismuth subsalicylate (used to treat infections of the digestive tract), which can cause poisoning after several doses.

DID YOU KNOW?

- A young child can die from swallowing less than 1 teaspoonful of oil of wintergreen.

Symptoms

The first symptoms of rapid aspirin poisoning are usually nausea and vomiting followed by rapid breathing, ringing in the ears, sweating, and sometimes fever. Later, if poisoning is severe, the child can develop light-headedness, drowsiness, confusion, seizures, and difficulty breathing.

The symptoms of gradual aspirin poisoning develop over days or weeks. Drowsiness, confusion, and hallucinations are the most common symptoms. Light-headedness, rapid breathing, and shortness of breath can develop.

Diagnosis and Treatment

A blood sample is taken to measure the precise level of aspirin in the blood. Measurement of the blood pH (acidity) and the level of carbon dioxide or bicarbonate in the blood also can help determine the severity of poisoning. Tests are usually repeated during treatment to reveal whether the child is recovering.

Activated charcoal reduces aspirin absorption. For moderate or severe poisoning, fluids containing sodium bicarbonate are given intravenously. Unless there is kidney damage, potassium is added to the fluid. This mixture moves aspirin from the bloodstream into the urine. If the child's condition is worsening despite other treatments, hemodialysis can remove aspirin from the blood. Vitamin K may be given to treat bleeding problems.

Carbon Monoxide Poisoning

- Carbon monoxide prevents blood from carrying oxygen and tissues from using it effectively.
- Carbon monoxide poisoning is common.
- Symptoms may include headache, nausea, and drowsiness.
- Adequate venting of furnaces and other sources of indoor combustion and carbon monoxide detectors help prevent carbon monoxide poisoning.

Carbon monoxide is a colorless, odorless gas that, when inhaled, prevents the blood from carrying oxygen and prevents the tissues from using oxygen effectively. Small amounts are not usually harmful, but poisoning occurs if levels of carbon monoxide in the blood become too high. Carbon monoxide disappears from the blood after several hours.

Smoke from fires commonly contains carbon monoxide, particularly when combustion of fuels is incomplete. If improperly vented, automobiles, boats, furnaces, hot water heaters, gas heaters, kerosene heaters, and stoves (including wood stoves and stoves with charcoal briquettes) can cause carbon monoxide poisoning. Inhaling tobacco smoke leads to carbon monoxide in the blood, but usually not enough to result in symptoms of poisoning.

_ DID YOU KNOW? _

- All homes should have carbon monoxide detectors.

Symptoms and Diagnosis

Mild carbon monoxide poisoning causes headache, nausea, vomiting, drowsiness, and poor coordination. Most children with mild carbon monoxide poisoning recover quickly when moved into fresh air. Moderate or severe carbon monoxide poisoning causes confusion, unconsciousness, chest pain, shortness of breath, and coma. Thus, most children are not able to move themselves and must be rescued. Severe poisoning is often fatal. Rarely, weeks after apparent recovery from severe carbon monoxide poisoning, symptoms such as memory loss, poor coordination, and uncontrollable loss of urine (which are referred to as delayed neuropsychiatric symptoms) develop.

Carbon monoxide is dangerous because children or their parents may not recognize drowsiness as a symptom of poisoning. Consequently, someone with mild poisoning can go to sleep and continue to breathe the carbon monoxide until severe poisoning or death occurs. Some children with long-standing, mild carbon monoxide poisoning caused by furnaces or heaters are thought to have another condition, such as the flu or other viral infections. Sometimes everyone in the household is affected.

Carbon monoxide poisoning is diagnosed by measuring the level of carbon monoxide in the blood.

Treatment and Prevention

For mild poisoning, fresh air may be all that is needed. For more severe poisoning, high concentrations of oxygen are given, usually through a face mask. Oxygen hastens the disappearance of carbon monoxide from the blood and relieves symptoms. The value of high-pressure oxygen treatment (in a hyperbaric chamber) remains uncertain.

For prevention, sources of indoor combustion, such as gas space heaters and wood stoves, require properly installed ventilation. If such ventilation is impractical, an open window can limit carbon monoxide accumulation by allowing it to escape from the building.

Exhaust pipes attached to furnaces and other heating appliances need periodic inspections for cracks and leaks. Chemical detectors that can sense carbon monoxide in the air and sound alarms when it is present are available for the home. Constant monitoring with such detectors can identify carbon monoxide before poisoning develops. Like smoke detectors, carbon monoxide detectors are recommended for all homes.

Poisoning With Caustic Substances

- Caustic substances, when swallowed, can burn all tissues they touch—from the lips to the stomach.
- Doctors may insert a flexible viewing tube into the esophagus and stomach to assess the damage.

Caustic substances (strong acids and alkalies), when swallowed, can burn the tongue, mouth, esophagus, and stomach. These burns may cause perforation (holes) of the esophagus or stomach. Food and saliva leaking from a perforation cause severe, sometimes deadly infection within the chest (mediastinitis or empyema) or abdomen (peritonitis). Burns that do not perforate can scar the esophagus and stomach.

Industrial products are usually the most damaging because they are highly concentrated. However, some common household products, including drain and toilet bowl cleaners and some dishwasher detergents, contain damaging caustic substances, such as sodium hydroxide and sulfuric acid.

Caustic substances are available as solids and liquids. The burning sensation of a solid particle sticking to a moist surface (such as the lips) may prevent a child from consuming much of the product. Because liquids do not stick, it is easier to consume more of the product, and the entire esophagus can be damaged.

DID YOU KNOW?

- A child that swallows a caustic substance should not be made to vomit.

Symptoms

Pain in the mouth and throat develops rapidly, usually within minutes, and can be severe, particularly during swallowing. Coughing, drooling, an inability to swallow, and shortness of breath may occur. In severe cases involving strong caustic substances, a child may develop very low blood pressure (shock), difficulty breathing, or chest pain, possibly leading to death.

Perforation of the esophagus or stomach may occur during the first week after ingestion, often after vomiting or severe coughing. Materials may leak from the esophagus into the area between the lungs (the mediastinum) or into the area surrounding the lungs (the pleural cavity). Either circumstance causes chest pain, fever, rapid heart rate, very low blood pressure, and an abscess (a collection of pus), which requires surgery. Peritonitis results in severe abdominal pain.

Scarring of the esophagus results in narrowing (stricture), which causes difficulty swallowing. Strictures usually develop weeks after the burn, sometimes in burns that initially caused only mild symptoms.

Diagnosis and Treatment

The mouth is examined for chemical burns. Because the esophagus and stomach may be burned without the mouth being burned, the doctor may insert an endoscope (a flexible viewing tube) down the esophagus to look for burns, particularly if the child drools or has difficulty swallowing. Directly inspecting the area allows the doctor to determine the severity of the injury and possibly to predict the risk of subsequent narrowing and the possible need for surgical repair of the esophagus.

The extent of damage determines treatment. Children with severe burns sometimes need immediate surgery to remove severely damaged tissue. Corticosteroids and antibiotics are used to try to prevent strictures and infections, but whether these drugs are helpful is not clear.

Because caustic substances can cause as much damage returning up the esophagus as they did when swallowed, a child who has swallowed a caustic substance should not be made to vomit.

If burns are mild, the child may be encouraged to begin drinking fluids fairly soon during recovery. Otherwise, fluids are given intravenously until drinking is possible. If strictures develop, a bypass tube (stent) may be placed in the narrowed portion of the esophagus to prevent esophageal closure and to allow for future widening (dilation). Repeated widening may be needed for months or years. For severe strictures, surgery to rebuild the esophagus may also be necessary.

Hydrocarbon Poisoning

- Swallowing gasoline, kerosene, paint thinners, some cleaning products, or furniture polish or sniffing glue can cause hydrocarbon poisoning.
- Hydrocarbon poisoning may cause pneumonia, fatal irregular heartbeats, and neurologic problems.

Petroleum products, cleaning products, and glues contain hydrocarbons (substances composed largely of hydrogen and carbon). Many children younger than age 5 are poisoned by swallowing petroleum products, such as gasoline, kerosene, and paint thinners, but most recover. At greater risk are teenagers who intentionally breathe the fumes of these products to become intoxicated, a type of drug abuse called huffing, sniffing, glue sniffing, or volatile substance use.

Swallowed hydrocarbons can enter and irritate the lungs— a serious condition in itself (chemical pneumonitis)— and can lead to severe pneumonia. Lung involvement is a particular problem with thin, easy-flowing hydrocarbons such as mineral seal oil, which is used in furniture polish. Serious poisoning also can affect the brain, heart, bone marrow, and kidneys.

Symptoms

A child usually coughs and chokes after swallowing hydrocarbons. A burning sensation can develop in the stomach, and the child may vomit. If the lungs are affected, the child continues to cough intensely. Breathing becomes rapid, and the skin may become bluish (cyanotic) because of low levels of oxygen in the blood.

Hydrocarbon ingestion also produces neurologic symptoms, including drowsiness, poor coordination, stupor or coma, and seizures. Inhalation of hydrocarbons may induce fatal irregular heartbeats or cardiac arrest, especially after exertion or stress.

DID YOU KNOW?

- Hydrocarbon, which has a petroleum-like odor, can often be smelled on the child's breath.
- Adolescents who get high breathing hydrocarbon fumes may die suddenly.

Diagnosis and Treatment

Hydrocarbon poisoning is diagnosed based on a description of the events and the characteristic odor of petroleum on the child's breath. Pneumonia and chemical pneumonitis are diagnosed with a chest x-ray and by measuring the level of oxygen in the blood.

Contaminated clothing should be removed, and the skin should be washed. If the child has stopped coughing and choking, particularly if the ingestion was small and accidental, treatment at home is possible. This situation should be discussed with someone at a poison center. Children with breathing problems are hospitalized. If pneumonia or chemical pneumonitis develops, hospital treatment can include oxygen, and, if severe, a ventilator. Antibiotics help if pneumonia develops. Recovery from pneumonia typically takes about a week.

Insecticide Poisoning

- Insecticides derived from nerve gases (organophosphates and carbamates) are the most poisonous.
- Several drugs are effective in treating serious poisonings.

The properties that make insecticides deadly to insects can sometimes make them poisonous to humans. Most serious insecticide poisonings result from the organophosphate and carbamate types of insecticides, particularly when used in suicide attempts. These compounds are derived from nerve gases. Pyrethrins and pyrethroids, which are commonly used insecticides derived from flowers, usually are not poisonous to humans.

Many insecticides can cause poisoning after being swallowed, inhaled, or absorbed through the skin. Some insecticides are odorless. Thus, the child is unaware of being exposed to them. Organophosphate and carbamate insecticides make certain nerves "fire" erratically, causing many organs to become overactive and eventually to stop functioning. Pyrethrins occasionally cause allergic reactions. Pyrethroids rarely cause any problems.

Symptoms

Organophosphates and carbamates cause eye tearing, blurred vision, salivation, sweating, coughing, vomiting, and frequent bowel movements and urination. Breathing may become difficult, and muscles twitch and become weak. Rarely, shortness of breath or muscle weakness is fatal. Symptoms last hours to days after exposure to carbamates but can last for weeks after exposure to organophosphates.

Pyrethrins can cause sneezing, eye tearing, coughing, and occasional difficulty breathing. Serious symptoms rarely develop.

DID YOU KNOW?

- Children may become poisoned without knowing that they were exposed to an insecticide.

Diagnosis and Treatment

The diagnosis of insecticide poisoning is based on the symptoms and on a description of the preceding events. Blood tests can confirm organophosphate or carbamate poisoning.

If an insecticide might have contacted the skin, clothing is removed and the skin is washed. Anyone with symptoms of organophosphate poisoning should see a doctor. Atropine, given intravenously, can relieve most of the symptoms. Pralidoxime, given intravenously, can speed up recovery of nerve function, eliminating the cause of the symptoms. Symptoms of carbamate poisoning are also relieved by atropine but usually not by pralidoxime. Symptoms of pyrethrin poisoning resolve without treatment.

Iron Poisoning

- Symptoms of iron poisoning develop in stages, beginning with vomiting, diarrhea, and abdominal pain.

Pills containing iron are commonly used to treat certain kinds of anemia. Iron also is included in many multiple vitamin supplements. Children—especially toddlers—who overdose on these pills may develop iron poisoning. Because many households contain multiple vitamin supplements with iron for adults, iron overdose is common. However, overdose of iron-containing vitamins, particularly children's chewable vitamins, usually does not involve enough iron to cause serious poisoning. Overdose of pure iron supplements, however, may cause serious iron poisoning.

Serious iron poisoning first irritates the stomach and digestive tract. Within hours, iron poisons the cells, interfering with their internal chemical reactions. Within days, the liver can be damaged. Weeks after recovery, the stomach, digestive tract, and liver can develop scars due to the previous irritation.

DID YOU KNOW?

- Usually, an overdose of vitamins with iron, particularly children's chewable vitamins, does not involve enough iron to cause serious poisoning.

Symptoms

Serious iron poisoning usually causes symptoms within 6 hours of the overdose. The symptoms of iron poisoning typically occur in four stages.

- **Stage 1** (within 6 hours after the overdose): Symptoms include vomiting, diarrhea, abdominal pain, drowsiness, unconsciousness, and seizures. The stomach may bleed. If poisoning is very serious, rapid breathing, a rapid heart rate, and low blood pressure may develop.
- **Stage 2** (8 to 24 hours after the overdose): The child's condition can appear to improve.
- **Stage 3** (6 to 48 hours after the overdose): Very low blood pressure (shock), bleeding, jaundice, liver failure, seizures, confusion, and coma can develop. Sugar levels in the blood can decrease.

- **Stage 4** (2 to 6 weeks after the overdose): The stomach or intestines can become blocked by constricting scars. Scarring in either organ can cause crampy abdominal pain and vomiting. Severe scarring of the liver (cirrhosis) can develop later.

Diagnosis and Treatment

The diagnosis of iron poisoning is based on the child's history, symptoms, and the amount of iron in the blood. If many pills have been swallowed, they can sometimes be seen on x-rays of the stomach or intestines.

Children with symptoms or high levels of iron in the blood need hospitalization. Gastric lavage may be necessary to remove any iron remaining in the stomach. However, a large amount of iron can remain in the stomach even after gastric lavage or vomiting. A special saltwater solution may be given by mouth or through a stomach tube to wash the contents of the stomach and intestines (whole bowel irrigation), although its effectiveness is unclear. Injections of deferoxamine, which binds iron in the blood, are given.

Lead Poisoning

- Extremely high levels of lead in the blood may cause personality changes, lethargy, headaches, loss of sensation, weakness, uncoordinated walking, seizures, and digestive system problems.
- More commonly, less elevated lead levels can cause subtle neurological damage that is not noticeable to parents teachers, or physicians.
- Lead poisoning is detected with a blood test; sometimes bone and abdominal x-rays reveal evidence of lead poisoning.
- Treatment includes stopping exposure to lead and giving chelation therapy to remove lead from the blood.

Although it is far less common since paint containing lead pigment was banned in 1977 and lead was eliminated from most gasoline, lead poisoning (plumbism) is still a major public health problem in U.S. cities on the East Coast. Children who live in older houses that contain peeling lead paint or lead pipes are at risk.

Young children may eat enough paint chips to develop symptoms of lead poisoning. Lead affects many parts of the body, including the brain, nerves, kidneys, liver, blood, digestive tract, and sex organs. Children are particularly susceptible because lead produces the most damage in nervous systems that are still developing.

If the level of lead in the blood is high for days, symptoms of sudden brain damage (encephalopathy) usually develop. Lower blood levels that are sustained for longer periods of time sometimes produce long-term intellectual deficits.

DID YOU KNOW?

- Lead poisoning is a major public health problem in some areas.
- Children are most at risk because lead causes the most damage in nervous systems that are still developing.
- Children living in communities where houses are old should be tested for lead poisoning, regardless of whether symptoms are present.
- Commercially available kits can be used to test household paint, ceramics, and water supplies for lead content.
- Lead poisoning can be prevented by repairing peeling lead-based paint, wiping affected windowsills weekly with a damp cloth, and using commercial home water filters.

Symptoms and Diagnosis

Most children with mild lead poisoning have no symptoms. Symptoms that do occur usually develop over months or years.

Typical symptoms of lead poisoning include personality changes, headaches, loss of sensation, weakness, a metallic taste in the mouth, uncoordinated walking, poor appetite, vomiting, constipation, crampy abdominal pain, bone or joint pains, and anemia. Kidney damage often develops without symptoms. Young children may become cranky and play less frequently over the course of several weeks. Encephalopathy can then begin suddenly and worsen over the next several days, resulting in persistent, forceful vomiting;

confusion; sleepiness; and, finally, seizures and coma. This acute lead poisoning is now rare, though it may occur when there is renovation in the home and the child is suddenly exposed to very high lead levels.

More commonly, children have slightly elevated blood lead levels. Although this does not cause noticeable symptoms in individual children, studies have demonstrated that children with mild to moderately elevated lead levels are at increased risk for subtle neurologic abnormalities, such as learning, behavioral, or processing problems. Thus all children who have any possible exposure should be tested at the point of peak risk. National advisory groups recommend universal screening with blood lead tests at ages 12 months and 24 months.

Some symptoms may diminish if exposure to lead is stopped, only to worsen again if exposure is resumed.

Lead poisoning is diagnosed with a blood test. Children living in communities with many older houses, where peeling lead-based paint is common, should undergo blood tests for lead. In children, bone and abdominal x-rays often show evidence of lead poisoning.

Treatment and Prognosis

Treatment of mild to moderate lead poisoning consists of stopping exposure to lead. Treatment of even more severe lead poisoning may involve removing accumulated lead from the body. Doctors remove lead from the body by giving drugs that bind with the lead (chelation therapy), allowing it to pass into the urine. All drugs that remove lead work slowly and can cause serious side effects. Children with certain levels of lead in the blood may be given succimer by mouth. Children with more serious lead poisoning are treated in the hospital with injections of chelating drugs, such as, dimercaprol, succimer, penicillamine, and edetate calcium disodium. Because chelating drugs also can remove beneficial minerals, such as zinc, copper, and iron, from the body, the person often is given supplements of these minerals.

Even after treatment, many children with encephalopathy develop some degree of permanent brain damage. Kidney damage is also sometimes permanent.

Prevention

Commercially available kits can be used to test household paint, ceramics, and water supplies for lead content. Dusting affected windowsills weekly with a damp cloth removes some dust that could contain lead from paint. Chipped leaded paint should be repaired. Larger renovation projects to remove leaded paint can release large quantities of lead into the house and should be done professionally. Commercially available faucet filters can remove most lead from drinking water.

CHAPTER 14

Injuries and First Aid

Children can have the same injuries as adults. Common ones include wounds, bumps, bruises, muscle strains, sprains, dislocations, fractures, bites, stings, burns, injuries to teeth, and near drowning. Rarely, an injury, illness, or poisoning leads to cardiac arrest in children. Keeping a first-aid kit handy can be helpful.

BASIC FIRST-AID SUPPLIES

A medicine chest or first-aid kit should always be kept well stocked. The following basic supplies may be useful:

- Activated charcoal (the poison center should be called before charcoal is used)
- Adhesive tape
- Antiseptic cream (such as bacitracin)
- Aspirin or acetaminophen
- Bandages or surgical tape
- Cold pack
- Cotton-tipped swabs
- First-aid manual

- Sharp scissors
- Soap or instant hand sanitizer
- Sterile adhesive or gauze bandages in several sizes
- Thermometer
- Thin, translucent gloves
- Tissues
- Tweezers

Wounds

Wounds include cuts or tears in tissue (lacerations), scrapes (abrasions), and puncture wounds.

- Wounds can be caused by bites or other injuries.
- Infection is more likely to develop in deep scrapes, puncture wounds, and wounds that contain foreign material.
- Thoroughly cleaning the wound is most important.

Wounds that are not caused by bites usually heal rapidly without any problems. However, some wounds cause extensive blood loss. Others become complicated by infection or injury to deeper structures, such as nerves, tendons, or blood vessels. A piece of foreign material can remain hidden inside a puncture wound.

Shallow cuts to most areas of the skin rarely bleed much and often stop bleeding on their own. Cuts to the hand and scalp as well as cuts to arteries and larger veins often bleed vigorously.

Infection can develop when a wound is contaminated with dirt and bacteria. Although any wound can become infected, infection is particularly likely in deep scrapes, which grind dirt into the skin, and in puncture wounds, which introduce contamination deep under the skin. Also, wounds that contain foreign material (such as splinters, glass, or clothing fragments) almost always become infected. The longer a wound remains contaminated, the more likely it is that infection will develop.

Wounds can be painful at first, but the pain usually lessens after the first day. If a cut affects a nerve or tendon, children may be unable to move the body part fully. Some nerve injuries cause numbness. If a foreign object remains inside a puncture wound, the part of the wound near the object is usually painful when touched.

Pain that worsens a day or more after the injury is often the first sign of infection. Later, an infected wound becomes red and swollen and may ooze pus. A fever may develop.

DID YOU KNOW?

- Pain that worsens a day or more after an injury is often the first sign of infection.
- Bleeding can almost always be stopped by applying pressure on the wound with a finger or hand.

First-Aid Treatment

The first step in treating a cut is to stop the bleeding. Visible bleeding can almost always be stopped by firmly compressing the bleeding area with a finger or hand for at least 5 minutes. Whenever possible, the bleeding part is elevated above the level of the heart—for example, by raising a limb. Because tourniquets shut off all blood flow to a body part and deprive it of oxygen, they are rarely used.

Dirt and particles are removed and the wound is washed to prevent infection. Large, visible particles are picked off. Smaller dirt and particles that cannot be seen are removed by washing with mild soap and tap water. Dirt and particles that remain after washing can often be removed with a more highly pressured stream of warm tap water. Harsher agents, such as alcohol, iodine, and peroxide, are not recommended. These solutions can damage tissue, impairing the capacity to heal. Scrubbing is required to clean deep scrapes. After cleaning, antibiotic ointment and a bandage are applied. If a wound is very small, it can be kept closed with certain commercially available tapes. Stitches may be needed for deep or large cuts.

The child should see a health care practitioner if any of following occurs:

- A cut is longer than $1/3$ inch, is on the face, appears deep, or has edges that separate.
- Bleeding does not stop within several minutes or after pressure is applied.
- There are symptoms of a nerve or tendon injury.
- A scrape is deep or contains dirt and particles that are difficult to remove.
- There is a puncture wound, particularly if a foreign object in the wound is likely.
- The child needs a tetanus vaccine.
- The child is anxious or in pain and thus cannot cooperate with the necessary first-aid treatment.

Health care practitioners can anesthetize wounds that require extensive or painful cleaning, sutures, or other procedures. They can surgically repair wounds that damage tendons, nerves, or blood vessels. They can give pain relievers or sedating drugs to children who otherwise cannot cooperate.

All wounds, whether treated at home or by health care practitioners, should be observed for signs of infection during the first several days after treatment. If any signs of infection develop, the child should be taken to a health care practitioner within several hours. Most small wounds heal within a few days.

Injuries to Limbs

Injuries to limbs include bumps and bruises (contusions, muscle tears (strains), tears of ligaments and tendons near joints (sprains), and fractures.

- Fractures in children often involve the part of the bone where growth occurs.
- Treatment usually includes *r*est, *i*ce, *c*ompression, and *e*levation (RICE).

- Children with severe symptoms should be evaluated by a health care practitioner.
- Severe injuries may require a cast or surgery.

Children often bump or bruise a limb, tear (strain) a muscle, tear (sprain) tendons or ligaments (which hold muscles and bones in place), injure joints, or break bones. Bones within a joint may become completely separated (dislocated) or partially separated (subluxated). If children are still growing, bones are most likely to break at the growth plate, an area of softer tissue where bone growth occurs. Some growth plate fractures prevent bones from growing normally. The growth plate hardens when growth is complete.

DID YOU KNOW?

- Splints can be made from readily available materials, such as a pillow, magazines, or sticks and cloth.
- If pain becomes much worse 24 hours or more after an injury, the child should be taken to a doctor at once.

Symptoms and Diagnosis

Bumps and bruises (contusions), mild strains, and mild sprains produce mild to moderate pain and swelling. The swollen area can become discolored, turning purple after a day and becoming yellow or brown days later. Usually, children can continue to use the body part. A mild strain or sprain may cause more severe symptoms, such as pain, deformity, or inability to walk or to use the injured part. However, these symptoms may indicate a more severe injury, such as a dislocation, subluxation, or fracture.

Regardless of the injury, pain tends to peak within 24 hours. Pain that becomes much worse 24 hours or more after an injury occasionally indicates compartment syndrome. Compartment syndrome is an uncommon, limb-threatening complication of limb injuries.

WHAT IS COMPARTMENT SYNDROME?

Compartment syndrome is an uncommon but serious complication of severe contusions, fractures, or, rarely, casts, splints, or snakebites.

Muscles are surrounded by a fibrous covering that forms a closed space (compartment). When injured, muscles swell. If they swell a lot, they press against their fibrous covering. This pressure reduces blood flow to the muscle. Thus, the muscle does not get enough oxygen. If the muscle is deprived of oxygen for too long, further injury occurs, and the muscle swells even more, increasing pressure. After a few hours, the muscle and sometimes other nearby tissues die.

A cast, if needed, confines swelling even more, putting more pressure on the muscle. Thus, a cast can contribute to compartment syndrome.

Doctors usually diagnose contusions, sprains, and strains by examining the child. X-rays are taken if a fracture, dislocation, or subluxation is suspected. Occasionally, magnetic resonance imaging (MRI) or computed tomography (CT) is needed.

Treatment

First Aid: Contusions, mild strains, and mild sprains can be treated at home with rest, ice, compression, and elevation (RICE), which speed recovery and reduce pain and swelling.

- **Rest:** Resting the injured part prevents the injury from worsening.
- **Ice:** Ice helps limit inflammation and reduces muscle spasms as well as pain and swelling. A commercial ice pack or a bag of crushed or chipped ice—which conforms to body contours better than ice cubes—can be placed on a towel over the injured part for 10 minutes. The ice is removed for 10 minutes, then reapplied for 10 minutes over a period of 1 to 1½ hours. This process can be repeated several times during the first 24 hours. Applying ice for too long can damage tissue. The skin may turn red, feel hot and itchy, and hurt.
- **Compression:** An elastic bandage can be wrapped around the injured part. An ice bag may be enclosed under the bandage.
- **Elevation:** The injured part is raised above the heart and is kept elevated.

Usually, children with severe symptoms need to see a health care practitioner. However, if a fracture, severe strain, severe sprain, subluxation, or dislocation is a possibility, a splint should be applied until a health care practitioner can be seen. A splint can be anything that prevents movement of a limb, such as a pillow, magazine, stack of newspapers, or a board. A splint should immobilize the joints above and below the injury. When an arm, a wrist, or the collarbone is injured, a sling may be used with a splint.

Commonly Used Splints

A splint is used to prevent movement of a limb and thus prevent further damage and limit pain. To be effective, a splint must immobilize the joints above and below the injury.

Splints can be made from readily available objects, such as a magazine or stack of newspapers. But splints usually consist of a rigid, straight object, such as a board, strapped to the limb. A sling may be used with a splint to support the forearm when an arm, a wrist, or the collarbone is injured.

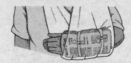

Splinted Arm in Sling

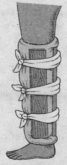

Splinted Leg

Medical Treatment: Severe injuries may require immobilization in a sling, splint, or cast. Crutches may be needed.

A sling by itself provides sufficient support for many shoulder and elbow fractures. A strap that passes around behind the back can be used to keep the arm from swinging outward, especially at night. Slings permit some use of the hand.

A cast is made by wrapping rolls of plaster or fiberglass strips that harden once wetted. Plaster is often chosen for the initial cast when the broken ends of a bone are separated or not aligned. Plaster molds well and is less likely to cause painful contact points between the body and cast. Otherwise, fiberglass is used because it is stronger, lighter, and more durable. In either case, the cast is lined with soft cottony material to protect the skin from pressure and rubbing, which can result in pressure sores. If the cast becomes wet, completely drying the lining is often impossible. A wet cast can make the skin soften and break down. For partially healed fractures, a special, less protective and more expensive waterproof lining is sometimes substituted.

After a cast is applied (especially for the first 24 to 48 hours), it should be kept elevated to the level of the heart, when possible, to control swelling. Regularly bending and extending the fingers or wiggling the toes helps blood drain from the limb and helps prevent swelling. If pain, pressure, or numbness remains constant or becomes much worse 24 hours or more after an injury, children should be taken to a doctor or another health care practitioner immediately. These symptoms may indicate developing compartment syndrome, which must be treated as soon as possible.

Severe sprains may require surgery. Dislocations, subluxations, and some fractures require bone realignment (a procedure called reduction). For reduction, pain relievers, an injection of a local anesthetic, a sedating drug, or sometimes general anesthesia may be required.

Treatment of most limb injuries (except fractures) is the same for children as for adults. However, the period of immobilization is often shorter for children because they heal more rapidly. Treatment of fractures in children is often different because their bones may still be growing, their bones heal more rapidly and perfectly, and surgery may damage the growth plate.

TAKING CARE OF A CAST

- When bathing, enclose the cast in a plastic bag and carefully seal the top with rubber bands or tape. Commercially available waterproof covers are convenient to use and are more reliable. If a cast becomes wet, the underlying padding may retain moisture. A hair dryer can be used to remove some dampness. Otherwise, the cast must be changed to prevent the breakdown of skin.

- Never push a sharp or pointed object down inside the cast (for example, to scratch the skin).

- Check the skin around the cast every day, and apply lotion to any red or sore area.

- When resting, position the cast carefully, possibly using a small pillow or pad, to prevent the edge from pinching or digging into the skin. Chafing or pressure sores may develop where the skin is in contact with the edge of the cast. If the edge of the cast feels rough, it can be padded with soft adhesive tape, moleskin, tissues, or cloth.

- Elevate the cast regularly, as directed by the doctor, to control swelling.

- Contact a doctor immediately if the cast causes persistent pain or feels too tight. Pressure sores or unexpected swelling may require immediate removal of the cast.

Severed or Constricted Limbs or Digits

Body parts such as fingers and toes (digits) can be severed. Also, tissue may die because blood flow has been cut off by rings or other constricting objects. An object cuts off blood flow when body parts near the object swell, often because they are injured or simply because the object constricts them.

Severed body parts, if properly preserved, can sometimes be reattached in the hospital. The severed part should be put in a sealed, dry plastic bag, and the bag should be put in a container with ice. These measures prolong tissue life. Dry ice should not be used.

DID YOU KNOW?

- If a limb or digit is injured or swells, a ring or other object that encircles any part, of the limb must be removed immediately.

If a limb or digit is injured or swells, a ring or other object that encircles the limb or digit must be removed immediately. As swelling increases, removal of a ring or object becomes more difficult. Sustained, gentle traction can be used to remove rings. Soap and water may reduce friction, easing removal. Otherwise, prompt medical care is needed.

Human Bites

Because children's teeth are not particularly sharp, most of their bites cause a bruise and only a shallow tear (laceration), if any. Human bite wounds may become infected, particularly if they are not cleaned and treated promptly. Sometimes the biting child transmits diseases, such as hepatitis, to the victim. HIV transmission, however, is extremely unlikely.

Bites are painful and usually produce a mark on the skin with the pattern of the teeth. Infected bites become very painful, red, and swollen.

DID YOU KNOW?

- All children with human bites that have broken the skin are given antibiotics to prevent infection.

Treatment

Human bites, like animal bites, are cleaned with sterile salt water (saline) or soap and water as soon as possible. All children with human bites that have broken the skin are given antibiotics by mouth to prevent infection. Tears, except those involving the hand, are surgically closed. However, a wound that is more than about several hours old is sometimes left open to be surgically closed a few days later. Infected bites are treated with antibiotics and often must be opened surgically to examine and clean the wound. If the biting person is known or suspected to have a disease that may be spread by biting, preventive treatment may be necessary.

Animal Bites

- In the United States, dogs account for most animal bites.
- A health care practitioner should clean and examine a bite wound as soon as possible.

Although any animal may bite, dogs account for most bites in the United States. Dogs usually bite when they are protecting their owners and territory. About 10 to 20 people, mostly children, die from dog bites each year. Cat bites are also common. However, cats do not defend territory and bite mainly when children restrain them for various reasons or attempt to intervene in a cat fight. Domestic animals, such as horses, cows, and pigs, bite infrequently, but their size and strength are such that serious wounds may result. Wild animal bites are rare.

Dog bites typically have a ragged, torn appearance. Cat bites are usually deep puncture wounds, which frequently become infected. Infected bites are painful, swollen, and red. Rabies may be transmitted from animals (most commonly bats) infected with that organism. Rabies is rare among pets in the United States because of vaccination.

DID YOU KNOW?

- In the United States, rabies is usually transmitted by infected bats.

Treatment

After receiving routine first-aid treatment for a bite wound, children should be taken to a health care practitioner immediately. If possible, the offending animal should be penned up by its owner. If the animal is loose, neither the child nor the child's parents should try to capture it. The police should be notified so that the proper authorities can observe the animal for signs of rabies.

A doctor cleans an animal bite with sterile saltwater (saline) or soap and water. Sometimes tissue is trimmed from the edge of the bite wound, particularly if the tissue is crushed or ragged. Facial bite wounds are surgically closed (sutured). However, minor wounds, puncture wounds, and bite wounds to the hands are not closed. Antibiotics are often given by mouth to prevent infection. Infected bites sometimes require antibiotics given orally, and if that is unsuccessful then intravenously.

Bee, Wasp, Hornet, and Ant Stings

- For bee stings, the stinger is removed, and ice and a cream are sometimes applied.
- A series of injections with small amounts of insect venom (desensitization) can sometimes prevent allergic reactions to a sting.
- Children who are allergic to stings should carry a preloaded syringe of epinephrine.

Stings by bees, wasps, and hornets are common throughout the United States. These insects puncture the skin with a hollow stinger and then inject venom. Some ants also sting. The average person can safely tolerate 10 stings for each pound of body weight. Thus, the average adult could withstand more than 1,000 stings, whereas 500 stings could kill a child. However, one sting can cause death from an anaphylactic reaction (a life-threatening allergic reaction in which blood pressure falls and the airway closes) in a person who is allergic to such stings. In the United States, 3 or 4 times more people die from bee stings than from snakebites. A more aggressive type of honeybee, called the Africanized killer bee, has reached some southern states as these bees travel north from South America. By attacking their victim in swarms, these bees cause a more severe reaction than do other bees.

In the South, particularly in the Gulf region, fire ants sting up to 40% of the people who live in infested areas each year, causing at least 30 deaths.

> **DID YOU KNOW?**
>
> - Death is more likely to result from an allergic reaction than from the venom's poisonous effects.
> - In the United States, 3 or 4 times more people die from bee stings than from snakebites.

Symptoms

Bee stings produce immediate pain and a red, swollen area about $1/2$ inch across. In some children, the area swells to a diameter of 2 inches or more over the next 2 or 3 days. This swelling is sometimes mistaken for infection, which is rare after bee stings.

The fire ant sting usually produces immediate pain and a red, swollen area, which disappears within 45 minutes. A blister then forms, rupturing in 2 to 3 days, and the area often becomes infected. In some cases, a red, swollen, itchy patch develops instead of a blister. Isolated nerves may become inflamed, and seizures may occur.

Treatment

A bee may leave its stinger in the skin. The stinger should be removed as quickly as possible without concern for the method of removal. An ice cube placed over the sting reduces the pain. A cream containing a combination of an antihistamine, an analgesic, and a corticosteroid is often useful. Children who are allergic to stings should always carry a preloaded syringe of epinephrine, which blocks anaphylactic or allergic reactions.

Children who have had a severe allergic reaction to a bee sting sometimes undergo desensitization (a series of injections with a small amount of insect venom, which gradually decrease or eliminate the allergic reaction). Desensitization may help prevent future allergic reactions.

Insect Bites

• Most insect bites cause only a small, itchy bump.

Among the more common biting and sometimes bloodsucking insects in the United States are sand flies, horseflies, deerflies, mosquitoes, fleas, lice, bedbugs, kissing bugs, and certain water bugs. The bites of these insects may be irritating because of the components of their saliva. But their saliva does not contain venom. Most bites result in nothing more than a small, red, itchy bump. Sometimes a child develops a large sore (ulcer), with swelling and pain. The most severe reactions occur in children who are allergic to the bites or who develop an infection after being bitten.

The bite should be cleaned, and an ointment containing a combination of an antihistamine, an analgesic, and a corticosteroid may be applied to relieve itching, pain, and inflammation. Children with multiple bites can take an antihistamine by mouth. Children who are allergic to the bite should be taken to a doctor or emergency department immediately and, if they have symptoms, be given an injection of epinephrine from a preloaded syringe.

Small, Shallow Burns

Most burns in children are small and shallow. Such burns can often be treated at home without a doctor. Simple first-aid measures may be all that is necessary if small, shallow burns are clean. In general, a clean burn affects only clean skin and does not contain any dirt particles or food. Running cold water over the burn can relieve pain. Covering the burn with an over-the-counter antibiotic ointment and a nonstick, sterile bandage can prevent infection.

Generally, a doctor's examination and treatment are recommended if a tetanus vaccination is needed or if the child is

Preventing Tick Bites

Ticks can transmit Rocky Mountain spotted fever and ehrlichiosis as well as Lyme disease. All are bacterial infections that can be serious.

Children should be encouraged to stay on paths and trails when walking in wooded areas and not to sit on the ground or on stone walls. These tactics help reduce the chances of picking up a tick. Wearing light-colored clothing makes ticks crawling on clothing easier to see. Applying an insecticide containing diethyltoluamide (DEET) to the skin and one containing permethrin to clothing may help protect against tick bites. Children who may have been exposed to ticks should inspect or have someone else inspect their whole body for ticks daily. Deer ticks, which transmit Lyme disease, are very small, much smaller than dog ticks. So the whole body should be inspected very carefully, especially hairy areas. Inspection is effective because ticks must be attached for more than a day to transmit Lyme disease.

To remove a tick, an adult should use fine-pointed tweezers to grasp the tick by the head or mouthparts right where they enter the skin and should pull the tick straight off. The tick's body should not be grasped or squeezed. Petroleum jelly, alcohol, lit matches, or any other irritants should not be used.

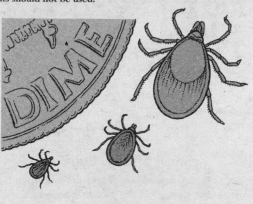

Actual size

Deer tick (nymph)   Deer tick (adult)   Dog tick (adult)

younger than 2 years. Also, a doctor should examine a burn if it has any of the following characteristics:

- Is larger than about the size of the child's palm
- Contains blisters
- Darkens or breaks the skin
- Involves the face, hand, foot, genitals, or skinfolds
- Is not completely clean
- Causes pain that is not relieved by acetaminophen
- Causes pain that does not decrease within one day after the burn occurred
- Was not accidental

Fractured, Loosened, or Knocked-Out Teeth

Baby (deciduous) teeth begin to appear at age 6 months, and all 20 are all in place by about age 30 months. Permanent teeth begin to appear at about age 6 years, and all 32 are all in place by about age 11.

Fractures: A child who has brief, sharp pain while chewing or while eating something cold may have an incomplete (greenstick) fracture of a tooth. If the fracture is incomplete and part of the tooth has not split off, the dentist can correct the problem with a filling.

The upper front teeth are prone to injury and fracture. If a tooth is not sensitive to air after an injury, most likely only the hard outer surface (enamel) has been harmed. Even if the enamel has a small chip, immediate treatment is not required. Fractures of the intermediate layer of the tooth (dentin) are usually painful when exposed to air and food. This pain usually motivates a prompt visit to the dentist. If the fracture affects the innermost part of the tooth (pulp), a red spot and often some blood appear in the fracture. Treatment by a dentist is needed.

Loosened Teeth: If an injury loosens a tooth in the socket or if the surrounding gum tissue bleeds a great deal, the child should be taken to a dentist immediately. If one or more very loose baby teeth are in the front of the mouth, they may be removed without losing space for the permanent teeth yet to come. Removing such teeth helps protect the permanent teeth.

DID YOU KNOW?

• If a permanent tooth is knocked out, it should be put in milk, then taken with the child to the dentist as soon as possible.

Knocked-Out Teeth: Knocked-out (avulsed) baby teeth should not be reimplanted because doing so may damage the permanent tooth bud. A knocked-out permanent tooth requires immediate treatment. The tooth should be rinsed off and placed back in its socket. If doing so is impossible, the tooth should be placed in a glass of milk (the milk provides a good medium for sustaining the tooth). In either case, the child and the tooth should be taken immediately to the nearest dentist.

If a tooth is reimplanted within 30 minutes, the likelihood that it will stay healthy is good. The longer the tooth is out of the socket, the worse the chance for long-term success. The dentist usually splints the tooth to the surrounding teeth for 7 to 10 days. If the bone around the tooth has also been fractured, the tooth may have to be splinted for 6 to 10 weeks. Reimplanted teeth eventually need root canal treatment.

Near Drowning

Near drowning is severe oxygen deprivation (suffocation) caused by submersion in water but not resulting in death. When death occurs, the event is called drowning.

• Children younger than 4 years are at highest risk.
• Prevention is essential and effective.
• Children who have been submerged in water should be taken to an emergency department.

When a person is submerged underwater, water enters the lungs. The vocal cords may go into severe spasm, temporarily preventing water from reaching the lungs. When filled with water, the lungs cannot efficiently transfer oxygen to the blood. The decrease in the level of oxygen in the blood that results may lead to brain damage and death. Water in the lungs, particularly water that is contaminated by bacteria, algae, sand, dirt, chemicals, or the person's vomit, can damage the lungs.

Children younger than 4 years are at greatest risk of near drowning because their energy and curiosity can easily lead them to fall into water, including bathtubs and large buckets, from which they cannot escape. For adolescents, near drowning is most common among those who are intoxicated, who have taken sedatives, who have had a seizure, who have attempted suicide, or who are physically impaired because of a medical condition. Spinal injuries and paralysis caused by diving accidents, which are likely to occur when diving into shallow water, increase the risk of near drowning. Children or adolescents who intentionally hold their breath under water for extended periods may pass out and be unable to surface, thus increasing the risk of near drowning.

DID YOU KNOW?

- Young children have survived after being submerged in cold water for as long as 40 minutes.

Submersion in cold water has both good and bad effects. It cools the muscles, making swimming difficult, and results in a dangerously low body temperature (hypothermia), which can impair judgment. Cold, however, protects tissues from the ill effects of oxygen deprivation. In addition, cold water may stimulate the mammalian diving reflex, which may prolong survival in cold water. The diving reflex slows the heartbeat and redirects the flow of blood from the hands, feet, and intestine to the heart and brain, helping preserve these vital organs. The diving reflex is more pronounced in children than in adults. Thus, children have a greater chance of surviving prolonged submersion in cold water than adults.

Symptoms and Diagnosis

Children and adolescents who are drowning and struggling to breathe are usually unable to call for help. Young children who cannot swim may become submerged in less than 1 minute compared with adolescents, who may struggle longer.

After rescue, symptoms may range from anxiety to near death. Children may be alert, drowsy, or comatose. Some may not be breathing. Those who are breathing may gasp for breath or vomit, cough, or wheeze. The skin may appear blue (cyanotic), indicating insufficient oxygen in the blood. Respiratory problems may not become evident for several hours after near drowning.

A doctor diagnoses near drowning based on the events and symptoms. Measurement of the level of oxygen in the blood and chest x-rays help reveal the extent of lung damage.

Prevention

Swimming pools should be adequately fenced because they are one of the most common sites of near-drowning accidents. In addition, all doors and gates leading to the pool area should be locked. Children in or near any body of water, including pools and bathtubs, need constant supervision, regardless of whether flotation devices are used. Because a child can drown in only a few inches of water, even water-filled containers, such as buckets or ice chests, can be hazardous.

Adolescents should not swim or boat when under the influence of alcohol or sedating drugs. Swimming should be curtailed if children or adolescents feel or look very cold. Those who have seizures that are well controlled need not avoid swimming but should be careful near water, whether they are boating, showering, or bathing.

To decrease the risk of drowning, a child or adolescent should not swim alone and should swim only in areas patrolled by lifeguards. Ocean swimmers should learn to escape rip currents (strong currents that pull away from the shore) by swimming parallel to the beach rather than by swimming toward the beach. Wearing life jackets when in boats is encouraged for everyone and is required for nonswimmers and for small children, who should also wear a life jacket when playing near bodies of water. Spinal injuries can be prevented by not diving into shallow water.

Treatment

Immediate on-site resuscitation is the key to increasing the chance of survival without brain damage. Resuscitation should be attempted even when the time under water is prolonged. Artificial respiration and cardiopulmonary resuscitation (CPR) should be provided as necessary (see page 266). The neck should be moved as little as possible if there is a chance of spinal injury. Anyone who nearly drowns must be transported to a hospital, by ambulance if possible.

In the hospital, most children need supplemental oxygen, and some need a ventilator. A ventilator can deliver oxygen using high pressures to reinflate collapsed sections of the lungs. If wheezing develops, bronchodilator drugs can help. Sometimes treatment with oxygen in a high-pressure (hyperbaric) chamber is tried.

If the water was cold, body temperature may be dangerously low, and warming with warm blankets, warmed oxygen, or other measures may be needed. Spinal injury requires special treatment.

If symptoms are mild, the child may be discharged home, but only after several hours of observation in the emergency department. If symptoms persist for a few hours or if the level of oxygen in the blood is low, the child needs to be admitted to the hospital.

Prognosis

The chances of survival without permanent brain and lung damage depend mostly on the duration of submersion, the water temperature (cold water accidents can have a better outcome), the child's age (young children are more likely to have a better outcome), and the timing of resuscitation (the sooner it begins, the better). Adolescents who have consumed alcoholic beverages before submersion are especially likely to die or develop brain or lung damage. Survival is possible after submersion for as long as 40 minutes. Almost all children and adolescents who are alert and conscious upon their arrival at the hospital recover fully. Many who need CPR also recover fully.

Choking

- Coughing may be the first symptom of choking, but children may turn blue, have a seizure, faint, or stop breathing.
- First-aid treatment is needed only if the child cannot cough or speak normally.
- For children, the Heimlich maneuver is used.
- For infants, back blows and chest thrusts are used.
- If the child loses consciousness, the airway is opened and artificial respiration is done.

How to treat choking is best learned through formal training. Maneuvers to relieve choking are frequently life saving. Infants do not have well-developed swallowing reflexes and may choke if given small, rounded foods such as peanuts or hard candies. Children, especially toddlers, may choke on toys, balloons, coins, or other inedible objects that they place in their mouths as well as foods (such as hot dogs, round candies, nuts, and grapes).

Coughing may be the first symptom and is often so severe that the child cannot ask for help. The child may grasp the throat with both hands. Breathing and speaking can become weak or stop. The child may make high-pitched or snoring sounds. The child can turn blue, have a seizure, or faint.

DID YOU KNOW?

- If a child who is choking has a strong cough or can speak normally, the Heimlich maneuver should not be done.
- Another maneuver, not the Heimlich maneuver, is used to relieve choking in infants.

First-Aid Treatment

Treatment for a child who is choking takes precedence over calling for emergency medical care.

A strong cough often expels the object from the airway. A child with a strong cough should be allowed to continue coughing. A child who can speak normally usually still has a strong cough. If a child who is choking cannot cough, the Heimlich maneuver should be performed. The Heimlich maneuver produces increased pressure in the abdomen and chest, which expels the object.

If the child is conscious, the rescuer approaches from behind, then the rescuer's arms encircle the child's waist. The rescuer forms a fist, with the thumb pointing inward, and places it between the breastbone and navel, toward the child. The other hand is then placed firmly over the fisted hand. With the arms kept off the child's ribs, the hands are then thrust inward and upward forcefully, 5 times in succession. Less force should be used for a child than for an adult. The series of thrusts should be repeated until the object is expelled. If the child loses consciousness, the rescuer should stop the thrusts.

Performing the Heimlich Maneuver

If the child is conscious, the rescuer encircles the child's waist with the arms. The rescuer forms a fist, with the thumb pointing inward, and places it between the breastbone and navel. The other hand is then placed firmly over the fisted hand. With the arms kept off the child's ribs, the hands are then thrust inward and upward forcefully, 5 times in succession.

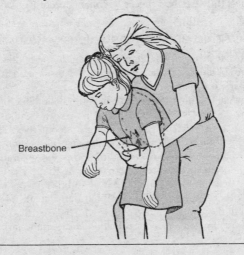

Breastbone

If a child loses consciousness, the rescuer should stop the thrusts and take steps to open the airway and provide artificial respiration (mouth-to-mouth resuscitation, or rescue breathing). The rescuer places the child face up, then removes any object visibly blocking the airway. Next, the rescuer tilts the child's head back slightly and lifts the chin. If breathing does not resume, the rescuer begins artificial respiration. With the rescuer's mouth covering the child's mouth, the rescuer slowly exhales air into the child's lungs. To prevent air from escaping from the child's nose, the rescuer pinches the nose shut while exhaling into the child's mouth.

If artificial respiration is done correctly but the chest does not rise, the child's airway is blocked. The rescuer again checks the airway for and removes any visible objects. Artificial respiration is then resumed.

For an infant, the Heimlich maneuver is not performed. Instead, the infant is turned face down, the chest resting on the rescuer's hand, with the head lower than the body. The rescuer then strikes the infant between the shoulder blades 5 times using the heel of the hand (back blows). The strikes should be firm but not hard enough to cause injury. The rescuer then checks the mouth, removing any visible objects. If the airway remains blocked, the rescuer turns the infant face up with the head down, thrusts his the second and third fingers inward and upward on the breastbone 5 times (chest thrusts), then checks the infant's mouth again.

Cardiac Arrest and Cardiopulmonary Resuscitation

- Cardiac arrest is what happens when the body dies.
- Cardiopulmonary resuscitation (CPR) can increase the chance for survival after cardiac arrest.
- Formal training is needed to become skilled in CPR.

Cardiac arrest is what happens when someone dies. The heart does not beat and breathing ceases, starving the body of oxygen. Sometimes a child can be revived during the first several minutes after cardiac arrest. However, the more time that passes, the less likely it is that the child can be revived and, if revived, the more likely it is that the child will have brain damage. In movies and television in the United States, people who have cardiac arrest are usually revived when a rescuer provides cardiopulmonary resusci-

Clearing a Blocked Airway in an Infant

The infant is held face down with the chest resting on the rescuer's hand. Then, the rescuer strikes the infant's back between the shoulder blades. The rescuer then checks the mouth, removing any visible objects.

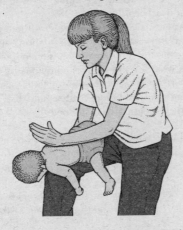

If the airway remains blocked, the infant is turned face up with the head lower than the body. Then, the rescuer places the second and third fingers on the infant's breastbone and thrusts inward and upward.

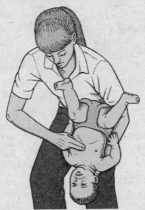

tation (CPR). However, in real life, most people, including children, are not revived.

In children, cardiac arrest is usually caused by an injury, poisoning, blockage of an airway, drowning, a respiratory infection, or sudden infant death syndrome (SIDS).

A child in cardiac arrest lies motionless without breathing and does not respond to questions or to stimulation, such as shaking. When someone who fits this description is encountered, a rescuer first determines whether the child is conscious by loudly asking, "Are you OK?" If there is no response, the rescuer places the child face up and uses the "look, listen, and feel" approach to determine whether breathing has stopped:

- Looking to see whether the chest moves up and down
- Listening for sounds of breathing
- Feeling for air movement over the child's mouth

If the child is not breathing, the rescuer checks for airway blockage by looking into the mouth and throat for any visible objects.

First-Aid Treatment

First aid for cardiac arrest should proceed as quickly as possible. The rescuer should call for professional medical assistance. Then, CPR should be started. CPR combines artificial respiration, which supplies oxygen to the lungs, with chest compressions, which circulate oxygen to the brain and other vital organs by forcing blood out of the heart.

Skill in CPR is best obtained through a training course. The American Heart Association, American Red Cross, and many local fire departments and hospitals offer CPR training courses. Because procedures may change over time, it is important to stay up to date on training and to repeat courses as recommended.

To begin CPR, the rescuer places the child face up, rolling the head, body, and limbs at the same time. The rescuer then removes any object visibly blocking the airway. Next, the rescuer tilts the child's head back slightly and lifts the chin. This maneuver sometimes opens a blocked airway. If breathing does not resume, artificial respiration (mouth-to-mouth resuscitation, or rescue breathing) is started. With the rescuer's mouth covering the child's mouth, the rescuer slowly exhales air into the child's lungs. To prevent air from escaping from the child's nose, the rescuer pinches the nose shut while exhaling into the child's mouth. For an infant, the rescuer's mouth should cover the infant's mouth and nose. To prevent damaging the infant's smaller lungs, the rescuer exhales with less force than with older children.

DID YOU KNOW?

- Cardiopulmonary resuscitation (CPR) is intense physical work.
- Survival after cardiac arrest and CPR is much less common in real life than in the movies and television.

If artificial respiration is done correctly but the chest does not rise, the child's airway is blocked. Then, the rescuer should attempt to clear the airway the same way as for a child who is choking (see page 264).

If the chest rises, the rescuer gives two deep, slow breaths. Next, chest compressions are performed. The rescuer kneels to one side and, with arms held straight, leans over the child and places both hands, one on top of the other, on the lower part of the breastbone. The rescuer compresses the chest to a depth of about 1 to 1 1/2 inches (2 1/2 to 4 cm) in a young child or 1 1/2 to 2 inches (4 to 5 cm) in an adolescent. For an infant, the rescuer places two fingers on the infant's breastbone just below the nipples and compresses the chest to a depth of 1/2 to 1 inch. CPR can be performed by one person (who alternately performs artificial respiration and chest compressions) or by two people (one to perform artificial respiration and one to perform chest compressions). The chest is compressed about 100 times per minute, and two breaths are given after each 30 compressions. Performing chest compressions can quickly tire a person, resulting in compressions that are too weak to be effective. Thus, if two rescuers are present, they should switch duties about every 2 minutes. CPR is continued until medical assistance arrives, a rescuer becomes too tired to continue, or the child recovers.

Part III

Medical Problems

CHAPTER 15

Bacterial Infections

Bacteria are microscopic, single-celled organisms; only some bacteria cause disease in people. The most common bacterial infections among children are skin infections (including impetigo), ear infections, and throat infections (strep throat). These disorders are treated similarly in adults and children. Other infections occur at all ages but have particular treatment considerations in children.

Certain children are at particular risk for bacterial infections. These children include infants younger than 2 months of age, children who have no spleen or who have an immune system disorder, and children who have sickle cell disease.

DID YOU KNOW?

- Infants younger than 2 months are at particular risk of serious bacterial infections.
- Culturing bacteria in a laboratory helps doctors determine which antibiotics will work against the bacteria.
- Many serious bacterial infections are becoming less common because of routine childhood vaccinations.
- Newborns with a serious infection may be irritable (particularly when they are held), feed poorly, or briefly stop breathing.
- Constant drooling or making a loud noise when inhaling may indicate a respiratory infection that could soon make breathing difficult or impossible.

Sometimes doctors diagnose bacterial infections by the typical symptoms they produce. Usually, however, bacteria must be identified in samples of tissue or body fluids, such as blood, urine, pus, or cerebrospinal fluid. Sometimes bacteria from these samples can be recognized under a microscope or identified with a rapid detection test. Usually, however, they are too few or too small to see, so doctors must try to grow them in the laboratory. It typically takes 24 to 48 hours to grow (culture) the organism. Cultures can also be used to test the susceptibility of a microorganism to various antibiotics; the results can help a doctor determine which drug to use in treating an infected child. Doctors may treat certain potentially serious childhood infections with antibiotics, preemptively while culture results are pending and then change or discontinue the antibiotics when results are obtained.

BACTERIAL INFECTIONS PREVENTABLE WITH ROUTINE IMMUNIZATION*

- Diphtheria
- Infection with *Haemophilus influenzae* type b (meningitis, epiglottitis, some severe eye infections, occult bacteremia)
- Infection with *Neisseria meningitidis* (meningitis, bloodstream infection)
- Infection with *Streptococcus pneumoniae* (pneumonia, meningitis, occult bacteremia, ear infections)
- Pertussis
- Tetanus

*Note: Many viral infections can also be prevented with routine immunization. (see page 32)

Occult Bacteremia

Occult (hidden) bacteremia is the presence of bacteria in the bloodstream of a child who has a fever but who may not appear particularly sick and who has no apparent other source of infection.

- Bacteria in the bloodstream can lead to other infections.
- If bacteremia is suspected in children younger than 3 years, a complete blood cell count and blood culture may be done, and a lumbar puncture may occasionally be performed to test for meningitis.

- Depending on how sick the child is, antibiotics are given by mouth at home or intravenously in the hospital.
- Vaccination against *Streptococcus pneumoniae* and *Haemophilus influenzae* type b greatly reduces the risk of bacteremia.

Children younger than 3 years commonly develop fevers. Most of the time, they have other symptoms, such as a cough and runny nose, which allow doctors to diagnose the cause. About one third of the time, children have no other symptoms besides fever. Most of these children have viral infections that go away without treatment. However, 2 to 4% of such children have bacteria circulating in the bloodstream (bacteremia). *Streptococcus pneumoniae* is the most common type of bacteria causing occult bacteremia. Circulating bacteria are almost never present in older children or adults with fever but no other symptoms. These circulating bacteria may attack various organs and result in serious illnesses, such as pneumonia or meningitis. Although only about 10 to 15% of children with occult bacteremia develop these serious problems, doctors perform blood cultures to identify the bacteria before such problems develop. An elevated white blood cell count indicates a higher risk of bacterial infection; in this case, a doctor may choose to start antibiotics before blood culture results are available.

Because doctors cannot tell with certainty which febrile children have bacteremia, doctors may perform complete blood cell counts and blood cultures on some children younger than 3 years whose temperature is higher than 102°F and who do not have an apparent reason for their fever. Because occult bacteremia is much less common in children older than 3, these children do not require blood cultures.

For children who may have occult bacteremia, doctors reevaluate them in 24 to 48 hours, when culture results are available. Children with positive culture results are given antibiotics by mouth at home if they do not appear very ill. Children who show signs of serious illness are typically given intravenous antibiotics in the hospital. Sometimes doctors treat certain children, such as those with an elevated white blood cell count, with a single injection of an antibiotic, such as ceftriaxone, while awaiting the results of blood cultures.

A new vaccine against *Streptococcus pneumoniae,* given to infants, has greatly reduced the chance of occult bacteremia in vaccinated children. The *Haemophilus influenzae* type b vaccine, now given to nearly all children in the United States, has nearly eliminated occult bacteremia due to *Haemophilus influenzae* type b.

Meningitis

Bacterial meningitis is infection of the layers of tissue covering the brain and spinal cord (meninges).

- Infection usually occurs in the birth canal for newborns and through contact with respiratory secretions for older children.
- Older children have a stiff neck with a fever, headache, and confusion.
- Infants rarely have a stiff neck but are usually irritable, stop eating, vomit, or have other symptoms.
- A spinal tap to obtain a sample of cerebrospinal fluid and blood tests are done.
- Vaccination against *Streptococcus pneumoniae, Haemophilus influenzae* type b, and *Neisseria meningitidis* helps prevent meningitis.
- Even with treatment, meningitis causes death in many children and serious damage in many others.
- High doses of antibiotics are given intravenously as soon as meningitis is suspected.

Meningitis can occur at any age. Meningitis is similar in older children, adolescents, and adults but different in newborns and infants.

Children at particular risk for meningitis include those with sickle cell disease and those lacking a spleen. Children with congenital deformities of the face and skull may have defects in the bones that allow bacteria access to the meninges. Children who have a weakened immune system, such as those with AIDS or those who have received chemotherapy, are more susceptible to meningitis.

Causes

Meningitis in newborns is typically caused by bacteria acquired from the birth canal. The most common such bacteria are group B streptococci, *Escherichia coli*, and *Listeria monocytogenes*. Older children usually develop infection from contact with respiratory secretions from infected people. Bacteria that infect older children include *Streptococcus pneumoniae* and *Neisseria meningitidis*. *Haemophilus influenzae* type b was the most common cause of meningitis, but the widespread use of vaccination against that organism has now made it a rare cause. A new, improved vaccine against *Streptococcus pneumoniae* also should make this organism a rare cause of childhood meningitis.

DID YOU KNOW?

- Meningitis may progress rapidly—children, particularly newborns, may go from having no symptoms to being near death in less than a day.

Symptoms and Diagnosis

Older children and adolescents with meningitis typically have a few days of increasing fever, headache, confusion, and a stiff neck. They may have an upper respiratory tract infection that is unrelated to the meningitis. Newborns and infants rarely develop a stiff neck and are unable to communicate specific discomfort. These younger children become fussy and irritable (particularly when they are held) and stop feeding—important signs that should alert parents to a possibly serious problem. Sometimes newborns and infants have fever, vomiting, or a skin rash. One third have seizures. The nerves controlling some eye and facial movements may be damaged, causing an eye to turn inward or outward or the facial expression to become lopsided. In about 25% of newborns with meningitis, increased pressure of the fluid around the brain may make the fontanelles (the soft spots between the skull bones) bulge or feel firm. These symptoms usually develop over at least 1 to 2 days, but some infants, particularly those between birth and 3 or 4 months old, become ill very rapidly, progressing from health to near death in less than 24 hours.

Pockets of pus (abscesses) may rarely form within the brain of infants with meningitis because of certain germs. As the abscesses grow, pressure on the brain increases, resulting in vomiting, head enlargement, and bulging fontanelles.

A doctor diagnoses bacterial meningitis by examining and culturing a sample of cerebrospinal fluid obtained through a spinal tap (lumbar puncture). Doctors also perform blood cultures to look for bacteria in the bloodstream. Ultrasound examination or computed tomography (CT) may be used to determine if an abscess is present.

Prevention, Prognosis, and Treatment

Health care practitioners can help prevent bacterial meningitis by ensuring that all children receive the *Haemophilus influenzae* type b, *Streptococcus pneumoniae*, and *Neisseria meningitidis* vaccines.

Even with timely, appropriate treatment, as many as 30% of newborns with bacterial meningitis die. In older infants and children, mortality varies from 3 to 5% when the cause is *Haemophilus influenzae* type b, 5 to 10% when the cause is *Neisseria meningitidis*, and 10 to 15% when the cause is *Streptococcus pneumoniae*. Nearly 25% of children with a brain abscess die.

Of the infants who survive, 10 to 20% develop serious brain and nerve damage, such as enlargement of the ventricles (hydrocephalus), deafness, cerebral palsy, and mental retardation. Up to 50% have mild residual problems, such as learning disorders, mild hearing loss, or occasional seizures.

Doctors give high doses of antibiotics intravenously as soon as they suspect meningitis. Very sick children receive antibiotics even before a spinal tap is performed. A doctor chooses an antibiotic based on the type of bacteria causing the meningitis. Children older than 6 weeks of age sometimes are given corticosteroids to help prevent permanent neurologic problems.

Diphtheria

Diphtheria is a contagious, sometimes fatal, infection of the upper respiratory tract caused by the bacterium Corynebacterium diphtheriae.

- Routine vaccination has made diphtheria rare in developed countries.
- A sore throat, general feeling of illness, and fever appear abruptly, sometimes with swollen lymph nodes, and a tough, gray pseudomembrane forms in the throat.
- Children are hospitalized and given antibodies and antibiotics.

Years ago, diphtheria was one of the leading causes of death among children. Today, diphtheria is rare in developed countries, primarily because of widespread vaccination. Fewer than five cases occur in the United States each year, but diphtheria bacteria still exist in the world and can cause outbreaks if vaccination is inadequate.

The bacteria that cause diphtheria are usually spread in droplets of moisture coughed into the air. Usually the bacteria multiply on or near the surface of the mucous membranes of the mouth or throat, where they cause inflammation. Some types of *Corynebacterium diphtheriae* release a potent toxin, which can damage the heart, nerves, kidneys, and brain.

Symptoms and Diagnosis

The illness begins 1 to 4 days after exposure to the bacteria. Symptoms begin abruptly with sore throat, a general feeling of illness (malaise), and a fever up to 103°F. The child also may have a fast heart rate, nausea, vomiting, chills, and a headache. The lymph nodes in the neck may swell. The inflammation may make the throat swell, narrowing the airway and making breathing extremely difficult.

Typically, the bacteria form a tough, gray pseudomembrane—a sheet of material composed of dead white blood cells, bacteria, and other substances—near the tonsils or other parts of the throat. The pseudomembrane narrows the airway and may suddenly become detached and block the airway completely, preventing the child from being able to breathe. The toxin produced by diphtheria bacteria generally affects certain nerves, producing symptoms, such as swallowing difficulty, weakness of eye muscles, and trouble moving the arms and legs. The bacterial toxin may also damage the heart muscle (myocarditis), sometimes causing heart failure and death.

A doctor suspects diphtheria in a sick child who has a sore throat with a pseudomembrane, particularly if there is paralysis of muscles of the face or throat, and if the child was not vaccinated. The diagnosis is confirmed by culture of material from the child's throat.

Prevention and Treatment

Children are routinely immunized against diphtheria. The diphtheria vaccine is usually combined with vaccines for tetanus and pertussis (whooping cough—see page 283).

A child with symptoms of diphtheria is typically hospitalized in an intensive care unit and given antibodies to neutralize the diphtheria toxin. Doctors also give antibiotics, such as penicillin or erythromycin, to kill the diphtheria bacteria.

Recovery from severe diphtheria is slow, and a child with the infection must avoid resuming activities too soon. Even normal physical exertion may harm an inflamed heart.

Retropharyngeal Abscess

A retropharyngeal abscess is a collection of pus in the lymph nodes at the back of the throat.

- Pain occurs during swallowing, a fever develops, and lymph nodes enlarge, sometimes causing drooling and making breathing difficult.
- X-rays and computed tomography (CT) scans can confirm the diagnosis.
- Antibiotics are given, and many abscesses need to be drained surgically.

Because the lymph nodes at the back of the throat disappear after childhood, a retropharyngeal abscess almost never occurs in adults. An abscess is usually caused by a bacterial infection that has spread from the tonsils, throat, sinuses, adenoids, nose, or middle ear. Many infections are caused by a combination of bacteria. An injury to the back of the throat from a sharp object, such as a fish bone, occasionally causes a retropharyngeal abscess. Rarely, tuberculosis can also cause a retropharyngeal abscess.

Symptoms and Diagnosis

The main symptoms are pain when swallowing, a fever, and enlargement of the lymph nodes in the neck. The voice is muffled, and the child drools. The abscess can block the airway, causing difficulty in breathing. The child tends to lie on his back, tilt his head and neck back, and raise his chin to make breathing easier.

Complications include bleeding around the abscess, rupture of the abscess into the airway (which can block the airway), and pneumonia. The larynx may go into spasm and further interfere with breathing. Blood clots may form in the jugular veins of the neck. Infection may spread down into the chest.

After observing the symptoms, a doctor orders x-rays and computed tomography (CT) scans of the neck to confirm the diagnosis.

Treatment and Prognosis

Retropharyngeal abscesses often need to be drained, which a doctor does surgically by cutting open the abscess and allowing the pus to drain out. Penicillin plus metronidazole, clindamycin, cefoxitin, or other antibiotics is given, at first intravenously, and then by mouth. Most children do well with prompt treatment.

Epiglottitis

Epiglottitis is a severe bacterial infection of the epiglottis, which can block the windpipe, obstructing air flow.

- Children suddenly develop a very sore throat, often with a high fever and drooling, and may have difficulty breathing.
- Routine vaccination helps prevent epiglottitis.
- If epiglottitis is suspected, children are hospitalized and are usually examined or have a breathing tube inserted in the operating room.

The epiglottis is the structure that closes the entrance to the voice box and windpipe (larynx and trachea) during swallowing. Epiglottitis is most common in children 2 to 5 years old. It is uncommon in children younger than 2 but may affect people of any age, including adults. In the past, most cases of childhood epiglottitis were caused by the bacterium *Haemophilus influenzae* type b. Now that most children are vaccinated against *Haemophilus influenzae* type b, the disease is quite rare and is typically caused by *Streptococcus pneumoniae*, other streptococci, and staphylococci. Children with epiglottitis often have bacteria in the bloodstream (bacteremia), which sometimes spreads the infection to the lungs, the joints, the tissues covering the brain (meninges), the sac around the heart, or the tissue beneath the skin.

Symptoms

The infection usually begins suddenly and progresses rapidly. A previously healthy child develops a sore throat and often a high fever. Difficulties in swallowing and breathing are common. The child usually drools, breathes rapidly, and has a loud noise while inhaling (called stridor). The difficulty in breathing often causes the child to lean forward while stretching the neck backward to try to increase the amount of air reaching the lungs. Labored breathing may lead to a buildup of carbon dioxide and low oxygen levels in the bloodstream, causing agitation and confusion followed by sluggishness (lethargy). The swollen epiglottis makes coughing up mucus difficult. Epiglottitis can quickly become fatal because swelling of the infected tissue may block the airway and cut off breathing.

Prevention, Diagnosis, and Treatment

Prevention of epiglottitis is better than treatment. Prevention is achieved by ensuring that all children receive the *Haemophilus influenzae* type b *and Streptococcus pneumoniae* vaccines.

Epiglottitis is an emergency, and a child is hospitalized immediately when a doctor suspects it. If the child does not have all of the typical symptoms of epiglottitis and does not appear seriously ill, the doctor sometimes takes an x-ray of the neck, which can show an enlarged epiglottis. The doctor does not hold the child down or use a tongue depressor to look in the throat, because these manipulations may cause throat spasm and complete airway blockage in a child with epiglottitis.

If an enlarged epiglottis is seen on x-ray or the child appears seriously ill, doctors examine the child under anesthesia in the operating room using a laryngoscope. If the examination shows epiglottitis or triggers throat spasm, the doctor inserts a plastic tube (endotracheal tube) into the airway to keep it open. If the airway is too swollen to allow placement of an endotracheal tube, the doctor cuts an opening through the front of the neck (tracheostomy) and inserts the tube. This tube is left in place for several days until the swelling of the epiglottis goes down. The child also receives antibiotics, such as ceftriaxone or ampicillin-sulbactam. Once the child's airway is opened, the prognosis is good.

Pertussis

Pertussis (whooping cough) is a highly contagious infection caused by the bacterium Bordetella pertussis, *which results in fits of coughing that usually end in a prolonged, high-pitched, deeply indrawn breath (the whoop).*

- Mild coldlike symptoms are followed by severe coughing fits, then gradual recovery.
- Children are routinely vaccinated against pertussis.
- Severely ill infants are usually hospitalized, and older children with milder infection are treated at home.
- An antibiotic is used to eradicate the bacteria.

Pertussis was once rampant in the United States but is now uncommon. However, pertussis remains a major problem throughout the world. Local epidemics among unimmunized people occur every 3 to 5 years. A person may develop pertussis at any age, although nearly two thirds of cases occur in children younger than 5 years. One attack of pertussis does not always give full immunity for life, but a second attack, if it occurs, is usually mild and not always recognized as pertussis. In fact, some adults with "walking pneumonia" actually have pertussis. Pertussis is most serious in children younger than 2 years.

An infected person spreads pertussis organisms into the air in droplets of moisture produced by coughing. Anyone nearby may inhale these droplets and become infected. Pertussis usually is not contagious after the third week of the infection.

Symptoms

The illness lasts about 6 weeks, progressing through three stages: mild coldlike symptoms, severe coughing fits, and gradual recovery. Coldlike symptoms include sneezing, runny nose, and a general feeling of illness (malaise). After 1 or 2 weeks, the person develops typical coughing fits. These fits typically consist of 5 to 15 or more rapid consecutive coughs followed by the whoop (a prolonged, high-pitched, deeply indrawn breath). After a fit, breathing is normal, but another coughing fit follows shortly thereafter. The cough often produces large amounts of thick mucus (usually swallowed by infants and children or seen as large bubbles from the nose). In younger children, vomiting often follows a prolonged fit of coughing. In infants, choking spells and pauses in breathing (apnea), possibly causing the skin to turn blue, can occur.

About one fourth of children develop pneumonia, resulting in difficulty breathing. Ear infections (otitis media) also frequently develop as a result of pertussis. Rarely, pertussis affects the brain of infants. Bleeding, swelling, or inflammation of the brain may cause seizures, confusion, brain damage, and mental retardation.

After several weeks, the coughing fits gradually subside, but for many weeks or even months the person has a lingering, persistent cough.

DID YOU KNOW?

- Pertussis is fatal in about 1 to 2% of children younger than 1 year.

Diagnosis and Prognosis

Doctors suspect pertussis because of the typical whooping cough or other symptoms and confirm the diagnosis by culture of a sample of mucus from the back of the nose or throat. Culture results often are negative after several weeks of illness; other diagnostic tests performed on samples from the nose or throat may be helpful (polymerase chain reaction or rapid detection test).

The majority of children with pertussis recover completely, although slowly. About 1 to 2% of the children younger than 1 year die.

Prevention and Treatment

Children are routinely vaccinated against pertussis. The pertussis vaccine is usually combined with vaccines for diphtheria and tetanus (see page 32). A pertussis vaccine has just been licensed in the United States for use in adolescents. The antibiotic erythromycin (or sometimes clarithromycin or azithromycin) is given as a preventive measure to children exposed to pertussis.

Severely ill infants are usually hospitalized because their breathing difficulty may become so severe that they require mechanical ventilation through a tube placed in their windpipe. Others may need extra oxygen and intravenous fluids. Older children who have mild disease are treated at home. Cough medicines are of questionable value and are not usually used.

The antibiotic erythromycin, clarithromycin, or azithromycin is usually used to eradicate the bacteria causing pertussis. Antibiotics are also used for infections that accompany the pertussis, such as pneumonia and ear infection.

Rheumatic Fever

Rheumatic fever is inflammation of the body's organ systems, especially the joints and the heart, resulting from a complication of streptococcal infection of the throat.

- Children may have joint pain, fever, chest pain, heart palpitations, jerky and uncontrollable movements, a rash, or small bumps under the skin.
- In a few children, the heart is permanently damaged.
- The diagnosis is based mainly on symptoms.
- Prompt, complete antibiotic treatment of any streptococcal throat infection can prevent rheumatic fever.
- Children are given penicillin to eliminate any residual streptococcal infection and aspirin to reduce inflammation, and their physical activity is limited.

Although rheumatic fever follows a streptococcal infection, it is not an infection. Rather, it is an inflammatory reaction to the infection. Most people with rheumatic fever recover, but the heart is permanently damaged in a small percentage of people.

In the United States, rheumatic fever rarely develops before age 4 or after age 18 and is much less common than in developing countries, probably because antibiotics are widely used to treat streptococcal infections at an early stage. However, the incidence of rheumatic fever sometimes rises and falls in a particular area for unknown reasons. Overcrowded living conditions seem to increase the risk of rheumatic fever, and heredity seems to play a part. In the United States, a child who has a streptococcal throat infection but is not treated has only a 0.4 to 1% chance of developing rheumatic fever. About half of the children who previously had rheumatic fever will develop it again with another streptococcal throat infection. Rheumatic fever follows streptococcal infections of the throat but not those of the skin (impetigo) or other areas of the body; the reasons are not known.

Symptoms

Rheumatic fever affects many parts of the body, such as the joints, heart, and skin. Symptoms of rheumatic fever vary greatly, depending on which parts of the body become inflamed. Typically, symptoms begin several weeks after the disappearance of strep throat. The most common symptoms of rheumatic fever are joint pain, fever, chest pain or palpitations caused by heart inflammation, jerky uncontrollable movements (Sydenham's chorea), a rash, and small bumps (nodules) under the skin. A child may have one symptom or several.

Joint pain and fever are the most common first symptoms. One or several joints suddenly become painful and feel tender when touched. They may also be red, hot, and swollen and may contain fluid. Ankles, knees, elbows, and wrists are commonly affected; the shoulders, hips, and small joints of the hands and feet also may be affected. As pain in one joint improves, pain in another starts (migratory pain). Joint pains may be mild or severe, and typically last 2 to 4 weeks. Long-term joint damage from rheumatic fever does not develop.

Sometimes, children with heart inflammation is recognized years later when heart damage is discovered. Some children feel their heart beating rapidly. Others have chest pain caused by inflammation of the sac around the heart. Heart failure may develop, causing the child to feel tired and short of breath, with nausea, vomiting, stomachache, or a hacking cough.

Heart inflammation disappears gradually, usually within 5 months. However, it may permanently damage the heart valves, resulting in rheumatic heart disease. The likelihood of rheumatic heart disease varies with the severity of the initial heart inflammation. About 1% of people who had no heart inflammation develop rheumatic heart disease, compared to 30% with mild inflammation and 70% with severe inflammation. In rheumatic heart disease, the valve between the left atrium and ventricle (mitral valve) is most commonly damaged. The valve may become leaky (mitral valve regurgitation), abnormally narrow (mitral valve stenosis), or both. Valve damage causes the characteristic heart murmurs that enable a doctor to diagnose rheumatic fever. Later in life, usually in middle age, the valve damage may cause heart failure and atrial fibrillation, an abnormal heart rhythm.

A flat painless rash with a wavy edge (erythema marginatum) may appear as the other symptoms subside. It lasts for only a short time, sometimes less than a day. In children with heart inflammation, small, hard nodules may form under the skin. The nodules are usually painless and disappear without treatment.

Jerky uncontrollable movements (Sydenham's chorea) may begin gradually in children with rheumatic fever, but usually only after all other symptoms have improved. A month may go by before the movements become so intense that the child is taken to a doctor. By then, the child typically has rapid, purposeless, sporadic movements that disappear during sleep. The movements may involve any muscle except those of the eyes. Facial grimacing is common. In mild cases, the child may seem clumsy and may have slight difficulties in dressing and eating. In extreme cases, the child may have to be protected from injuring himself with his flailing arms or legs. The chorea lasts between 4 and 8 months.

DID YOU KNOW?

- Rheumatic fever follows a streptococcal infection, but it is not an infection.

Diagnosis

A doctor bases the diagnosis of rheumatic fever mainly on the characteristic combination of symptoms. Blood tests showing high levels of antibodies to streptococci may be helpful, but low levels of these antibodies are present in many children who do not have rheumatic fever. Abnormal heart rhythms caused by heart inflammation can be seen on an electrocardiogram (ECG—a recording of the heart's electrical activity). An echocardiogram (an image of structures in the heart produced by ultrasound waves) may be used to diagnose abnormalities of the heart valves.

Prevention and Treatment

The best way to prevent rheumatic fever is with prompt and complete antibiotic treatment of any streptococcal throat infection. In addition, children who have had rheumatic fever should be given penicillin by mouth every day, or by monthly injections into the muscle, to help prevent another streptococcal infection. This preventive treatment should be continued until adulthood, and some doctors feel that it should be continued for life.

Treatment of rheumatic fever has three goals: curing any residual streptococcal infection; reducing inflammation, particularly in the joints and heart; and limiting physical activity that might aggravate the inflamed structures.

Doctors give children with rheumatic fever an injection of a long-acting penicillin to eliminate any remaining infection. Aspirin is given in high doses to reduce inflammation and pain, particularly if inflammation has reached the joints and heart. It is unclear whether other nonsteroidal anti-inflammatory drugs (NSAIDs) are as effective as aspirin. Analgesics, such as codeine, are sometimes used in addition to aspirin. If heart inflammation is severe, corticosteroids such as prednisone may be given to further reduce inflammation.

Bed rest may help by avoiding stress on the painful, inflamed joints. When the heart is inflamed, more rest is generally suggested.

If the heart valves become damaged, the risk of developing a valve infection (endocarditis) remains throughout life. Those who have heart damage must always take an antibiotic before undergoing any surgery, including dental surgery, even in adulthood.

Impetigo

Impetigo is a skin infection, caused by Staphylococcus aureus, Streptococcus pyogenes, or both, that leads to the formation of scabby, yellow-crusted sores and, sometimes, small blisters filled with yellow fluid.

Impetigo is common. It affects mostly children. Impetigo can occur anywhere on the body but most commonly occurs on the face, arms, and legs. The blisters that may form (bullous impetigo) can vary from pea-sized to large rings and can last for days to weeks. Impetigo often affects normal skin but may follow an injury or a condition that causes a break in the skin, such as a fungal infection, sunburn, or an insect bite.

Impetigo is itchy and slightly painful. The itching often leads to extensive scratching in children, which serves to spread the infection. Impetigo is very contagious—both to other areas of the person's own skin and to other people.

The infected area should be washed gently with soap and water several times a day to remove any crusts. Small areas are treated with bacitracin ointment or mupirocin cream or ointment. If large areas are involved, an antibiotic taken by mouth, such as a cephalosporin or dicloxacillin, may be needed.

Urinary Tract Infection

A urinary tract infection (UTI) is a bacterial infection of the urinary bladder (cystitis) or the kidneys (pyelonephritis).

- In some newborns and infants, the only symptom is a fever.
- Older children may have pain or burning during urination and pain near the bladder or the affected kidney.
- Doctors examine and culture a urine sample, and tests may be done to check for structural abnormalities in the urinary tract.
- Good hygiene may help prevent infections.
- Antibiotics can eliminate the infection, but children with structural abnormalities may need surgery.

Urinary tract infections (UTIs) are common in childhood. Nearly all UTIs are caused by bacteria that enter the urethral opening and move upward to the urinary bladder and sometimes the kidneys. Among infants, boys are more likely to develop UTIs; after infancy, girls are much more likely to develop them. UTIs are more common in girls because their short urethras make passage of bacteria easier. Uncircumcised infant boys (who tend to accumulate bacteria under the foreskin) and young children with severe constipation also are more prone to UTIs.

UTIs in older school-aged children and adolescents differ little from UTIs in adults. Younger infants and children who have UTIs, however, more commonly have various developmental abnormalities of their urinary system that make them more susceptible to urinary infection. These abnormalities include vesicoureteral reflux (an abnormality of the tube connecting the kidney to the bladder that allows urine to pass backward from the bladder up to the kidney) and a number of conditions that produce obstruction to the flow of urine. Such abnormalities occur in as many as 50% of newborns and infants with a UTI, and in 20 to 30% of school-aged children with a UTI.

Up to 65% of infants and preschool children with a UTI—particularly those with fever—have both bladder and kidney infections. If the kidney is infected and there is severe reflux, up to 50% of children go on to have some scarring of the kidneys. If there is little or no reflux, very few children have scarring of the kidneys. Scarring is a concern because it may lead to high blood pressure and poor kidney function in adulthood.

DID YOU KNOW?

- About half of newborns and infants and one fourth of school-aged children with a urinary tract infection also have a structural abnormality in the urinary tract.
- To get a urine sample in newborns and infants, doctors usually insert a catheter into the urethra.

Symptoms and Diagnosis

Newborns and infants with a UTI may have no symptoms other than a fever. Sometimes they do not eat well and have sluggishness (lethargy), vomiting, or diarrhea. Older children with bladder infections usually have pain or burning with urination, increased urinary frequency, and pain in the bladder region. Children with kidney infections typically have pain in the side or back over the affected kidney, fever, and a general feeling of illness (malaise).

A doctor diagnoses a UTI by examining the urine. Toilet-trained children may provide a urine sample by urinating into a cup after thoroughly cleaning the urethral opening. Doctors obtain urine from younger children and infants by inserting a thin, flexible, sterile tube (catheter) through the urethral opening into the bladder. Urine collected in plastic bags taped to the child's genital region is not helpful because it is often contaminated with bacteria and other material from the skin.

To detect white blood cells and bacteria in the urine, which occur in UTI, the laboratory examines the urine under a microscope and performs several chemical tests. The laboratory also performs a culture of the urine to grow and identify any bacteria present. The culture is the most significant of these tests.

In general, boys of all ages and girls younger than 2 to 3 years who develop even a single UTI need further tests to look for structural abnormalities of the urinary system. Such tests are also performed on older girls who have had recurring infections. The tests include ultrasound, which identifies kidney abnormalities and obstruction; and voiding cystourethrography, which further identifies abnormalities of the kidneys, ureters, and bladder and can also identify when the flow of urine is partially reversed (reflux). For voiding cystourethrography, a catheter is passed through the urethra into the bladder, a dye is instilled through the catheter, and x-rays are taken before and after urinating. Another test, radiocontrast cystourethrography, is similar to voiding cystourethrography, except that a radioactive agent is placed in the bladder and images are taken using a nuclear scanner. This procedure exposes the child's ovaries or testes to less radiation than voiding cystourethrography. However, radiocontrast cystourethrography is much more useful for following the healing of reflux rather than in its initial diagnosis, because it does not outline the structures as well. Another type of nuclear scan may be used to confirm the diagnosis of pyelonephritis and identify scarring of the kidneys.

Prevention and Treatment

Prevention of UTIs is difficult, but proper hygiene may help. Girls should be taught to wipe themselves from front to back (as opposed to back to front) after passing a bowel movement to minimize the chance of bacteria entering the urethral opening. Frequent bubble baths may irritate the skin around the urethral opening of both boys and girls at risk for UTIs. Circumcision of boys lowers their risk of UTIs during infancy by about 10 times, although it is not clear that this improvement by itself is a sufficient reason for circumcision. Regularly urinating and regular bowel movements may lessen the risk of UTIs.

Children with UTIs are given antibiotics. Children who are very ill and all newborns receive antibiotics by injection either intramuscularly or intravenously. Other children are given antibiotics by mouth. Treatment typically lasts 7 to 14 days. Children who require tests to diagnose developmental abnormalities often continue antibiotic treatment at a lower dose until tests are complete.

Some children with structural abnormalities of the urinary tract require surgery to correct the problem. Others need to take antibiotics daily to prevent infection. Certain mild abnormalities go away on and require no treatment.

CHAPTER 16

Viral Infections

A number of viral infections are common in children. Most childhood viral infections are not serious, and most children get better without treatment. Many viral infections are so distinctive that a doctor can diagnose them based on their symptoms. A doctor usually does not need to have a laboratory identify the specific virus involved.

DID YOU KNOW?

- Most viral infections in children are not serious and resolve on their own.
- Many viral infections can be diagnosed without any laboratory testing.
- Antibiotics are not useful for treating viral infections.
- Children should not usually take aspirin because of the risk of Reye's syndrome.

Most viral infections result in fever and body aches or discomfort. Aspirin is not given to children or adolescents with these symptoms, because it increases the risk of Reye's syndrome in those who might have a viral infection; acetaminophen or ibuprofen is given instead. Viral infections range from mild (for example, a cold) to a life-threatening infection (for example, encephalitis).

Some Viral Infections at a Glance

INFEC-TION	PERIOD OF INCUBA-TION	PERIOD OF CONTA-GIOUS-NESS	SITE OF RASH	NATURE OF RASH
Measles (rubeola)	7 to 14 days	From 2 to 4 days before the rash appears until 2 to 5 days after	Starts around the ears and on the face and neck; in more severe cases, spreads over the trunk, arms, and legs	Irregular, flat, red areas that soon become raised; begins 3 to 5 days after the onset of symptoms; lasts 4 to 7 days
Rubella (German measles)	14 to 21 days	From shortly before the onset of symptoms until the rash disap-pears; infected newborns are usually contagious for many months	Starts on the face and neck; spreads to the trunk, arms, and legs	Fine, pinkish, flat rash; begins 1 or 2 days after the onset of symp-toms; lasts 1 to 3 days
Roseola infantum	About 5 to 15 days	Unknown	The chest and abdo-men, with moderate involve-ment of the face, arms, and legs	Red and flat, possi-bly with raised areas; begins on about the 4th day, appearing as body temperature drops suddenly to nor-mal; lasts 1 or 2 days
Erythema infectio-sum (fifth disease)	4 to 14 days	From before the onset of the rash until a few days after	Starts on the cheeks; spreads to the arms, legs, and trunk	Red and flat with raised areas, often blotchy and with lacy patterns; begins shortly after the onset of symp-toms; lasts 5 to 10 days; may recur for several weeks

Some Viral Infections at a Glance (Continued)

INFEC-TION	PERIOD OF INCUBA-TION	PERIOD OF CONTA-GIOUS-NESS	SITE OF RASH	NATURE OF RASH
Chicken-pox (vari-cella)	4 to 21 days	From a few days before the onset of symptoms until all spots have crusted	Usually appears first on the trunk; later on the face, neck, arms, and legs; infrequently on the palms and soles	Small, flat, red sores that become raised and form round, fluid-filled blisters against a red background before finally crusting; appears in crops, so various stages are present simultaneously; begins shortly after the onset of symptoms; lasts a few days to 2 weeks

Generally, parents can discern if their child is ill with a potentially serious infection and needs immediate medical care. This is particularly true for children beyond infancy.

Central Nervous System Infections

Central nervous system infections are extremely serious infections; **meningitis** *affects the membranes surrounding the brain and spinal cord;* **encephalitis** *affects the brain itself.*

- The first symptom is usually a fever.
- Newborns may have no other symptoms, but infants and older children may vomit or may be irritable and refuse to eat.
- A spinal tap is needed to detect viral infections of the central nervous system.
- Supportive care is needed until the infection resolves.
- Many infections are mild, and the child recovers quickly.

Viruses that infect the central nervous system (brain and spinal cord) include herpesviruses, arboviruses, coxsackieviruses, echoviruses, and enteroviruses. Some of these infections primarily affect the meninges (the tissues covering the brain) and result in meningitis; others primarily affect the brain and result in encephalitis; many affect both the meninges and brain and result in meningoencephalitis. Meningitis is far more common in children than is encephalitis.

Viruses affect the central nervous system in two ways. They directly infect and destroy cells during the acute illness. After recovery from the infection, the body's immune response to the infection sometimes causes secondary damage to the cells around the nerves. This secondary damage (**postinfectious encephalomyelitis**) results in the child having symptoms several weeks after recovery from the acute illness.

DID YOU KNOW?

- Meningitis is a worry in every newborn that has a fever, so doctors ask parents to report any fever in a newborn.

Children become infected through various routes. Newborns can develop herpesvirus infections through contact with infected secretions in the birth canal. Other viral infections are acquired by breathing air contaminated with virus-containing droplets exhaled by an infected person. Arbovirus infections are acquired from bites by infected insects.

The symptoms and treatment of viral meningitis and encephalitis in older children and adolescents are similar to those in adults. Because the immune system is still developing in newborns and infants, different infections can occur, and the inability of infants to communicate directly makes it difficult to understand their symptoms. Usually, however, infants with central nervous system infections have some of the symptoms described below.

Symptoms

Viral central nervous system infections in newborns and infants usually begin with fever. Newborns may have no other symptoms and may initially not otherwise appear ill. Infants older than a month or so typically become irritable and fussy and refuse to eat. Vomiting is common. Because irritation of the meninges is worsened by movement, an infant with meningitis may cry more, rather than calm down, when he is picked up and rocked. Some infants develop a strange, high-pitched cry. Infants with encephalitis often have seizures or bizarre movements. An infection with herpes simplex virus, which often concentrates in only one part of the brain, may lead to seizures or weakness appearing in only one part of the body. Infants with severe encephalitis may become lethargic and comatose and then die.

In older children and adolescents, viral meningitis can cause fever, headache, vomiting, weakness, and a stiff neck. Viral encephalitis may cause personality changes, limb paralysis, confusion, and sleepiness that can progress to coma and death. Encephalitis caused by the herpes simplex virus causes headache, fever, and flu-like symptoms.

Postinfectious encephalomyelitis may produce many neurologic problems, depending on the part of the brain that is damaged. Children may have weakness of an arm or leg, vision or hearing loss, mental retardation, or recurring seizures. These symptoms may not be apparent until the child is old enough for the problem to appear on testing. Often the symptoms resolve with time; occasionally they are permanent.

Diagnosis

Doctors are concerned about the possibility of meningitis or encephalitis in every newborn who has a fever, as well as in an older infant who has a fever, is irritable, or is otherwise not acting normally. These infants undergo a spinal tap (lumbar puncture) to obtain cerebrospinal fluid (CSF) for laboratory analysis. In viral infections, the number of lymphocytes (a type of white blood cell) is increased in the cerebrospinal fluid, and no bacteria are seen. Immunologic tests that detect antibodies against viruses in samples of cerebrospinal fluid may be performed, but these tests take days to complete. Polymerase chain reaction (PCR) techniques are used to identify organisms such as herpesviruses and enteroviruses.

A test of brain waves (electroencephalogram) can be used to help diagnose encephalitis caused by herpesvirus. Very rarely, a biopsy of brain tissue is needed to determine whether herpesvirus is the cause.

Prognosis and Treatment

Prognosis varies greatly with the type of infection. Many types of viral meningitis and encephalitis are mild, and the child recovers quickly and completely. Other types are severe. Infection with herpes simplex virus is particularly grave. Even with treatment, 15% of newborns with herpes simplex infection of the brain die.

If the herpes infection involves other parts of the body as well as the brain, mortality is as high as 50%. Nearly two thirds of the survivors have permanent neurologic disability of some kind.

Most infants require only supportive care—they need to be kept warm and given plenty of fluids. Antiviral drugs are not effective for most central nervous system infections. However, infections caused by herpes simplex virus can be treated with acyclovir given intravenously.

Chickenpox

Chickenpox (varicella) is a highly contagious infection with the varicella-zoster virus that produces a characteristic itchy rash, consisting of small, raised, blistered or crusted spots.

- In addition to the characteristic rash, children have a mild headache, fever, loss of appetite, and malaise.
- Diagnosis is usually based on the characteristic appearance of the rash.
- Chickenpox can be prevented with a vaccine.
- Usually, only treatment of symptoms is needed.

Chickenpox is a highly contagious disease of childhood. Before the introduction of a vaccine in 1995, about 90% of children developed chickenpox by age 15. Now, the use of the vaccine has decreased the number of cases of chickenpox per year dramatically. The disease is spread by airborne droplets of moisture containing the varicella-zoster virus. A person with chickenpox is most contagious just after symptoms start but remains contagious until the last blisters have crusted.

Although most people with chickenpox simply have sores on the skin and in the mouth, the virus sometimes infects the lungs, brain, heart, or joints. Such serious infections are more common in newborns, adults, and people with an impaired immune system.

A person who has had chickenpox develops immunity and cannot contract it again. However, the varicella-zoster virus remains dormant in the body after an initial infection with chickenpox, sometimes reactivating in later life, causing shingles.

Symptoms and Diagnosis

Symptoms begin 10 to 21 days after infection. They include mild headache, moderate fever, loss of appetite, and a general

WHAT IS REYE'S SYNDROME?

Reye's syndrome is a very rare but life-threatening disorder that causes inflammation and swelling of the brain and degeneration of the liver.

The cause of Reye's syndrome is unknown, although it typically occurs after infection by certain viruses, such as influenza or varicella (chickenpox), particularly in children who take aspirin. Because of this increased risk of Reye's syndrome, aspirin is not recommended for children, except for the treatment of a few specific diseases. Now that aspirin use has declined—in large part because of the possibility of triggering Reye's syndrome—fewer than a dozen children a year develop this disorder. The condition occurs mainly in children between the ages of 4 and 12 years, in late fall and winter.

Reye's syndrome begins with the symptoms of a viral infection, such as an upper respiratory tract infection, influenza, or chickenpox. After 4 or 5 days, the child suddenly develops very severe nausea and vomiting. Within a day, the child becomes confused, followed by disorientation, agitation, and sometimes seizures, coma, and death. Degeneration of the liver may lead to blood clotting problems and bleeding. The severity of illness varies greatly.

The child's prognosis depends on the amount of swelling in the brain. The overall chances that the child will die are about 20%, but range from less than 2% among children with mild disease to more than 80% among those in a deep coma.

Children who survive the acute phase of the illness usually recover fully. Those with more severe symptoms may later show some evidence of brain damage, such as mental retardation, a seizure disorder, abnormal muscle movement, or damage to specific nerves. Reye's syndrome rarely affects a child twice.

There is no specific treatment for Reye's syndrome. Children are placed in intensive care. Vitamin K or fresh frozen plasma is given to help prevent bleeding. Drugs such as mannitol, corticosteroids, or barbiturates may be used to help reduce the pressure within the brain.

feeling of illness (malaise). Younger children often do not have these symptoms, but symptoms are often severe in adults.

About 24 to 36 hours after the first symptoms begin, a rash of small, flat, red spots appears. The spots usually begin on the trunk and face, later appearing on the arms and legs. Some children have only a few spots; others have them almost everywhere, including on the scalp and inside the mouth. Over 6 to 8 hours, each spot becomes raised; forms an itchy, round, fluid-filled blister against a red background; and finally crusts. Spots continue to develop and crust for several days. The spots may become infected by bacteria, causing erysipelas, pyoderma, cellulitis, or bullous impetigo. New spots usually stop appearing by the fifth day, the majority are crusted by the sixth day, and most disappear in fewer than 20 days.

DID YOU KNOW?

- Children with chickenpox are contagious from the time symptoms begin until the last blisters have crusted.
- After chickenpox resolves, the virus remains dormant in the body, sometimes reactivating later in life to cause shingles.

Spots in the mouth quickly rupture and form raw sores (ulcers), which often make swallowing painful. Raw sores may also occur on the eyelids and in the upper airways, rectum, and vagina. Spots in the voice box (larynx) and upper airways may occasionally cause severe difficulty in breathing. Lymph nodes at the side of the neck may become enlarged and tender. The worst part of the illness usually lasts 4 to 7 days.

Lung infection occurs in about 1 out of 400 people, especially adolescents and adults, resulting in cough and difficulty breathing. Brain infection (encephalitis) is less common and produces unsteadiness in walking, headache, dizziness, confusion, and seizures. Heart infection sometimes causes a heart murmur. Joint inflammation produces joint pain.

Reye's syndrome, a rare but very severe complication that occurs almost only in those younger than 18, may begin 3 to 8 days after the rash begins.

A doctor is usually certain of the diagnosis of chickenpox because the rash and the other symptoms are so typical. Measurement of the levels of antibodies in the blood and laboratory identification of the virus are rarely needed.

Prevention

In the United States, children are routinely vaccinated against varicella-zoster beginning at 12 months of age (see page 33). Anyone without immunity may also be vaccinated. Susceptible people who are at high risk of complications—such as those with an impaired immune system and pregnant women—and have been exposed to someone with chickenpox may be given antibodies against the varicella virus (varicella-zoster immune globulin). Isolation of an infected person helps prevent the spread of infection to people who have not had chickenpox.

Prognosis and Treatment

Healthy children nearly always recover from chickenpox without problems; only about 2 of 100,000 children die. However, even this low rate means that before routine immunization, 100 children died annually in the United States because of complications of chickenpox. Chickenpox is fatal in up to 15% of people with an impaired immune system.

Mild cases of chickenpox require only the treatment of symptoms. Wet compresses on the skin help soothe itching, which may be intense, and prevent scratching, which may spread the infection and cause scars. Because of the risk of bacterial infection, the skin is bathed often with soap and water, the hands are kept clean, the nails are clipped to minimize scratching, and clothing is kept clean and dry. Drugs that relieve itching, such as antihistamines, are sometimes given by mouth. If a bacterial infection develops, antibiotics may be needed.

Doctors may use antiviral drugs, such as acyclovir, valacyclovir, and famciclovir, for adolescents as well as for groups at high risk of complications—premature infants and children with immune system disorders. The drugs must be given within 24 hours of onset of disease to be effective. These antiviral drugs are not given to pregnant women.

Erythema Infectiosum

Erythema infectiosum (fifth disease) is a contagious viral infection that causes a blotchy or raised red rash with mild illness.

- Some children have no symptoms, but usually the child has a low fever and red cheeks and is mildly ill before the rash appears on the arms, legs, and trunk.
- Diagnosis is based on the appearance of the rash.
- Treatment aims to relieve fever and pain.

Erythema infectiosum is caused by human parvovirus B19 and occurs most often during the spring months, often in geographically limited outbreaks among children and adolescents. Infection is spread mainly by breathing in small droplets that have been breathed out by an infected person. The infection can also be transmitted from mother to fetus during pregnancy; it rarely causes stillbirth or severe anemia and excess fluid and swelling (edema) in the fetus (hydrops).

Symptoms begin about 4 to 14 days after infection. Symptoms can vary, and some children have none. However, a child with erythema infectiosum typically has a low fever, feels mildly ill, and develops red cheeks that often look like they have been slapped. Within a day or two, a rash appears, especially on the arms, legs, and trunk but not usually on the palms or soles. The rash can be itchy and consists of raised, blotchy red areas and lacy patterns, particularly on areas of the arms not covered by clothing, because the rash may be worsened by exposure to sunlight.

The illness generally lasts 5 to 10 days. Over the next several weeks, the rash may temporarily reappear in response to sunlight, exercise, heat, fever, or emotional stress. In adolescents, mild joint pain and swelling may remain or come and go for weeks to months.

Erythema infectiosum can also present in a different way, particularly in children with sickle cell disease, or immunodeficiency diseases, such as acquired immunodeficiency syndrome (AIDS). The virus can affect the bone marrow and produce severe anemia.

A doctor makes the diagnosis based on the characteristic appearance of the rash. Blood tests can help identify the virus, although these are rarely performed. Treatment is aimed at relieving the fever and pain.

Human Immunodeficiency Virus Infection

Human immunodeficiency virus (HIV) infection is a viral infection that progressively destroys the white blood cells and causes acquired immunodeficiency syndrome (AIDS).

- Most young children who become infected acquire infection before they are born, during the birth process, or during breastfeeding.
- The first signs are usually slowed growth, recurring diarrhea, lung infections, or a fungal infection of the mouth.
- Special blood tests are used to diagnose HIV infection in children younger than 18 months.
- Children are treated with the same anti-HIV drugs used in adults.

Only about 2% of the people infected with HIV in the United States are children or adolescents. Worldwide, HIV is a much more common problem in children.

The two human immunodeficiency viruses—HIV-1 and HIV-2—progressively destroy certain types of white blood cells called lymphocytes, which are an important part of the body's immune defenses. When these lymphocytes are destroyed, the body becomes susceptible to attack by many other infectious organisms. Many of the symptoms and complications of HIV infection, including death, are the result of these other infections and not of the HIV infection itself. HIV infection may lead to various troublesome infections with organisms that do not ordinarily infect healthy people. These are termed opportunistic infections; these infections may result from viruses, parasites, and—in children, unlike in adults—bacteria.

Acquired immunodeficiency syndrome (AIDS) is the most severe form of HIV infection. A child with HIV infection is considered to have AIDS when at least one complicating illness develops or there is a significant decline in the body's ability to defend itself from infection.

Transmission of Infection

In young children, HIV infection is nearly always acquired from the mother. Only a small percentage of children now living with AIDS acquired the infection from other sources, including blood transfusion (from blood products used to treat hemophilia) or sexual abuse. Because of improved safety measures in blood and blood products, very few current infections result from these mechanisms.

Thousands of HIV-infected women give birth each year in the United States. Without preventive measures, one fourth to one third of them would transmit the infection to their baby. The risk is highest in mothers who acquire the infection during pregnancy, who have more virus in their bodies, or who are severely ill. Transmission often takes place during labor and delivery.

The virus also can be transmitted in breast milk; 10 to 15% of babies not infected at birth acquire HIV infection if they breastfeed from an HIV-infected mother. Most often, transmission occurs in the first few weeks or months of life, although transmission may occur later. Transmission is more likely in mothers who acquire the infection while breastfeeding or who have infection of the breast (mastitis).

In adolescents, transmission is the same as in adults: through sexual intercourse—both heterosexual and homosexual—and through sharing of infected needles while injecting drugs.

The virus is *not* transmitted through food, water, household articles, or social contact in a home, workplace, or school. In very rare cases, HIV has been transmitted by contact with infected blood on the skin. In almost all such cases, the skin surface was broken by scrapes or open sores. Although saliva may contain the virus, transmission of infection by kissing or biting has never been confirmed.

DID YOU KNOW?

- A pregnant woman who is infected can minimize her chance of transmitting HIV infection to her infant if she takes anti-HIV drugs during pregnancy.
- HIV is not transmitted through food, water, household articles, or social contact, so a child with HIV infection is able to attend school.
- Nearly all HIV-infected children should receive most routine childhood vaccinations.

Symptoms

Children born with HIV infection rarely have symptoms for the first few months. If the children remain untreated, only about 20% develop problems during the first or second year of life; for the remaining 80% of children, problems may not appear until age 3 or later even without treatment. With the use of effective anti-HIV drugs, children with HIV infection do not necessarily develop any signs or symptoms of HIV infection.

The first signs of HIV infection in children are usually slowed growth and a delay of maturation, recurring diarrhea, lung infections, or a fungal infection of the mouth (thrush). Sometimes children have repeated episodes of bacterial infections, such as otitis media, sinusitis, or pneumonia.

A variety of symptoms and complications can appear as the child's immune system deteriorates. About one third of HIV-infected children develop lung inflammation (lymphocytic interstitial pneumonitis), with cough and difficulty breathing.

Children born with HIV infection commonly have at least one episode of *Pneumocystis* pneumonia in the first 15 months of life if they are not receiving anti-HIV drugs. More than half of untreated children infected with HIV develop pneumonia at some time. *Pneumocystis* pneumonia is a major cause of death among children and adults with AIDS.

In a significant number of HIV-infected children, progressive brain damage prevents or delays developmental milestones, such as walking and talking. These children also may have impaired intelligence and a head that is small in relation to their body size. Up to 20% of untreated infected children progressively lose social and language skills and muscle control. They may become partially paralyzed or unsteady on their feet, or their muscles may become somewhat rigid.

Anemia (a low red blood cell count) is common in HIV-infected children; because of anemia, they become weak and tire easily. About 20% of untreated children develop heart problems, such as rapid or irregular heartbeat, or heart failure.

Less commonly, untreated children develop inflammation of the liver (hepatitis) or kidneys (nephritis). Cancers are uncommon in children with AIDS, but non-Hodgkin's lymphoma and lymphoma of the brain may occur somewhat more often than in uninfected children. Kaposi's sarcoma, an AIDS-related cancer that affects the skin and internal organs, is extremely rare in children.

The symptoms of HIV infection acquired during adolescence are similar to those in adults. In adolescents, fever, rashes, swollen lymph nodes, and fatigue may develop within a few weeks of HIV infection and last a few weeks. A person can have HIV infection for years before AIDS develops. The symptoms of AIDS are those of the specific infections and cancers that develop.

Diagnosis

The diagnosis of HIV infection among children begins with the identification of HIV infection in pregnant women through routine prenatal screening. Newborns of mothers with HIV infection or of mothers who are at risk for HIV infection because of lifestyle should be tested. Such infants should be tested at frequent intervals—typically in the first 2 days of life, at 2 weeks of age, between 1 and 2 months, and between 3 and 6 months. Such frequent testing identifies most HIV-infected infants by 6 months of age.

In infants, the standard adult blood tests for HIV antibodies are not helpful, because an infant's blood almost always contains HIV antibodies if the mother is HIV-infected (even if the infant is not). To definitively diagnose HIV infection in children younger than 18 months of age, special blood tests that identify the virus in the blood are used. The standard blood tests are used to diagnose HIV infection in children older than 18 months and in adolescents.

Prevention

The most effective means of preventing infection in newborns is for HIV-infected women to avoid pregnancy. If an infected woman does become pregnant, anti-HIV drugs are fairly effective at minimizing transmission. Women not already taking drugs are given zidovudine (AZT) by mouth during the 2nd and 3rd trimesters (last 6 months) of pregnancy; zidovudine is also given intravenously during labor and delivery. Zidovudine is then given daily to the newborn for 6 weeks. This treatment reduces the rate of transmission from about 33% to about 8%. The rate may be as low as 1 to 2% in women receiving combination therapy with three anti-HIV drugs. Also, delivery by cesarean section reduces the baby's risk of acquiring HIV infection.

In countries where good infant formulas and clean water are readily available, HIV-infected mothers should bottle-feed their babies. In countries where the risks of malnutrition or infectious diarrhea from unclean water are high, the benefits of breastfeeding outweigh the risk of HIV transmission.

Because a child's HIV status may not be known, all schools and day care centers should adopt special procedures for handling accidents, such as nosebleeds, and for cleaning and disinfecting surfaces contaminated with blood. During cleanup, personnel are advised to avoid having their skin come in contact with blood. Latex gloves should be routinely available, and hands should be washed after the gloves are removed. Contaminated surfaces should be cleaned and disinfected with a freshly prepared bleach solution containing 1 part of household bleach to 10 to 100 parts of water.

Prevention for adolescents is the same as for adults. All adolescents should be taught how HIV is transmitted and how it can be avoided, including abstaining from sex, using safe-sex practices, and avoiding contaminated needles.

Treatment and Prognosis

Children are treated with most of the same anti-HIV drugs as adults, typically a combination of two or more reverse-transcriptase inhibitors and a protease inhibitor. However, not all of the drugs used for adults are available to small children, in part because some are not available in liquid form. It may be difficult for parents and children to follow complicated drug regimens, which can limit the effectiveness of therapy. In general, children develop the same types of side effects as adults but usually at a much lower rate; however, the side effects of drugs may also limit the treatment. A doctor monitors the effectiveness of treatment by regularly measuring the amount of virus present in the blood and the child's CD4+ count. Increased numbers of virus in the blood may be a sign of the development of resistance of HIV to the drugs or a lack of taking the drugs. In either case, the doctor may need to change the drugs.

To prevent *Pneumocystis* pneumonia, trimethoprimsulfameth-oxazole is given to infants older than 1 month who were born to HIV-infected women and children with a significantly impaired immune system. Children with serious allergic reactions to this drug may be given dapsone or atovaquone. Children with a significantly impaired immune system also are given azithromycin or clarithromycin to prevent *Mycobacterium avium* complex infection. Children with recurring bacterial infections may be given intravenous immune globulin once a month.

Nearly all HIV-infected children should receive the routine childhood vaccinations, except usually the measles-mumps-rubella and varicella vaccines. Both of these vaccines contain live virus and can cause a severe or fatal illness in the most immunologically compromised children with HIV, but they are recommended for children with HIV infection whose immune system is not severely compromised. However, the effectiveness of any vaccination will be less in children with HIV infection.

For children who need foster care, childcare, or schooling, a doctor can help assess the child's risk of exposure to infectious diseases. In general, transmission of infections, such as chickenpox, to the HIV-infected child (or to any child with an impaired immune system) is more of a danger than is transmission of HIV from that child to others. A young child with HIV infection who has open skin sores or who engages in potentially dangerous behavior, such as biting, should not attend childcare.

HIV-infected children should participate in as many routine childhood activities as their physical condition allows. Interaction with other children enhances social development and self-esteem. Because of the stigma associated with the illness and the fact that transmission of the infection to other children is extremely unlikely, there is no need for anyone other than the parents, the doctor, and perhaps the school nurse to be aware of the child's HIV status.

As a child's condition worsens, treatment is best given in the least restrictive environment possible. If home health care and social services are available, the child can spend more time at home rather than in a hospital.

With current drug therapy, 75% of children born today with HIV infection are alive at 5 years, and 50% are alive at 8 years.

The average age at death is still about 10 years for HIV-infected children, but more and more children are surviving well into adolescence and early adulthood.

Measles

Measles (rubeola, 9-day measles) is a highly contagious viral infection that produces various symptoms and a characteristic rash.

- Symptoms include fever, runny nose, sore throat, hacking cough, and red eyes.
- Tiny white spots appear inside the mouth 2 to 4 days after symptoms begin, and a mildly itchy rash develops.
- Diagnosis is based on the symptoms and characteristic appearance of the rash.
- Immunization of young children helps prevent measles.

Children become infected with measles by breathing in small airborne droplets of moisture coughed out by an infected person or by touching items contaminated by such droplets. Measles is contagious from 2 to 4 days before the rash appears until the rash disappears.

Before vaccination became widely available, measles epidemics occurred every 2 or 3 years, particularly in preschool-aged and school-aged children, with small localized outbreaks during intervening years. Although measles is still common in other countries, only about 100 people a year in the United States develop measles. A woman who has had measles or has been vaccinated passes immunity (in the form of antibodies) to her child; this immunity lasts most of the first year of life. Thereafter, however, susceptibility to measles is high unless vaccination is given. A person who has had measles develops immunity and cannot contract it again.

Symptoms and Diagnosis

The symptoms of measles begin about 7 to 14 days after infection. The infected child first develops a fever, runny nose, sore throat, hacking cough, and red eyes. Sometimes, the eyes are

ENTEROVIRAL INFECTIONS: COMMON IN CHILDHOOD

The enteroviruses include numerous strains of coxsackievirus, echovirus, and others. These viruses are responsible for illness in 10 to 30 million people each year in the United States, primarily in the summer and fall. Infections are highly contagious and typically affect many people in a community, sometimes reaching epidemic proportions. Enteroviral infections are most common in children, particularly those living in conditions of poor hygiene.

The infection begins when material contaminated with the virus is swallowed; the virus then reproduces in the digestive tract. The body's immune defenses stop many infections at this stage; the result is few or no symptoms. Sometimes, the virus survives and spreads into the bloodstream, resulting in fever, headache, sore throat, and vomiting. People often refer to such illnesses as the "summer flu," although they are not influenza. Some strains of enterovirus also produce a generalized, nonitchy rash on the skin or sores inside the mouth. This type of illness is by far the most common enteroviral infection. Rarely, an enterovirus will progress from this stage to attack a particular organ. The virus can attack many different organs, and the symptoms and severity of disease depend on the specific organ infected. Several diseases are caused by enteroviruses:

- **Hand-foot-and-mouth disease** affects the skin and mucous membranes; painful sores appear inside the mouth and on the hands and feet.

- **Herpangina** also affects the skin and mucous membranes, producing painful sores on the tongue and the back of the throat.

- **Aseptic meningitis** affects the central nervous system, causing severe headache, stiff neck, and sensitivity to light.

- **Encephalitis** causes confusion, weakness, seizures, and coma.

- **Paralytic Illness** leads to weakness of various muscles.

- **Myocarditis** affects the heart, causing weakness and shortness of breath with exertion.

- **Epidemic pleurodynia** affects the muscles, leading to intermittent painful spasms of muscles in the wall of the lower chest or upper abdomen.

- **Acute hemorrhagic conjunctivitis** affects the eyes, causing painful, red, runny eyes; bleeding under the conjunctiva; and swollen eyelids.

Enteroviral infections usually resolve completely, but infections of the heart or central nervous system are occasionally fatal. There is no cure. Treatment is directed at relieving symptoms.

sensitive to bright light. Tiny white spots (Koplik's spots) appear inside the mouth 2 to 4 days later.

A mildly itchy rash appears 3 to 5 days after the start of symptoms. The rash begins in front of and below the ears and on the side of the neck as irregular, flat, red areas that soon become raised. The rash spreads within 1 to 2 days to the trunk, arms, and legs, as it begins to fade on the face.

At the peak of the illness, the child feels very sick, the rash is extensive, and the temperature may exceed 104°F. In 3 to 5 days, the temperature falls, the child begins to feel better, and any remaining rash quickly fades. The diagnosis is based on the typical symptoms and characteristic rash. No special tests are performed.

Brain infection (encephalitis) occurs in about 1 of 1,000 children with measles. If encephalitis occurs, it often starts with a high fever, seizures, and coma, usually 2 days to 3 weeks after the rash appears. The illness may be brief, with recovery in about 1 week, or it may be prolonged, resulting in brain damage or death.

Secondary bacterial infections, such as pneumonia (especially in infants) or a middle ear infection (otitis media), occur fairly often, and children with measles are especially susceptible to infection with streptococci bacteria. Rarely, blood platelet levels become so low that the child bruises and bleeds.

DID YOU KNOW?

- Although measles is rare in the United States, it is still common in other countries.

Prognosis, Prevention, and Treatment

In healthy, well-nourished children, measles is rarely serious. However, secondary bacterial infections, particularly pneumonia, can occasionally be fatal. In rare cases, subacute sclerosing panencephalitis—a serious complication of measles—occurs months to years later, resulting in brain damage (see page 326).

Measles vaccine, one of the routine immunizations of childhood, is given between 12 and 15 months of age (see page 33), with a booster at age 4 to 5 years. Children (and adults) who are exposed to measles and do not have immunity may be protected by vaccination within 2 days of the exposure. Pregnant women and infants younger than 1 year should not receive the vaccine and are given measles immune globulin for protection.

There is no specific treatment for measles. Some doctors in the United States give vitamin A to children aged 6 months to 2 years hospitalized with measles, because vitamin A has reduced the number of deaths from measles in countries where vitamin A deficiency is common. A child with measles is kept warm and comfortable. Acetaminophen or ibuprofen may be given to reduce fever. If a secondary bacterial infection develops, an antibiotic is given.

Mumps

Mumps is a contagious viral infection that causes painful enlargement of the salivary glands; the infection may also affect the testes, brain, and pancreas, especially in adults.

- Mumps causes chills, headache, poor appetite, and a feeling of illness, followed about a day later by swelling of the salivary glands.
- Beginning at age 12 to 15 months, children are vaccinated against mumps, and they receive a booster at age 4 to 5 years of age.
- Children with mumps get better on their own, but may be given acetaminophen to relieve headache and pain.

Children become infected with mumps by breathing in small airborne droplets of moisture coughed out by an infected person or by having direct contact with objects contaminated by infected saliva. Mumps is less contagious than measles or chickenpox. In heavily populated areas, it occurs year-round but is most frequent in late winter and early spring. Epidemics may occur when people without immunity are crowded together. Although the infection may occur at any age, most cases occur in children 5 to 15 years old. The infection is unusual in children younger than 2 years. One infection with the mumps virus usually provides lifelong immunity.

Symptoms and Diagnosis

Symptoms begin 14 to 24 days after infection. Most children develop chills, headache, poor appetite, a general feeling of illness (malaise), and a low to moderate fever. These symptoms are followed in 12 to 24 hours by swelling of the salivary glands, which is most prominent on the second day. Some children simply have swelling of the salivary glands without the other symptoms; this results in pain when chewing or swallowing, particularly when swallowing acidic liquids, such as citrus fruit juices. The glands are tender when touched. At this stage, the temperature usually rises to 103 or 104°F.

Young men who become infected after puberty may develop inflammation of one or both testes (orchitis). Inflammation of the testes produces severe pain. On healing, the affected testis may be smaller. If both testes are damaged, sterility may result.

DID YOU KNOW?

- Infection can be more serious in older children and adults, especially in boys or men.

Mumps leads to viral inflammation of the brain or its covering (meningoencephalitis) in 10% of people. Meningoencephalitis causes headache, stiff neck, drowsiness, coma, or seizures. Most people recover completely, but some have permanent nerve or brain damage, such as nerve deafness or paralysis of the facial muscles, usually affecting only one side of the body.

Inflammation of the pancreas (pancreatitis) may occur toward the end of the first week of infection. This disorder causes abdominal pain, nausea, and vomiting, which varies from mild to severe. These symptoms disappear in about a week, and the person recovers completely.

Doctors diagnose mumps based on the typical symptoms, particularly when they occur during an outbreak of mumps. Laboratory tests can identify the mumps virus and its antibodies, but such tests are rarely needed to make the diagnosis.

Prognosis, Prevention, and Treatment

Almost all children with mumps recover fully without problems, but in rare cases symptoms may worsen again after about 2 weeks.

Vaccination against mumps is routine in childhood, beginning at 12 to 15 months of age (see page 33), and fewer than 1,000 cases occur each year. Once the infection has started, it just has to run its course. To minimize discomfort, children should avoid foods that require much chewing or are acidic. Analgesics, such as acetaminophen and ibuprofen, may be used for headache and discomfort.

Young men with inflammation of the testes need bed rest. The scrotum may be supported with an athletic supporter or by an adhesive tape bridge connected between the thighs. Ice packs may be applied to relieve pain.

If pancreatitis causes severe nausea and vomiting, intravenous fluids may be given, and intake by mouth should be avoided for a few days. Children with meningoencephalitis may need intravenous fluids and acetaminophen or ibuprofen for a fever or headache. If seizures develop, anticonvulsant drugs may be needed.

Polio

Polio (poliomyelitis) is a highly contagious, sometimes fatal, viral infection that affects nerves and can produce permanent muscle weakness, paralysis, and other symptoms.

- Most infected children have no symptoms.
- Sometimes mild symptoms develop, such as fever, headache, sore throat, and a general feeling of illness.

- Occasionally, severe symptoms develop, such as stiff neck and back and muscle pain.
- Diagnosis is based on symptoms.
- Polio can be prevented by vaccination.
- Polio cannot be cured, and existing antiviral drugs do not affect the course of the disease.

Polio is caused by poliovirus, an enterovirus, which is spread by swallowing material contaminated by the virus. The infection spreads from the intestine to the parts of the brain and spinal cord that control the muscles.

In the early 20th century, polio was widespread throughout the United States. Today, because of extensive vaccination polio outbreaks have largely disappeared, and most doctors have never seen a new polio infection. The last case of wild poliovirus infection in the United States occurred in 1979. The Western Hemisphere was certified polio-free in 1994. A global polio eradication program is under way. Unimmunized people of all ages are susceptible to polio. In the past, polio outbreaks occurred mainly in children and adolescents, because many older people had already been exposed to the virus and developed immunity.

Symptoms and Diagnosis

Fewer than 1 of 100 infected people develop any symptoms. Of those with symptoms, 80 to 90% simply have fever, mild headache, sore throat, and a general feeling of illness (malaise). This mild illness resolves completely in 24 to 72 hours. The remaining 10 to 20% of people have more serious symptoms (major polio). Major polio is more likely in older children and adults. The symptoms, which usually appear 7 to 14 days after infection, include fever, severe headache, a stiff neck and back, and deep muscle pain. Sometimes areas of skin develop odd sensations, such as pins and needles or unusual sensitivity to pain. Depending on which parts of the brain and spinal cord are affected, the disease may progress no further, or weakness or paralysis may develop in certain muscles. The person may have difficulty in swallowing and may choke on saliva, food, or fluids. Sometimes fluids go up into the nose, and the voice may develop a nasal quality. Sometimes the part of the brain responsible for breathing is affected, causing weakness or paralysis of the chest muscles. Some people are completely unable to breathe.

A doctor can diagnose polio from its symptoms. Diagnosis is confirmed by identifying poliovirus in a stool sample and by detecting high levels of antibodies to the virus in the blood.

DID YOU KNOW?

- Adults who were not vaccinated as children should receive polio vaccine before they travel to areas where polio is still a health risk.

Prevention

Polio vaccine is included among the routine childhood immunizations (see page 32). Two types of vaccine are available worldwide: an inactivated poliovirus vaccine (Salk vaccine) given by injection and a live poliovirus vaccine (Sabin vaccine) taken by mouth. The live oral vaccine provides better immunity but can mutate and cause polio in about 1 in every 2.4 million children. Although this is very uncommon, because live polio was eradicated in the United States, doctors recommend only the injected vaccine for children in this country. The oral vaccine is used for rapid treatment of unprotected people in local outbreaks in other parts of the world.

Prognosis and Treatment

About 50% of people with major polio recover without paralysis. Another 25% have mild permanent disability, and 25% have permanent severe paralysis. Some children, even those who apparently recovered completely, develop a return or worsening of muscle weakness 15 or more years after an attack of polio. This condition (postpolio syndrome) often results in severe disability.

Polio cannot be cured, and available antiviral drugs do not affect the course of the disease. A ventilator may be needed if the muscles used in breathing are weakened. Often, the need for a ventilator is temporary.

Primary Oral Herpes Simplex

Primary herpes simplex is infection of the mouth with herpes simplex virus, causing mouth sores.

- Primary herpes simplex predisposes to eventual development of recurring sores (often called cold sores).
- Mouth rinses can help relieve pain.

The first eruption of sores due to infection with oral herpes simplex virus is called primary herpes. It is usually contracted in childhood. Primary herpes may be mild or severe, but it often affects large areas of the mouth and always the gums. Any subsequent eruption of the sores is called secondary herpes. Secondary herpes is a reactivation of the virus rather than a new infection. There are at least two forms of herpes simplex virus. In the past, herpes simplex virus type 1 only caused sores above the waist, and type 2 only below the waist (genital herpes). Now, however, either type can cause sores anywhere on the body. Herpes simplex virus type 2 tends to be more severe than type 1.

Typically, a previously uninfected child acquires the virus from contact with an adult who has a cold sore.

A person is capable of spreading the infection (contagious) from the time the tingling sensation that precedes the development of a sore (the prodrome) is experienced to the time at which the sore has completely crusted over. It is unknown whether herpes can be spread by sharing a glass or touching something that an infected person has touched.

Symptoms

When primary herpes is acquired in childhood, the infection causes gum inflammation and extensive mouth soreness. Fever, swollen lymph nodes in the neck, and general discomfort may develop. A child may be cranky and cry continually. However, many cases are mild and go unrecognized. Parents often mistake the problem for teething or another illness. In more severe cases, small blisters form in the child's mouth. These blisters may not be noticed because they rupture within a day or two, leaving many ulcers. The ulcers may occur anywhere in the mouth but always include the gums. Though the child gets better in a week to 10 days, the herpes simplex virus never leaves the body.

DID YOU KNOW?

- Cold sores are caused by reactivation of the virus that caused primary oral herpes simplex.

Treatment

Treatment for primary herpes aims to relieve the pain so that the child can sleep, eat, and drink comfortably. Pain may keep a child from eating and drinking, which, combined with a fever, can quickly lead to dehydration. Thus, a child should drink as much fluids as possible. An older child can use a prescribed anesthetic mouth rinse such as lidocaine to reduce pain. A mouth rinse containing baking soda may also be soothing.

Respiratory Tract Infections

Respiratory tract infections affect the nose, throat, and airways and may be caused by any of several different viruses.

- Symptoms can include nasal congestion, a runny nose, scratchy throat, and cough, which may last up to 14 days; fever is common.
- Usually, respiratory infections are recognized because of their symptoms.
- Good hygiene, including frequent hand washing, can help prevent the spread of respiratory viruses.
- Unless a child has trouble breathing, is not drinking, or has a fever that lasts longer than a day or two, a visit to a doctor is not usually needed.

Children develop on average six viral respiratory tract infections each year. Viral respiratory tract infections include the common cold and influenza. Doctors often refer to these as upper respiratory infections (URIs), because they produce symptoms mainly in the nose and throat. In small children, viruses also commonly cause infections of the lower respiratory tract—the windpipe, airways, and lungs. These infections include croup, bronchiolitis, and pneumonia. Children sometimes have infections involving both the upper and lower respiratory tracts.

In children, rhinoviruses, influenza viruses (during annual winter epidemics), parainfluenza viruses, respiratory syncytial virus (RSV), and certain strains of adenovirus are the main causes of viral respiratory infections.

Most often, viral respiratory tract infections spread when a child's hands come into contact with nasal secretions from an infected person. These secretions contain viruses. When the child touches his mouth, nose, or eyes, the viruses gain entry and produce a new infection. Less often, infections spread when a child breathes air containing droplets that were coughed or sneezed out by an infected person. For various reasons, nasal or respiratory secretions from children with viral respiratory tract infections contain more viruses than those from infected adults. This increased output of viruses, along with typically lesser attention to hygiene, makes children more likely to spread their infection to others. The possibility of transmission is further enhanced when many children are gathered together, such as in childcare centers and schools. Contrary to what people may think, other factors, such as becoming chilled, wet, or tired, do not cause colds or increase a child's susceptibility to infection.

DID YOU KNOW?

- Even moderate nasal congestion in a young infant can create difficulty breathing and feeding.
- Influenza is the only respiratory viral infection that is preventable by vaccination.
- Infants and younger children are particularly sensitive to the side effects of decongestants, so these drugs should be avoided in them.

Symptoms and Complications

When viruses invade cells of the respiratory tract, they trigger inflammation and production of mucus. This situation leads to nasal congestion, a runny nose, scratchy throat, and cough, which may last up to 14 days. Fever, with a temperature as high as 101 to 102°F, is common. The child's temperature may even rise to 104°F. Other typical symptoms in children include decreased appetite, lethargy, and a general feeling of illness (malaise). Headaches and body aches develop, particularly with influenza. Infants and young children are usually not able to communicate their specific symptoms and just appear cranky and uncomfortable.

Because newborns and young infants prefer to breathe through their nose, even moderate nasal congestion can create difficulty breathing. Nasal congestion leads to feeding problems as well, because infants cannot breathe while suckling from the breast or bottle. Because infants are unable to spit out mucus that they cough up, they often gag and choke.

The small airways of young children can be significantly narrowed by inflammation and mucus, making breathing difficult. These children breathe rapidly and may develop a high-pitched noise heard on breathing out (wheezing) or a similar noise heard on breathing in (stridor). Severe airway narrowing may cause children to gasp for breath and turn blue (cyanosis). Such airway problems are most common with infection caused by parainfluenza viruses and RSV; affected children need to be seen urgently by a doctor.

Some children with a viral respiratory tract infection also develop an infection of the middle ear (otitis media) or the lung tissue (pneumonia). Otitis media and pneumonia may be caused by the virus itself or by a bacterial infection that develops because the inflammation caused by the virus makes tissue more susceptible to invasion by other germs. In children with asthma, respiratory tract infections often lead to an asthma attack.

Diagnosis

Doctors and parents recognize respiratory tract infections by their typical symptoms. Generally, otherwise healthy children with mild upper respiratory tract symptoms do not need to see a doctor unless they have trouble breathing, are not drinking, or have a fever for more than a day or two. X-rays of the neck and chest may be taken in children who have difficulty breathing, stridor, wheezing, or audible lung congestion. Blood tests and tests of respiratory secretions are rarely helpful.

Prevention and Treatment

The best preventive measure is practicing good hygiene. A sick child and the people in the household should wash their hands frequently. In general, the more intimate physical contact (such as hugging, snuggling, or bed sharing) that takes place with an ill child, the greater the risk of spreading the infection to other family members. Parents must balance this risk with the need to comfort an ill child. Children should stay home from school or childcare until the fever is gone and they feel well enough to attend.

Influenza is the only viral respiratory infection preventable by vaccination. Children with heart or lung disease (including asthma), diabetes, kidney failure, or sickle cell disease should receive the vaccine. Additionally, children whose immune system is compromised (including children with HIV infection and those undergoing chemotherapy) should receive the vaccine.

Antibiotics are not necessary to treat viral respiratory tract infections. Children with respiratory tract infections need additional rest and increased fluids. Acetaminophen or nonsteroidal anti-inflammatory drugs (NSAIDs), such as ibuprofen, can be given for fever and aches. School-aged children may take a non-prescription decongestant for bothersome nasal congestion, although the drug often does not help. Infants and younger children are particularly sensitive to the side effects of decongestants and may experience agitation, confusion, hallucinations, lethargy, and rapid heart rate. In infants and young children, congestion may be relieved somewhat by using a cool-mist vaporizer to humidify the air and by suctioning the mucus from the nose with a rubber suction bulb.

Doctors may give certain children at high risk of developing a severe RSV infection monthly injections of palivizumab, which contains antibodies against RSV. Children who receive palivizumab are less likely to need hospitalization, but doctors are not sure whether this treatment prevents death or serious complications.

Children who have difficulty breathing are taken to a hospital. Depending on their condition, doctors may treat them with oxygen and drugs, such as albuterol or epinephrine, to open the airways (bronchodilators). Ribavirin is sometimes given to children with severe RSV pneumonia; however, the benefit of this drug is not clear.

Roseola Infantum

Roseola infantum is a contagious viral infection of infants or very young children that causes a high fever followed by a rash.

- Roseola infantum is diagnosed on the basis of symptoms.
- The fever is treated with acetaminophen or ibuprofen.
- Seizures and rash do not need treatment.

Roseola infantum occurs most often in the spring and fall, sometimes in local outbreaks. The usual cause is herpesvirus 6, one of the many herpesviruses. Most children who develop roseola infantum are between 6 months and 3 years old.

Symptoms begin about 5 to 15 days after infection. A fever of 103 to 105°F begins abruptly and lasts for 3 to 5 days. In 5 to 15% of children, seizures occur as a result of high fever, particularly as the fever begins and rises quickly. Despite the high fever, the child is usually alert and active. A few children have a mild runny nose, sore throat, or an upset stomach. The lymph nodes at the back of the head, the sides of the neck, and behind the ears may be enlarged. The fever usually disappears on the fourth day.

DID YOU KNOW?

- Seizures develop in 5 to 15% of children with roseola infantum.

About 30% of children develop a rash within a few hours to at most a day after the temperature falls. The rash is red and flat, but it may have raised areas, mostly on the chest and abdomen and less extensively on the face, arms, and legs. The rash is not itchy and may last from a few hours to 2 days.

A doctor makes the diagnosis based on the symptoms. Antibody tests and a culture of the virus are rarely needed.

Fever is treated with acetaminophen or ibuprofen. The seizures and rash do not require any specific treatment. But since they are frightening, most parents bring their child to the doctor for evaluation.

Rubella

Rubella (German measles, 3-day measles) is a contagious viral infection that produces mild symptoms, such as joint pain and a rash.

- Often the first sign of illness is swollen lymph nodes.
- Children may also have rose-colored spots on the roof of the mouth, and they develop a characteristic rash.
- Diagnosis is usually based on symptoms, but a blood test is needed to confirm the infection in a pregnant woman who may have rubella.
- Prevention is with routine vaccination at age 12 to 15 months and a booster at age 4 to 5 years.
- Usually, no treatment is needed.

Rubella is a typically mild childhood infection that may, however, have devastating consequences for infants infected prior to birth. A woman infected during the first 16 weeks (particularly the first 8 to 10 weeks) of pregnancy often passes the infection to the fetus. This fetal infection causes miscarriage, stillbirth, or severe birth defects.

Rubella was once common during the springtime, with major epidemics every 6 to 9 years infecting millions of people. The disease is now rare in the United States because of widespread vaccination. Nonetheless, some young adult women have never had rubella or rubella vaccination and are thus at risk of having children with serious birth defects if they become infected during early pregnancy.

Rubella is spread mainly by breathing in small virus-containing droplets of moisture that have been coughed into the air by an infected person. Close contact with an infected person can also spread the infection. The infection is contagious from 1 week before the rash appears until 1 week after the rash disappears. An infant infected before birth can spread the infection for many months after birth.

DID YOU KNOW?

- Rubella is generally a mild illness, but the consequences for infants infected before birth may be devastating.

Symptoms and Diagnosis

Symptoms begin about 14 to 21 days after infection. Some children feel mildly ill for a few days, with a runny nose, cough, and painless, rose-colored spots on the roof of the mouth. These spots later merge with one another into a red blush extending over the back of the throat. In most children, particularly older ones, the first sign of illness is the development of swollen lymph nodes in the neck and back of the head. A characteristic rash develops about a day later and lasts about 3 days. The rash begins on the face and neck and quickly spreads to the trunk, arms, and legs. As the rash appears, a mild reddening of the skin (flush) occurs, particularly on the face.

Up to one third of older girls and women develop arthritis or joint pain with rubella. In rare instances, a middle ear infection (otitis media) develops. Brain infection (encephalitis) is a very rare but occasionally fatal complication.

The diagnosis is based on the typical symptoms. A definite diagnosis, necessary during pregnancy, can be made by measuring levels of antibodies to rubella virus in the blood.

Prevention and Treatment

Rubella vaccine, one of the routine immunizations of childhood, is given beginning at 12 months of age (see page 33), with a

WHAT IS KAWASAKI SYNDROME?

Kawasaki syndrome produces inflammation in the walls of blood vessels throughout the body. The cause is unknown, but evidence suggests a virus or other infectious organism. Inflammation of blood vessels in the heart causes the most serious problems.

Most children with Kawasaki syndrome range from 2 months to 5 years old, although adolescents can be affected. Roughly twice as many boys as girls are affected. The illness is more common in children of Asian descent. Several thousand cases of Kawasaki syndrome are estimated to occur in the United States every year.

The illness begins with fever—usually above 102°F—which rises and falls over 1 to 3 weeks. Within a day, a red, patchy rash usually appears over the trunk and around the diaper area.

Within several days, the rash appears on mucous membranes, such as the lining of the mouth or vagina. The child has a red throat; reddened, dry, cracked lips; and a strawberry-red tongue. The eyes become red but without any discharge. Also, the palms and soles turn red or purplish red, and the hands and feet often swell. The skin on the fingers and toes begins to peel 10 to 20 days after the illness starts. The lymph nodes in the neck are often swollen and slightly tender.

About 50% of children develop problems involving the heart, such as a rapid or irregular heart beat, usually beginning 2 to 4 weeks after the onset of illness. Half of the children with heart problems develop the most serious heart problem, coronary artery aneurysm (a bulge in the wall of the coronary artery). These aneurysms can rupture or provoke a blood clot, leading to a heart attack and sudden death. Other problems include inflammation of the tissues lining the brain (meningitis), joints, and gallbladder. These symptoms eventually resolve without causing permanent damage. Doctors perform ultrasound of the heart to detect coronary artery aneurysms.

Children recover completely if their coronary arteries are not affected within the first 8 weeks of illness. For those with coronary artery problems, survival varies with the severity of disease, but overall between 0.05% and 0.1% of children with Kawasaki syndrome die, even with treatment. Of these, most die in the first few months, but death can occur decades afterward. About half of the aneurysms resolve within 1 to 2 years. The remaining half are

(Continued)

WHAT IS KAWASAKI SYNDROME? (Continued)

permanent. Even the ones that resolve may lead to an increased risk of heart problems in adulthood.

Treatment given within 10 days of symptoms significantly reduces the risk of coronary artery damage and speeds the resolution of fever, rash, and discomfort. For 1 to 4 days, high doses of immunoglobulin are given intravenously, and high doses of aspirin are given by mouth. Once the fever is gone, a lower dose of aspirin is usually continued for several weeks to months. If the child contracts influenza or chickenpox, dipyridamole is sometimes used temporarily instead of aspirin to lessen the risk of Reye's syndrome.

Children with large coronary aneurysms may be treated with anticoagulant drugs. Some children may even require coronary artery angioplasty, stent placement, or coronary artery bypass grafting.

booster at age 4 to 5 years of age. A person who has had rubella develops immunity and cannot contract it again.

Most children with rubella recover fully without treatment. A middle ear infection (see page 402) can be treated with antibiotics. No treatment is available for encephalitis, which must just run its course with supportive care.

Subacute Sclerosing Panencephalitis

Subacute sclerosing panencephalitis, a progressive and usually fatal disorder, is a rare complication of measles that appears months or years later and produces mental deterioration, muscle jerks, and seizures.

- The first symptoms are usually poor school performance, forgetfulness, temper outbursts, distractibility, sleeplessness, and hallucinations.
- The disorder is diagnosed on the basis of symptoms and may be confirmed when a blood test shows high levels of antibodies to the measles virus.

- The disorder is progressive and usually fatal within three years.
- Drugs can be taken to help control the seizures.

Subacute sclerosing panencephalitis results from a long-term brain infection with the measles virus. The virus sometimes enters the brain during a measles infection. It may cause immediate symptoms of brain infection (encephalitis), or it may remain in the brain for a long time without causing problems.

Subacute sclerosing panencephalitis occurs because the measles virus reactivates; in the United States for reasons that are not known, the disorder occurs in about 1 or 2 people per 1 million who previously had measles. In very rare cases, a person who never had measles but received live measles vaccine may develop subacute sclerosing panencephalitis.

The number of people with subacute sclerosing panencephalitis is declining in the United States and Western Europe. Males are affected more often than females.

Symptoms and Diagnosis

The disorder usually begins in children or young adults, generally before age 20. The first symptoms may be poor performance in schoolwork, forgetfulness, temper outbursts, distractibility, sleeplessness, and hallucinations. Sudden muscular jerks of the arms, head, or body may occur. Eventually, seizures may occur, together with abnormal uncontrollable muscle movements. Intellect and speech continue to deteriorate. Later, the muscles become increasingly rigid, and swallowing may become difficult. The swallowing difficulty sometimes causes the person to choke on his saliva, resulting in pneumonia. The person may become blind. In the final phases, the body temperature may rise, and the blood pressure and pulse become abnormal.

A doctor makes the diagnosis based on the symptoms. The diagnosis may be confirmed by a blood test that reveals high levels of antibody to the measles virus, by an abnormal electroencephalogram (EEG), or by magnetic resonance imaging (MRI) or computed tomography (CT) scans that show brain abnormalities.

Prognosis and Treatment

The disease is nearly always fatal within 1 to 3 years. Although the cause of death is usually pneumonia, the pneumonia results from the extreme weakness and abnormal muscle control caused by this disease.

Nothing can be done to halt progression of the disease. Anticonvulsant drugs may be taken to control or reduce seizures.

CHAPTER 17

Allergic Reactions

Allergic reactions (hypersensitivity reactions) are inappropriate immune responses to a normally harmless substance.

Normally, the immune system—which includes antibodies, white blood cells, mast cells, complement proteins, and other substances—defends the body against foreign substances (called antigens). However, in susceptible children, the immune system can overreact to certain antigens (called allergens), which are harmless in most people. The result is an allergic reaction. Some children are allergic to only one substance; others are allergic to many.

Allergens may cause an allergic reaction when they land on the skin or in the eye, are inhaled, are eaten, or are injected. An allergic reaction can occur as part of a seasonal allergy (such as hay fever), caused by exposure to such substances as grass or ragweed pollen. Or an allergic reaction can be triggered by taking a drug, eating certain foods, or breathing in dust or animal dander.

In most allergic reactions, the immune system, when first exposed to an allergen, produces a type of antibody called immunoglobulin E (IgE). IgE binds to a type of white blood cell called basophils in the bloodstream and to a similar type of cell called mast cells in the tissues. The first exposure may make a child sensitive to the allergen but does not cause symptoms. When the sensitized child subsequently encounters the allergen, the cells that have IgE on their surface release substances (such as histamine, prostaglandins, and leukotrienes) that cause swelling or inflammation in the surrounding tissues. Such substances begin a cascade of reactions that continue to irritate and harm tissues. These reactions range from mild to severe.

DID YOU KNOW?

- Identifying an allergen may require a lot of detective work.
- Allergen immunotherapy (allergy shots or injections), which is one option in the treatment of allergies, usually takes a few years to complete.
- Every child who has a severe allergic reaction should go to a hospital emergency department for treatment and observation.

Symptoms and Diagnosis

Most allergic reactions are mild, consisting of watery, itchy eyes, a runny nose, itchy skin, and some sneezing. Rashes (including hives) are common and often itch. Swelling may occur in small areas of the skin (with hives) or in larger areas under the skin (as angioedema—see page 344). Swelling is caused by fluids leaking from blood vessels. Depending on which areas of the body are affected, angioedema may be serious. Allergies may trigger attacks of asthma. Certain allergic reactions, called anaphylactic reactions (see page 342), can be life threatening. The airways can constrict (causing wheezing), and blood vessels can dilate (causing a fall in blood pressure).

Doctors first determine whether a reaction is allergic. They may ask whether the child has close relatives with allergies, because a reaction is more likely to be allergic in such cases. Blood tests are usually performed to detect a type of white blood cell called eosinophils. Eosinophils are produced in large numbers as a result of an allergic reaction.

Because each allergic reaction is triggered by a specific allergen, the main goal of diagnosis is to identify that allergen. Often, the parent and doctor can identify the allergen based on when the allergy started and when and how often the reaction occurs (for example, during certain seasons or after eating certain foods).

Skin tests are the most useful way to identify specific allergens. Usually, a skin prick test is performed first. Dilute solutions are made from extracts of pollens (from trees, grasses, weeds, or fungal spores), dust, animal dander, insect venom, foods, and some drugs. A drop of each solution is placed on the child's skin, which is then pricked with a needle. If the child is allergic to one or more of these substances, a wheal and flare reaction develops: A pale, slightly elevated swelling—the wheal—appears at the pinprick site within 15 to 20 minutes. The wheal is surrounded by a well-defined area of redness—the flare. The resulting area is about $1/2$ inch in diameter. The skin prick test can identify most allergens. If no allergen is identified, a tiny amount of each solution can be injected into the child's skin. This type of skin test is more likely than the skin prick test to detect a reaction to an allergen. Antihistamines should not be taken before skin tests, because they may suppress a reaction to the tests.

The radioallergosorbent test (RAST) is used when skin tests cannot be used—for example, when a skin rash is widespread. This test measures blood levels of different types of IgE that are specific to particular allergens and thus helps doctors identify the allergen.

Prevention

Avoiding an allergen, if possible, is the best approach. Avoiding an allergen may involve discontinuing a drug, keeping a pet out of the house, installing high-efficiency air filters, or not eating a particular food. A child with severe seasonal allergies may benefit from moving to an area that does not have the allergen. Items that collect dust should be removed from the home if the child has an allergy to house dust.

Allergen Immunotherapy

Because some allergens, especially airborne allergens, cannot be avoided, allergen immunotherapy, commonly called allergy shots or injections, can be given to desensitize a child to the allergen. With allergen immunotherapy, allergic reactions can be prevented or reduced in number or severity. However, allergen immunotherapy is not always effective. Some children and some allergies tend to respond better than others. Immunotherapy is used most often for allergies to pollens, house dust mites, insect venoms, and animal dander. Immunotherapy for food allergies is usually not advised because it can cause severe reactions and is less effective. Also, foods can usually be avoided.

In immunotherapy, tiny amounts of the allergen are injected under the skin. The dose is gradually increased until a dose adequate to control symptoms (maintenance dose) is reached. A gradual increase is necessary because exposure to a high dose of the allergen too soon can produce an allergic reaction. Injections are usually given once or twice a week until the maintenance dose is reached. Then injections are usually given every 2 to 6 weeks. The procedure is most effective when maintenance injections are continued throughout the year, even for seasonal rhinitis. Allergen immunotherapy may take 3 to 4 years to complete.

Because immunotherapy injections occasionally cause dangerous allergic reactions, the child remains in the doctor's office for at least 20 minutes afterward. If the child has mild reactions to immunotherapy (such as sneezing, coughing, flushing, tingling sensations, itching, chest tightness, wheezing, and hives), a drug—usually an antihistamine, such as diphenhydramine or loratadine—may help. For more severe reactions, epinephrine (adrenaline) is injected.

Allergen immunotherapy may be used to prevent anaphylactic reactions (see page 342) in people who are allergic to unavoidable allergens, such as insect stings. Immunotherapy is not used when the allergen, such as penicillin and other drugs, can be avoided. However, for children who need to take a drug they are allergic to, immunotherapy, closely monitored by a doctor, can be rapidly performed to desensitize them.

Treatment

Antihistamines: The drugs most commonly used to relieve the symptoms of allergies are antihistamines. Antihistamines block the effects of histamine rather than stop its production. Taking antihistamines partially relieves the itching and reduces the swelling due to hives or mild angioedema. Older antihistamines, such as diphenhydramine, are very effective. These antihistamines, which normally have a sedating effect, can paradoxically cause excitement in children, especially infants. A number of newer antihistamines have been developed that are both longer lasting and less sedating. Many of these newer antihistamines, as well as the tried and true diphenhydramine, are available over the counter;

others require a prescription. Parents should discuss choices with their primary care practitioner.

Cromolyn: Cromolyn is occasionally used to help control allergic symptoms. It is available by prescription for use with an inhaler or nebulizer (which delivers the drug to the lungs) or as eye drops. It is available without a prescription as a nasal spray. Cromolyn usually affects only the areas where it is applied, such as the back of the throat, lungs, eyes, or nose. When taken by mouth, cromolyn is not absorbed into the bloodstream, but it can relieve the digestive symptoms of mastocytosis. Cromolyn inhibits mast cells from releasing substances that damage nearby tissues.

Corticosteroids: When antihistamines cannot control allergy symptoms, a corticosteroid may help. Corticosteroids can be taken as a nasal spray to treat nasal symptoms or through an inhaler, usually to treat asthma. If symptoms are very severe or widespread, taking a corticosteroid (such as prednisone) by mouth may be necessary. If taken by mouth for more than 3 to 4 weeks, corticosteroids have many, sometimes serious side effects. Therefore, corticosteroids taken by mouth are prescribed only for severe symptoms when all other treatments are ineffective, and they are given for as short a time as possible.

Leukotriene modifiers: This new class of drugs is being increasingly used in adults and now children for chronic allergic diseases, including both seasonal and year-round allergies and asthma that is related to allergies. These drugs are taken by mouth.

Emergency Treatment: Severe allergic reactions, such as an anaphylactic reaction, require prompt emergency treatment. Children who have severe allergic reactions should always have with them a special syringe of epinephrine which is designed specifically for use in emergencies and is easy to use. Such children often also should have with them antihistamine tablets, which are also taken as quickly as possible. Usually, the combination of epinephrine and an antihistamine stops the reaction. Nonetheless, children who have had a severe allergic reaction should be taken to the hospital emergency department where they can be closely monitored and treatment can be repeated or adjusted as needed.

Seasonal Allergies

Seasonal allergies result from exposure to airborne substances (such as pollens) that appear only during certain times of the year.

- Itching of the nose, mouth, and eyes is common, as is sneezing and a runny or stuffy nose.
- A doctor bases the diagnosis on the symptoms and on the circumstances under which they occur.
- Antihistamines, decongestants, nasal sprays, and eye drops are some of the many available treatments.

Seasonal allergies are common. Seasonal allergies (commonly called hay fever) occur only during certain times of the year—particularly the spring, summer, or fall—depending on what the child is allergic to. Symptoms involve primarily the membrane lining the nose, causing allergic rhinitis, or the membrane lining the eyelids and covering the whites of the eyes (conjunctiva), causing allergic conjunctivitis. (Rhinitis and conjunctivitis may be caused by other disorders.)

The term hay fever is somewhat misleading, because symptoms do not occur only in the summer when hay is traditionally gathered and never include fever. Hay fever is usually a reaction to pollens and grasses. Different parts of the country have very different pollen seasons. In the eastern, southern, and midwestern United States, the pollens that cause hay fever in the spring usually come from trees, such as oak, elm, maple, alder, birch, juniper, and olive. In the early summer, pollens come from grasses, such as bluegrasses, timothy, redtop, and orchard grass; in the late summer, pollens come from ragweed. In the western United States, mountain cedar (a juniper) is one of the main sources of tree pollen from December to March. In the arid Southwest, grasses pollinate for much longer, and in the fall, pollen from other weeds, such as sagebrush and Russian thistle, can cause hay fever. Children may react to one or more pollens, so a child's pollen allergy season may be from early spring to late fall. Seasonal allergy is also caused by mold spores, which can be airborne for long periods of time during the spring, summer, and fall.

Allergic conjunctivitis may result when airborne substances, such as pollens, contact the eyes directly.

DID YOU KNOW?

- Seasonal allergies are reactions to grass, weed, and tree pollens and to mold spores.
- Many children who have a seasonal allergy also have asthma.
- Using decongestant nose drops or sprays for more than a few days at a time may worsen or prolong nasal congestion.

Symptoms and Diagnosis

Hay fever can cause itching of the nose, roof of the mouth, back of the throat, and eyes. Itching may start gradually or abruptly. The nose runs, producing a clear watery discharge, and may become stuffed up. Sneezing is common.

Hay fever causes the eyes to water, sometimes profusely, and itch. The whites of the eyes and the eyelids may become red and swollen. Wearing contact lenses can irritate the eyes further. The lining of the nose may become swollen and bluish red. Other symptoms include headache, coughing, wheezing, and irritability. More rarely, depression, loss of appetite, and insomnia develop.

Many children who have a seasonal allergy also have asthma (which results in wheezing), caused by the same allergens that contribute to allergic rhinitis and conjunctivitis.

The diagnosis is based on symptoms plus the circumstances under which they occur—that is, during certain seasons. This information can also help doctors identify the allergen. Rarely, the nasal discharge may be examined to see if it contains eosinophils (a type of white blood cell produced in large numbers as a result of an allergic reaction). Skin tests can help confirm the diagnosis and the identity of the allergen (see page 330).

Treatment

Nondrug treatments include shutting windows to keep out the allergens, using an air conditioner, and placing a hepafilter in the child's bedroom. A hepafilter can remove pollen, dust, animal dander, smoke, and other harmful allergens from the air.

For allergic rhinitis, antihistamines are usually used first. Sometimes a decongestant, such as pseudoephedrine, is taken by mouth with the antihistamine to help relieve a stuffy nose. Many antihistamine-decongestant combinations are available as a single tablet. Nonprescription decongestant nose drops or sprays should not be used for more than a few days at a time, because using them continually for a week or more may worsen or prolong nasal congestion. This reaction is called a rebound effect, which may eventually result in chronic congestion.

Cromolyn, which is available as a nonprescription nasal spray, may be useful. To be effective, it must be used regularly. Its effects are usually limited to the areas where it is applied.

When antihistamines cannot control allergy symptoms, doctors may prescribe a corticosteroid nasal spray. Corticosteroid nasal sprays are very effective, and most have minimal side effects. Occassionally, these sprays can cause nosebleeds and a sore nose. Azelastine, an antihistamine taken as a nasal spray, may be effective. But it can cause side effects similar to those of antihistamines taken by mouth, especially drowsiness.

When these treatments are ineffective, a corticosteroid may be taken by mouth or by injection for a short time (usually for fewer than 10 days). If taken by mouth or injection for a long time, corticosteroids can produce serious side effects. Sometimes leukotriene modifiers may be used.

Certain children can benefit from allergen immunotherapy (see page 331). They include children who have severe side effects from taking drugs usually used to treat allergic rhinitis, who need to take corticosteroids by mouth to control allergic rhinitis, or who also develop asthma. Allergen immunotherapy for hay fever should be started after the pollen season to prepare for the next season. Immunotherapy is most effective when continued year-round.

For allergic conjunctivitis, bathing the eyes with plain eyewashes (such as artificial tears) can help reduce irritation. Any substance that may be causing the allergic reaction should be avoided. Contact lenses should not be worn during episodes of conjunctivitis.

For allergic conjunctivitis, antihistamines are usually taken as eye drops, although they can be effective when taken by mouth, and many children absolutely refuse eye drops. Usually, nonprescription antihistamine eye drops also contain a drug that causes blood vessels to narrow (a vasoconstrictor) and thus reduces the redness. However, something in the eye drops—the antihistamine or another component—sometimes makes the allergic reaction worse. Also, long-term use of a vasoconstrictor may worsen or prolong the inflammation. Prescription eye drops may be more effective.

Eye drops containing cromolyn, available by prescription, are used to prevent rather than relieve allergic conjunctivitis. They can be used when exposure to the allergen is anticipated. Eye drops containing olopatadine, available by prescription, can be very effective. This drug is an antihistamine and, like cromolyn, inhibits mast cells from releasing damaging substances.

If symptoms are very severe, eye drops containing corticosteroids, available by prescription, may be used as a last resort. During treatment with corticosteroid eye drops, eye pressure should be checked regularly, because use of these eye drops can lead to glaucoma. Eyes should also be checked for infection, because corticosteroids suppress the immune system and thus increase the risk of infection. Use of these eye drops is best supervised by an ophthalmologist. If other treatments are ineffective, allergen immunotherapy may be beneficial.

Year-Round Allergies

Year-round (perennial) allergies result from exposure to airborne substances, such as house dust.

- Itching of the nose, mouth, and eyes is common, as is sneezing and a runny or stuffy nose.
- A doctor diagnoses year-round allergies based on symptoms plus the circumstances under which they occur.
- Modifying the household environment and frequent cleaning to reduce or eliminate the source of symptoms are needed.

Perennial allergies may occur at any time of year—unrelated to the season—or may last year-round. Perennial allergies are often a reaction to house dust. House dust may contain mold and fungal spores, fibers of fabric, animal dander, dust mites, and bits of insects. Substances in and on cockroaches are often the cause of allergic symptoms. These substances are present in houses year-round but may cause more severe symptoms during the cold months when more time is spent indoors.

Usually, perennial allergies cause nasal symptoms (allergic rhinitis) but not eye symptoms (allergic conjunctivitis). However, allergic conjunctivitis can result when certain substances are purposely or inadvertently placed in the eyes. These substances include drugs used to treat eye disorders, cosmetics such as eyeliner and face powder, and hair dye. The cleaning solutions for contact lenses can cause a chemical allergic reaction.

DID YOU KNOW?

- House dust, which may contain mold spores, fabric fibers, animal dander, dust mites, and much more, is a common cause of year-round allergies.
- "Roach dust," made up of cockroach body parts and droppings, can trigger allergic symptoms as well as asthma.
- Year-round allergies can cause hearing impairment and recurring sinus infections.
- Exposure to cigarette smoke can cause allergies throughout the year.

Symptoms and Diagnosis

Perennial allergies can cause itching of the nose, roof of the mouth, back of the throat, and eyes. Itching may start gradually or abruptly. The nose runs, producing a clear watery discharge, and may become stuffed up. Sneezing is common. The nose may become chronically stuffy. The eustachian tube, which connects the middle ear and the back of the nose, may become swollen. As a result, hearing can be impaired, especially in children. Some children also have recurring sinus infections (chronic sinusitis) and growths inside the nose (nasal polyps).

When affected, the eyes water and itch. The whites of the eyes and the eyelids may become red and swollen.

Many children who have a perennial allergy also have asthma, caused by the same allergens that contribute to the allergic rhinitis and allergic conjunctivitis.

Diagnosis is based on symptoms plus the circumstances under which they occur—that is, in response to certain activities—for example, when petting a cat.

Prevention and Treatment

Avoiding the allergen, if possible, is recommended, thus preventing the development of symptoms. If a child is allergic to house dust, removing items that collect dust, such as knickknacks, magazines, and books, may help. Upholstered furniture can be replaced or vacuumed frequently. Draperies and shades can be replaced with blinds, and carpets can be removed or replaced with throw rugs. Mattresses and pillows can be covered with finely woven fabrics that cannot be penetrated by dust mites and allergen particles. Frequently dusting and wet-mopping rooms may help. Air conditioners can reduce the high indoor humidity that encourages the breeding of dust mites, and high-efficiency air filters can be installed. If the child is allergic to animal dander, the family pet may be limited to certain rooms of the house or, if possible, kept out of the house. Washing the pet weekly can also help. A hepafilter to remove dust and other allergens, particularly if placed in the child's bedroom, may be helpful. A total ban on cigarette or other smoke within the house and in the car is extremely important for children exposed to these toxins.

Drug treatment is similar to that for seasonal allergies.

Food Allergy

A food allergy is an allergic reaction to a particular food.

- Symptoms may include a rash, nausea, vomiting, and diarrhea.
- Skin tests with extracts from various foods may be performed to confirm a suspected food allergy.
- An elimination diet is another option to identify a specific food or ingredient as the cause of symptoms.

- Avoiding the food or ingredient that causes an allergic reaction is important.
- Children with severe food allergies must have epinephrine available to them at all times.

Many different foods can cause allergic reactions. However, food allergies are most commonly triggered by certain nuts, peanuts, shellfish, fish, milk, eggs, wheat, and soybeans. Allergic reactions to foods may be severe and sometimes include an anaphylactic reaction (see page 342).

Food allergies may start during infancy. They are most common among children whose parents have food allergies, allergic rhinitis, or allergic asthma. Children with food allergies tend to be allergic to the most common allergens, such as those in eggs, milk, peanuts, and soybeans.

Food allergies are sometimes blamed for such disorders as hyperactivity in children, chronic fatigue, arthritis, poor athletic performance, and depression. However, these associations have not been substantiated.

Some reactions to food are not an allergic reaction. For example, food intolerance differs from a food allergy because it does not involve the immune system. Instead it involves a reaction in the digestive tract that results in digestive upset. For example, some children lack an enzyme necessary for digesting the sugar in milk (lactose). Other reactions to a food may result from contamination or deterioration of the food.

In some children, food additives can cause a reaction that resembles but is not an allergic reaction. For example, monosodium glutamate (MSG), some preservatives (such as metabisulfite), and dyes (such as tartrazine, a yellow dye used in candies, soft drinks, and other foods) can cause symptoms such as asthma and hives.

DID YOU KNOW?

- Many common reactions to food are not allergies.
- Elimination diets can be very complicated.
- Desensitization is not effective for food allergies.
- Many children outgrow food allergies.

Symptoms

In infants, the first symptom of a food allergy may be a rash such as eczema (atopic dermatitis) or a rash that resembles hives. The rash may be accompanied by nausea, vomiting, and diarrhea. By about age 1 year, the rash often lessens. By about age 10, food allergies—most commonly to milk and less commonly to eggs and peanuts—tend to subside. Allergies to airborne substances, such as allergic asthma and hay fever, may develop as food allergies subside.

In severe reactions, a rash may cover the entire body, the throat may swell, and the airways may narrow, making breathing difficult. Occasionally, this reaction is a life-threatening anaphylactic reaction. For some children, allergic reactions to food occur only if they exercise immediately after eating the food.

Diagnosis

Doctors suspect a food allergy primarily on the basis of the child's history. Then skin tests with extracts from various foods may be performed. A reaction to a food tested does not necessarily mean that the child is allergic to that food, but no skin reaction means that an allergy to that food is unlikely. If the child reacts to the food tested, an oral challenge test may be performed to confirm the diagnosis. In this test, the suspected food is given in a carrier food such as milk or applesauce, and the doctor observes as the child eats the food. If no symptoms develop, the child is not allergic to the food.

Another way to identify the food allergy is an elimination diet. The child stops eating all foods that may be causing the symptoms for about 1 week. The doctor prescribes the diet the child is to follow. Only the foods or fluids specified in the diet may be eaten, and only pure products should be used. Following such a diet is not easy, because many food products have ingredients that are not obvious or expected. For example, many rye breads contain some wheat flour. Eating in restaurants is not advisable, because the parent and the doctor need to know the ingredients of every meal eaten. If no symptoms occur, foods are added back one at a time. Each added food is given for several days or until symptoms appear, and thus the allergen is identified.

Treatment

Children with food allergies must eliminate from their diet the foods that trigger their allergies. Desensitization by first eliminating the food, then eating small amounts of the food or placing drops of food extracts under the tongue is not effective. Antihistamines are useful only for relieving hives and swelling. Children with severe food allergies often must have antihistamines with them to take immediately if a reaction starts. They should also have available a syringe of epinephrine to use when needed for severe reactions.

Anaphylactic Reactions

Anaphylactic reactions (anaphylaxis) are sudden, widespread, potentially severe and life-threatening allergic reactions.

- Anaphylactic reactions begin quickly, within 1 to 15 minutes, of exposure to the allergen.
- Symptoms may include a rapid heart beat, a drop in blood pressure, tingling sensations, itchy skin, and difficulty breathing.
- Rapid treatment with an epinephrine injection is essential.
- Observation and further treatment in a hospital emergency department are also important.

Anaphylactic reactions are most commonly caused by drugs (such as penicillin), insect stings, certain foods, and allergy injections (allergen immunotherapy). But they can be caused by any allergen. Like other allergic reactions, an anaphylactic reaction does not usually occur after the first exposure to an allergen but may occur after a subsequent exposure. However, many parents do not recall a first exposure. Any allergen that causes an anaphylactic reaction in a child is likely to cause that reaction with subsequent exposures, unless measures are taken to prevent it.

DID YOU KNOW?

- An anaphylactic reaction can progress so rapidly that it can lead to loss of consciousness within 1 to 2 minutes.
- Children with severe allergic reactions should always have epinephrine available to them for prompt treatment.

ANAPHYLACTOID VERSUS ANAPHYLACTIC

Anaphylactoid reactions resemble anaphylactic reactions. However, anaphylactoid reactions may occur after the first exposure to a substance—for example, after the first injection of certain drugs, such as polymyxin, pentamidine, opioids, or the radiopaque dyes sometimes used with x-ray procedures. Anaphylactoid reactions are not allergic reactions because IgE, the class of antibodies involved in allergic reactions, does not cause them. Rather, the reaction is caused by the substance itself. Aspirin and other nonsteroidal antiinflammatory drugs (NSAIDs) can occasionally cause anaphylactoid reactions in some children.

If possible, doctors avoid using dyes with x-ray procedures in children who have anaphylactoid reactions to such dyes. However, some disorders cannot be diagnosed without dyes. In such cases, special dyes that reduce the risk of reactions are used. In addition, drugs that block anaphylactoid reactions, such as prednisone, diphenhydramine, or ephedrine, are usually given before the dye is injected.

Symptoms

Anaphylactic reactions begin within 1 to 15 minutes of exposure to the allergen. Rarely, reactions begin after 1 hour. The heart beats quickly. The child may feel uneasy and become agitated. Blood pressure may fall, causing fainting. Other symptoms include tingling (pins-and-needles) sensations, itchy and flushed skin, throbbing in the ears, coughing, sneezing, hives, and swelling (angioedema). Breathing may become difficult and wheezing may occur because the windpipe (upper airway) constricts or becomes swollen.

An anaphylactic reaction may progress so rapidly that it leads to collapse, cessation of breathing, seizures, and loss of consciousness within 1 to 2 minutes. The reaction may be fatal unless emergency treatment is given immediately.

Prevention and Treatment

Children who are allergic to unavoidable allergens (such as insect stings) may benefit from long-term allergen immunotherapy (see page 331).

If an anaphylactic reaction occurs, an epinephrine injection should be given immediately. Children who have these reactions should always have with them a syringe of epinephrine and antihistamine tablets for prompt treatment. Usually, this treatment stops the reaction. Nonetheless, after a severe allergic reaction, such children should be taken to the hospital emergency department, where they can be closely monitored and treatment can be adjusted as needed.

Hives and Angioedema

Hives, also called urticaria, is a skin reaction characterized by pale, slightly elevated swellings (wheals) surrounded by an area of redness with clearly defined borders. Angioedema is swelling of larger areas of tissue under the skin, sometimes affecting the face and throat.

- Itching, then wheals, develop, typically in crops that disappear then reappear elsewhere.
- Angioedema can cause swelling of the airways and make breathing difficult.
- For hives and mild angioedema, antihistamines can relieve the itching and swelling.
- Corticosteroids are given when symptoms are severe and other treatments are ineffective.

Hives and angioedema, which may occur together, can be severe. Common triggers are drugs, insect stings or bites, allergy injections (allergen immunotherapy), and certain foods—particularly eggs, shellfish, nuts, and fruits. Eating even a tiny amount of some foods can suddenly result in hives or angioedema. But with other foods (such as strawberries), these reactions occur only after a large amount is eaten. Also, hives sometimes follow viral infections such as hepatitis, infectious mononucleosis, and German measles.

Hives or angioedema can be chronic, recurring over weeks or months. In most cases, no specific cause is identified. The cause may be habitual, unintentional intake of a substance—for example, a food additive, such as a preservative or food dye. In some children, antibodies to thyroid hormone may be the cause. Use of certain drugs, such as aspirin or other nonsteroidal anti-inflammatory drugs (NSAIDs), can also cause chronic hives or angioedema. Chronic angioedema that occurs without hives may be hereditary angioedema.

DID YOU KNOW?

- In many cases, the cause of hives cannot be found.
- If the cause of hives is not apparent, parents should avoid giving their child any nonessential drug until the hives subside.

Symptoms and Diagnosis

Hives usually begin with itching. Then wheals quickly develop. The wheals usually remain small (less than $1/2$ inch across). Wheals that are larger (up to 4 inches across) may look like rings of redness with a pale center. Typically, crops of hives come and go. One spot may remain for several hours, then disappear, and later, another may appear elsewhere. After the hive disappears, the skin usually looks completely normal.

Angioedema may affect part or all of the hands, feet, eyelids, lips, or genitals. Sometimes the membranes lining the mouth, throat, and airways swell, making breathing difficult.

In children, when hives appear suddenly, disappear quickly, and do not recur, an examination by a doctor is usually unnecessary, because the cause is usually a viral infection. If the cause is a bee sting, seeing a doctor is important. A parent can obtain advice about treatment if another bee sting occurs. When angioedema or hives recur without an obvious cause, an examination by a doctor is recommended.

Treatment

Usually, if hives appear suddenly, they subside without any treatment within days and sometimes within minutes. If the cause is not obvious, the child should stop taking all nonessential drugs until the hives subside.

For hives and mild angioedema, taking antihistamines partially relieves the itching and reduces the swelling. Corticosteroids are prescribed only for severe symptoms when all other treatments are ineffective, and they are given for as short a time as possible.

When taken by mouth for more than 3 to 4 weeks, they cause many, sometimes serious side effects.

In about half of the people with chronic hives, the hives disappear without treatment within 2 years. If severe angioedema results in difficulty swallowing or breathing or in collapse, prompt emergency treatment is necessary. Affected children should always have with them a syringe of epinephrine and antihistamine tablets to be used immediately if a reaction occurs. After a severe allergic reaction, such children should be taken to the hospital emergency department, where they can be checked and treated as needed.

Henoch-Schönlein Purpura

Henoch-Schönlein purpura (allergic purpura) is a disease in which blood vessels in the skin, joints, digestive tract, or kidneys may become inflamed and leak.

- Small, bluish purple bruises appear on the feet, legs, arms, and buttocks.
- Joints are swollen and achy.
- Symptoms may recur, but most children recover completely within a month.
- In some cases, treatment includes corticosteroid drugs such as prednisone.

Henoch-Schönlein purpura, an uncommon disease, affects mainly young children but can rarely affect older children and adults. The disease is believed to be the result of an autoimmune reaction, in which the body attacks its own tissues. Usually, allergic purpura develops after a respiratory tract infection, but it can be caused by an allergic reaction to drugs. The rate at which the disease develops and its duration vary.

Symptoms and Diagnosis

The disease may begin with the appearance of small, bluish purple bruises (purpura)—most often on the feet, legs, arms, and buttocks—as blood leaks from vessels in the skin. Over several days, the purpura may become raised and hard; crops of new purpura may break out for several weeks after the first one appears. Swollen, achy joints are common, usually accompanied by fever. Bleeding in the digestive tract may cause abdominal cramps and pain. Blood in the urine (hematuria) may develop. Most children recover completely within a month, but symptoms may recur several times. Bleeding in the kidneys may cause kidney damage.

The diagnosis is based on the symptoms.

Treatment

A drug that may be causing an allergic reaction is discontinued immediately. Corticosteroids (for example, prednisone) may help relieve swelling, joint pain, and abdominal pain, but they do not prevent or reverse kidney damage. Drugs that reduce the activity of the immune system (immunosuppressive drugs), including azathioprine or cyclophosphamide, are sometimes used if kidney damage develops, but it is not known if they are helpful.

CHAPTER 18

Immunodeficiency Disorders

Immunodeficiency disorders involve malfunction of the immune system, resulting in infections that develop and recur more frequently, are more severe, and last longer than usual.

Immunodeficiency disorders impair the immune system's ability to defend the body against foreign or abnormal cells that invade or attack it (such as bacteria, viruses, fungi, and cancer cells). As a result, unusual bacterial, viral, or fungal infections and rare cancers may develop.

An immunodeficiency disorder may be present at birth (congenital, or primary) or may develop later in life, often as a result of another disorder (acquired, or secondary). Congenital immunodeficiency disorders are usually hereditary. They typically become evident during infancy or childhood. There are more than 70 congenital immunodeficiency disorders; all are relatively rare. Acquired immunodeficiency disorders are much more common. Some immunodeficiency disorders shorten lifespan, others persist throughout life but do not affect lifespan, and a few resolve with or without treatment.

Immunodeficiency disorders are grouped by which part of the immune system is affected. They may involve problems with antibodies (due to abnormalities in B lymphocytes, a type of white blood cell), T lymphocytes (a type of white blood cell that helps

Some Congenital Immunodeficiency Disorders

CLASSIFICATION	DISORDER
Problems with antibodies (due to abnormalities in B lymphocytes)	Common variable immunodeficiency
	Selective antibody deficiency (such as IgA deficiency)
	Transient hypogammaglobulinemia of infancy
	X-linked agammaglobulinemia
Problems with T lymphocytes	Chronic mucocutaneous candidiasis
	DiGeorge anomaly
Problems with B and T lymphocytes	Ataxia-telangiectasia
	Severe combined immunodeficiency disease
	Wiskott-Aldrich syndrome
	X-linked lymphoproliferative syndrome
Problems with the movement or killing activity of phagocytes	Chédiak-Higashi syndrome
	Chronic granulomatous disease
	Hyperimmunoglobulinemia E syndrome
	Leukocyte adhesion defects
	Leukocyte glucose-6-phosphate dehydrogenase deficiency
	Myeloperoxidase deficiency
Problems with complement proteins	Complement component 1 (C1) inhibitor deficiency (hereditary angioedema)
	C3 deficiency
	C6 deficiency
	C7 deficiency
	C8 deficiency

identify and destroy foreign or abnormal cells), both B and T lymphocytes, phagocytes (cells that ingest and kill microorganisms), or complement proteins. The affected component of the immune system may be missing, reduced in number, or abnormal and malfunctioning.

Causes

Congenital immunodeficiency disorders are caused by a genetic abnormality, which is often X-linked. That is, boys are more likely to be affected than girls. As a result, about 60% of affected people are male.

Acquired immunodeficiency disorders may result from almost any prolonged serious disorder. Examples are cancer, blood disorders (such as aplastic anemia, leukemia, and myelofibrosis), kidney failure, diabetes, liver disorders, and spleen disorders. Diabetes can result in an immunodeficiency disorder because white blood cells do not function well when the blood sugar level is high. Infections can also cause immunodeficiency disorders. Human immunodeficiency virus (HIV) infection results in acquired immunodeficiency syndrome (AIDS), the most common severe acquired immunodeficiency disorder.

Undernutrition—whether of all nutrients or only one—can impair the immune system. When undernutrition causes weight to decrease to less than 80% of recommended weight, the immune system is usually impaired. A decrease to less than 70% usually results in severe impairment.

Use of certain drugs called immunosuppressants may result in an acquired immunodeficiency disorder. These drugs are intentionally used to suppress the immune system. For example, immunosuppressants are used to prevent rejection of a transplanted organ or tissue, and corticosteroids, a type of immunosuppressant, are used to suppress inflammation due to various disorders. However, immunosuppressants also suppress the body's ability to fight infections and perhaps to destroy cancer cells. Chemotherapy and radiation therapy can also result in immunodeficiency disorders.

DID YOU KNOW?

- One common disorder that causes splenic damage in childhood is sickle cell disease.
- Use of immunosuppressant drugs, undernutrition, hereditary disorders, and almost any prolonged serious disorder can cause immunodeficiency.
- Stem cell transplantation can cure severe combined immunodeficiency disease.
- Stem cell transplantation is life-saving in Wiskott-Aldrich syndrome.

Symptoms

Children with an immunodeficiency disorder tend to have one infection after another. Usually, respiratory infections develop first and recur often. Most children eventually develop severe bacterial infections that persist, recur, or lead to complications. For example, sore throats and head colds may progress to pneumonia. However, having many colds does not suggest an immunodeficiency disorder.

Infections of the skin and the membranes lining the mouth, eyes, and digestive tract are common. Thrush, a fungal infection of the mouth, may be an early sign of an immunodeficiency disorder. Skin infections by bacteria or viruses are also common. Bacterial infections (with staphylococci, for example) may cause pyoderma, in which the skin is covered with pus-filled sores. Warts (caused by viruses) may occur.

Children tend to develop slowly or even lose weight. Other symptoms vary depending on the severity and duration of the infections.

Diagnosis

Doctors first establish that an immunodeficiency exists. Then they identify the abnormality in the immune system.

Doctors suspect immunodeficiency when a severe or an unusual infection recurs often or when an organism that normally does not cause infection causes infection. The results of a physical examination may also suggest immunodeficiency. Evidence of recurring infections—such as rashes, hair loss, many skin infections, chronic cough, weight loss, and an enlarged liver and spleen—is often present.

To help identify the type of immunodeficiency disorder, doctors ask at what age the child began to have recurring or unusual infections. Infections in infants younger than 6 months usually indicate an abnormality in T lymphocytes. Infections in older children usually indicate an abnormality in B lymphocytes and antibody production. The type of infection may also help doctors identify the type of immunodeficiency disorder.

Doctors ask the parent about risk factors, such as diabetes, use of certain drugs, exposure to toxic substances, and the possibility of having close relatives with immunodeficiency disorders (family history). These ask questions to determine whether HIV infection could be the cause.

Laboratory tests are needed to confirm the diagnosis of immunodeficiency and identify the type of immunodeficiency disorder. A blood sample is taken and analyzed to determine the total number of white blood cells and the percentages of each main type of white blood cell. The white blood cells are examined under a microscope for abnormalities. Antibody levels, the number of red blood cells and platelets, and the levels of complement proteins are determined. If any results are abnormal, additional tests are usually performed.

A laboratory test using a chemical to stimulate lymphocytes or skin tests may be performed if the immunodeficiency is thought to be due to a T-lymphocyte abnormality. The skin test resembles the tuberculin skin test, which is used to screen for tuberculosis: Small amounts of proteins from common infectious organisms such as yeast are injected under the skin. If a reaction (redness, warmth, and swelling) occurs within 48 hours, the T lymphocytes are functioning normally. No reaction suggests a T-lymphocyte abnormality. These skin tests are not useful in children younger than 2 years.

People whose families are known to carry a gene for a hereditary immunodeficiency disorder may wish to have genetic testing to learn whether they carry the gene for the disorder and what the chances are of having an affected child. Genetic counseling before testing is helpful. Several immunodeficiency disorders, such as X-linked agammaglobulinemia, Wiskott-Aldrich syndrome, severe combined immunodeficiency disease, and chronic granulomatous disease, can be detected in a fetus by testing a sample of the fluid around the fetus (amniotic fluid) or the fetus's blood.

Prevention and Treatment

Some of the disorders that can cause immunodeficiency disorders can be prevented or treated. For example, successful treatment of cancer usually restores the function of the immune system. Treatment with antiviral drugs can help improve white blood cell function, thus preventing additional infections due to immunodeficiency. Good control of diabetes can help white blood cells function better and thus prevent infections.

Strategies for reducing the risk of and for treating infections depend on the type of immunodeficiency disorder. For example, children who have an immunodeficiency disorder due to a deficiency of antibodies are at risk of bacterial infections. Periodic treatment with immune globulin given intravenously and good personal hygiene (including conscientious dental care) reduce this risk, as does not eating undercooked food, drinking bottled water and avoiding contact with people who have infections. Antibiotics are given as soon as a fever or another sign of an infection develops and before surgical and dental procedures, which may introduce bacteria into the bloodstream.

For children who have an immunodeficiency disorder that increases the risk of viral infections, antiviral drugs, such as amantadine for influenza or acyclovir for herpes, are promptly given at the first sign of infection.

Children who can produce antibodies are vaccinated. However, children who have a B- or T-lymphocyte abnormality are given only killed viral and bacterial vaccines rather than live vaccines. Live viruses may cause an infection in such children. Live vaccines include oral poliovirus vaccine, measles-mumps-rubella vaccine, chicken pox (varicella) vaccine, and bacille Calmette-Guérin (BCG) vaccine. An influenza vaccine given once a year is recommended for children who can produce antibodies and for their immediate family members.

Stem cell transplantation can correct some immunodeficiency disorders, particularly severe combined immunodeficiency disease. Stem cells are usually obtained from bone marrow but occasionally from blood (including umbilical cord blood). Stem cell transplantation, which is available at some major medical centers, is usually reserved for severe disorders.

Transplantation of thymus tissue is sometimes helpful. Gene therapy for a few congenital immunodeficiency disorders is being studied.

X-Linked Agammaglobulinemia

X-Linked agammaglobulinemia (Bruton's agammaglobulinemia) is a hereditary immunodeficiency disorder due to an abnormality in the X chromosome and resulting in few or no B lymphocytes and very low levels of antibodies.

X-Linked agammaglobulinemia affects only boys. For about the first 6 months after birth, antibodies from the mother protect against infection. At about age 6 months, affected infants start having recurring infections of the ears, sinuses, lungs, and bones, usually due to bacteria such as pneumococcus, haemophilus, and streptococcus. Some unusual viral infections of the brain may develop. The risk of cancer is increased.

Infusions of immune globulin are given throughout life to help prevent infections. Antibiotics are promptly given to treat bacterial infections and may be given continuously. Despite these measures, chronic sinus and lung infections often develop. With treatment, lifespan may be unaffected.

Selective Antibody Deficiency

Selective antibody deficiency is a usually acquired but sometimes hereditary immunodeficiency disorder resulting in a low level of a specific class of antibody, even though the total level of antibodies is normal.

There are several classes of antibodies (immunoglobulins). Each helps protect the body from infection in a different way. The level of any class of antibody may be low, but the most commonly affected class is immunoglobulin A (IgA). Selective IgA deficiency usually persists throughout life. The disorder sometimes results from a chromosomal abnormality or from taking phenytoin, an anticonvulsant.

Most children with selective IgA deficiency have few or no symptoms. Others develop chronic respiratory infections, allergies, chronic diarrhea, or autoimmune disorders. If given blood transfusions or immune globulin that contains IgA, some children with selective IgA deficiency produce antibodies against IgA. Such children may have a severe allergic (anaphylactic) reaction (see page 342) the next time they are given a blood transfusion or immune globulin. They should wear a medical identification bracelet or tag to alert doctors to take precautions against such reactions.

Usually, no treatment of selective IgA deficiency is needed. Antibiotics are given to children who have recurring infections. Lifespan is usually unaffected. Selective IgA deficiency that results from taking phenytoin may resolve if the drug is discontinued.

Common Variable Immunodeficiency

Common variable immunodeficiency is an acquired immunodeficiency disorder resulting in very low antibody levels despite a normal number of B lymphocytes.

Common variable immunodeficiency usually develops between the ages of 10 and 20. In some children with this disorder, T lymphocytes malfunction. Recurring lung infections, particularly pneumonia, are common. Autoimmune disorders, including Addison's disease, thyroiditis, and rheumatoid arthritis, often develop. Diarrhea may occur, and food may not be absorbed well from the digestive tract.

Infusions of immune globulin are given throughout life, and antibiotics are promptly given to treat infections. Lifespan may be shortened.

Transient Hypogammaglobulinemia of Infancy

Transient hypogammaglobulinemia of infancy is an immunodeficiency disorder in which antibody production by an infant is delayed.

At birth, the immune system is not fully developed. Most of the antibodies in infants are those produced by the mother and transferred via the placenta before birth. Antibodies from the mother protect infants against infection until infants start to produce their own antibodies, usually by age 6 months. Infants who have transient hypogammaglobulinemia of infancy do not start producing antibodies until later. As a result, antibody levels become low starting at age 3 to 6 months and return to normal at about age 12 to 36 months. This disorder is more common among premature infants, because they receive fewer antibodies from the mother. Although the disorder is present at birth, it is not hereditary.

Most infants with the disorder have some antibodies. Therefore, they do not have a problem with infections and need no treatment. However, some infants, particularly those born prematurely, develop infections frequently. Immune globulin can prevent and help treat infections. It is usually given for about 6 to 12 months. Antibiotics are given when needed. Lifespan is unaffected.

Chronic Mucocutaneous Candidiasis

Chronic mucocutaneous candidiasis is a hereditary immunodeficiency disorder in which T lymphocytes malfunction.

Because the T lymphocytes malfunction, the body is less able to fight fungal infections, including yeast infections. The ability to fight other infections is not reduced. Infections with the *Candida* fungus (candidiasis develop and persist, usually beginning during infancy but sometimes during early adulthood. The fungus may cause mouth infections (thrush) as well as infections of the scalp; skin; nails; and membranes lining the mouth, eyes, digestive tract, and reproductive tract. Severity varies: The disorder may affect one nail or cause a disfiguring rash that covers the face and scalp. Hair may fall out. Hepatitis and chronic lung disorders sometimes develop. Many children also have endocrine disorders, such as underactive parathyroid glands (hypoparathyroidism).

Usually, the infections can be treated with an antifungal drug—nystatin or clotrimazole—applied to the skin. Severe infections, which are rare, require a stronger antifungal drug, such as itraconazole given by mouth. Usually, this disorder is chronic but does not affect lifespan.

DiGeorge Anomaly

DiGeorge anomaly is a congenital immunodeficiency disorder in which the thymus gland is absent or underdeveloped at birth.

Usually, DiGeorge anomaly is due to a chromosomal abnormality but is not usually hereditary. The fetus does not develop normally, and abnormalities of the heart, parathyroid gland, face, and thymus gland often result. The thymus gland is necessary for the normal development of T lymphocytes. Consequently, children with this disorder have a low number of T lymphocytes, limiting their ability to fight many infections. Infections begin soon after birth and recur often. However, the degree to which the immune system is affected varies considerably.

Typically, children with DiGeorge anomaly also have symptoms that are unrelated to immunodeficiency, such as congenital heart disease and unusual facial features, with low-set ears, a small jawbone that recedes, and wide-set eyes. They also are born without parathyroid glands, which help regulate the calcium levels in the blood. The resulting low calcium levels lead to muscle spasms (tetany).

For children who have some T lymphocytes, the immune system may function adequately without treatment. Infections that develop are treated promptly. For children who have very few or no T lymphocytes, transplantation of stem cells or thymus tissue can cure the immunodeficiency.

A low calcium level is treated with calcium supplements to prevent muscle spasms. Sometimes the heart disease is worse than the immunodeficiency, and surgery to prevent severe heart failure or death may be needed. The prognosis usually depends on the severity of the heart disease.

Ataxia-Telangiectasia

Ataxia-telangiectasia is a hereditary disorder characterized by incoordination, dilated capillaries, and increased susceptibility to infections.

The increased susceptibility to infections in children with ataxia-telangiectasia results from malfunction of B and T lymphocytes. Often, levels of the antibody classes IgA and IgE are also deficient. Sinus and respiratory infections recur, often leading to pneumonia and chronic lung disorders such as bronchitis. The risk of cancer, especially leukemia, brain tumors, and stomach cancer, is increased.

Abnormalities in the cerebellum (which are unrelated to the immunodeficiency disorder) lead to incoordination (ataxia). Incoordination usually develops when the child begins to walk but may be delayed until age 4. Speech becomes slurred, and muscles progressively weaken, leading to severe disability. Mental retardation may develop and progress. Between the ages of 1 and 6, capillaries in the skin and eyes become dilated and visible. The dilated capillaries (telangiectasia), called spider veins, are usually most obvious on the eyeballs and ears. The endocrine system may be affected, resulting in small testes (in boys), infertility, and diabetes.

Antibiotics and immune globulin help prevent infections but do not relieve the problems with the nervous system. Ataxia-telangiectasia usually progresses to paralysis, dementia, and death, usually by age 30.

Severe Combined Immunodeficiency Disease

Severe combined immunodeficiency disease is a congenital immunodeficiency disorder resulting in low levels of antibodies and a low number and malfunction of T lymphocytes.

Severe combined immunodeficiency disease is the most serious immunodeficiency disorder. It can be caused by several different genetic defects, most of which are hereditary. One form of the disorder is due to a deficiency of the enzyme adenosine deaminase. In the past, children with this disorder were kept in strict isolation, sometimes in a plastic tent, leading to the disorder being called "bubble boy syndrome."

Most infants with severe combined immunodeficiency disease develop pneumonia, thrush, and diarrhea, usually by age 3 months. More serious infections, including pneumocystis pneumonia, can also develop. If not treated, these children usually die before age 2.

Treatment with antibiotics and immune globulin is helpful. The best treatment is transplantation of stem cells from bone marrow or umbilical cord blood; stem cell transplantation can provide a cure. For a deficiency of adenosine deaminase, replacement of that enzyme can be effective.

Wiskott-Aldrich Syndrome

Wiskott-Aldrich syndrome is a hereditary immunodeficiency disorder characterized by abnormal antibodies and T lymphocytes, a low platelet count, and eczema.

Wiskott-Aldrich syndrome affects only boys. The number of platelets is low. Consequently, bleeding problems, usually bloody diarrhea, may be the first symptom. Eczema also develops at an early age. Susceptibility to infections, particularly of the respiratory tract, is increased because the antibody levels are low and T lymphocytes malfunction. The risk of developing cancers such as lymphoma and leukemia is increased.

Stem cell transplantation is necessary to preserve life. Without it, most boys with this disorder die by age 15. Surgical removal of the spleen may relieve the bleeding problems. Antibiotics are given continuously to prevent infections, and immune globulin may help.

Hyperimmunoglobulinemia E Syndrome

Hyperimmunoglobulinemia E syndrome (hyper-IgE syndrome, or Job-Buckley syndrome) is a hereditary immunodeficiency disorder with very high levels of IgE and normal levels of other antibody classes, resulting in recurring infections.

In most children with hyperimmunoglobulinemia E syndrome, neutrophils—a type of white blood cell that is also a phagocyte—are abnormal. (Phagocytes are cells that ingest and kill bacteria.) The cause is unknown. The skin, joints, lungs, or other organs may be infected, usually with *Staphylococcus* bacteria. Many children with this disorder have weak bones and therefore many fractures. Some children have symptoms of allergy, such as eczema, nasal stuffiness, and asthma. Facial features may be coarse.

Antibiotics, often trimethoprim-sulfamethoxazole, are given continuously or intermittently for the staphylococcal infections. Lifespan depends on the severity of the lung infections.

Chronic Granulomatous Disease

Chronic granulomatous disease is a hereditary immunodeficiency disorder in which phagocytes (neutrophils, eosinophils, monocytes, and macrophages) malfunction.

In this disorder, neutrophils, eosinophils, monocytes, and macrophages do not produce hydrogen peroxide, superoxide, and other substances that kill certain bacteria and fungi. Chronic granulomatous disease usually affects boys.

Symptoms usually first appear during early childhood but sometimes not until adolescence. Chronic infections occur in the skin, lungs, lymph nodes, mouth, nose, and intestines. Pockets of pus (abscesses) can develop around the anus and in the lungs, bones, and liver. The lymph nodes tend to fill with bacteria and enlarge. The skin over the lymph nodes may break down. As a result, the abscess drains. The liver and spleen enlarge. Children may grow slowly.

Antibiotics are given continuously or intermittently. Interferon-gamma, injected 3 times a week, can reduce the number and severity of infections. Stem cell transplantation has been successful in some children but because of the risks is not usually recommended.

Spleen Disorders and Immunodeficiency

The spleen is crucial to the function of the immune system: The spleen traps and destroys bacteria and other infectious organisms in the bloodstream and produces antibodies. For children whose spleen is absent at birth, damaged, or removed because of disease, the risk of developing severe bacterial infections is increased. One common disorder that causes splenic damage in adolescence is sickle cell disease.

Children who do not have a spleen are given pneumococcal and meningococcal vaccines in addition to the usual childhood vaccines. Children who have a spleen disorder or no spleen are given antibiotics at the first sign of infection. Children who do not have a spleen should take antibiotics continuously until at least age 5. An antibiotic, usually penicillin or ampicillin, is often given to prevent an infection in the bloodstream.

CHAPTER 19

Respiratory Disorders

Respiratory disorders commonly affect children. The most serious and common are asthma, bronchiolitis, and croup.

> **DID YOU KNOW?**
>
> - Children with a respiratory problem should be taken to the hospital immediately if they do any of the following:
>   - Appear anxious or struggle to breathe.
>   - Have difficulty eating or drinking.
>   - Have sweaty, pale, or blue-tinged skin.
>   - Sit upright and lean forward to breathe.
>   - Gasp for breath or make a noise when breathing in.

Asthma

Asthma is a recurring condition in which certain stimuli trigger the airways to temporarily narrow, resulting in difficulty breathing.

- Difficulty breathing is often accompanied by a high-pitched sound made when the child breathes out (wheezing).
- Symptoms suggest the diagnosis, especially in children who have family members with asthma.

- Avoiding triggers, using inhaled drugs before exercising, and using inhaled drugs to open the airways during an attack can help.
- If an attack is very severe, children should be treated in a hospital.
- There are two types of drugs for asthma:
    - One type, taken when needed, stops an asthma attack or is used before exercise.
    - The second type, taken daily, help prevent asthma attacks.
    - Some children take drugs every day to prevent attacks.

Although asthma can develop at any age, it most commonly begins in children, particularly in the first 5 years of life. Some children continue to have asthma into the adult years; in others, it resolves. More children than ever have asthma. Doctors are not sure why this is so, although there are theories. More than 6% of children in the United States have been diagnosed with asthma, a 75% increase in recent decades. The rate soars to 40% among some populations of urban children.

Most children with asthma are able to participate in normal childhood activities, except during flare-ups. A smaller number of children have moderate or severe asthma and need to take daily preventive drugs to enable them to engage in sports and normal play.

For unknown reasons, children with asthma respond to certain stimuli (triggers) in ways that children without asthma do not. There are many potential triggers, and most children respond to only a few. Triggers include indoor irritants, such as strong odors and irritating fumes (perfume, tobacco smoke); outdoor pollution; cold air; exercise; emotional distress; viral respiratory infections; and various substances to which the child is allergic, such as animal dander, dust or house dust mites, molds, and outdoor pollen. In some children, specific triggers for flare-ups cannot be identified.

These triggers all result in a similar response; certain cells in the airways release chemical substances. These substances cause the airways to become inflamed and swollen and stimulate the muscle cells in the walls of the airways to contract. Repeated stimulation by these chemical substances increases mucus production in the airways, causes shedding of the cells lining the airways, and enlarges the muscle cells in the walls of the airways. Each of these responses contributes to a sudden narrowing of the airways (asthma attack). In most children, the airways return to normal between asthma attacks.

DID YOU KNOW?

- Asthma usually begins by age 5 years.
- The percentage of children with asthma in the United States is increasing.
- One half or more children with asthma outgrow it by adulthood.
- Children of mothers who smoked cigarettes during pregnancy are more likely to develop asthma.
- Having bronchiolitis with wheezing during subsequent viral infections does not increase the risk of developing asthma during adolescence.
- Mild asthma may cause only a cough (particularly during exercise or at night).
- Most children with asthma can exercise without restriction.

Risk Factors

Doctors do not completely understand why some children develop asthma, but a number of risk factors are recognized. A child with one asthmatic parent has a 25% risk of developing asthma; if both parents have asthma, the risk increases to 50%. Children whose mothers smoked during pregnancy are more likely to develop asthma. In the United States, children in urban environments are more likely to develop asthma, particularly if they are from lower socioeconomic groups. Although asthma affects a higher percentage of black children than white, the role that genetic aspects of race play in the increasing rate of asthma is controversial because black children are also more likely to live in urban areas. Children who are exposed to high concentrations of allergens, such as dust mites or cockroach feces, at an early age are more likely to develop asthma. Children who have bronchiolitis (see page 366) at an early age often wheeze with subsequent viral infections. The wheezing may at first be interpreted as asthma, but these children are no more likely than others to have asthma during adolescence.

Symptoms and Diagnosis

As the airways narrow in an asthma attack, the child develops difficulty breathing, typically accompanied by wheezing. Wheezing is a high-pitched noise heard when the child breathes out. Not all asthma attacks produce wheezing, however. Mild asthma, particularly in very young children, may result only in a cough; some older children with mild asthma tend to cough only when exercising or when exposed to cold air. Some children with asthma cough a lot at night but don't have obvious wheezing. Also, children with extremely severe asthma may not wheeze because there is too little air flowing to make a noise. In a severe attack, breathing becomes visibly difficult, wheezing usually becomes louder, the child breathes faster and with greater effort, and the ribs stand out when the child breathes in (inspiration). With very severe attacks, the child gasps for breath and sits upright, leaning forward. The skin is sweaty and pale or blue-tinged.

Children with frequent severe attacks sometimes have a slowing of their growth, but their growth usually catches up to that of other children by adulthood.

A doctor suspects asthma in children who have repeated episodes of wheezing, particularly when family members are known to have asthma or allergies. Children with frequent wheezing episodes who do not improve with asthma treatment may be tested for other disorders, such as cystic fibrosis or gastroesophageal reflux. Older children sometimes undergo pulmonary function tests, although in most children, pulmonary function is normal between flare-ups.

Prognosis, Prevention, and Treatment

One half or more of children with asthma outgrow the condition. Those with more severe disease are more likely to have asthma as adults.

Asthma flare-ups can often be prevented by avoiding whatever triggers a particular child's attacks. Parents of children with allergies usually are advised to remove feather pillows, carpets, drapes, upholstered furniture, stuffed toys, and other potential sources of dust and allergens from the child's room. Secondhand tobacco smoke often worsens symptoms in children with asthma and a smoking ban in the house and car is critical. If a particular allergen cannot be avoided, a doctor may try to desensitize the child using allergy shots, although the benefits of allergy shots for asthma are not well known. Because exercise is so important for a child's development, doctors usually recommend that a child not avoid exercise, but rather use an asthma drug immediately before exercising if needed.

Older children or adolescents known to have asthma often use a peak flow meter—a small device that records how fast a person can blow out air—to measure the degree of airway obstruction. This measurement can be used as an objective assessment of the child's condition.

Treatment of an acute attack consists of opening the airways (bronchodilation) and stopping inflammation. The treatment depends on the severity of the asthma. Children with mild asthma (often called "mild intermittent asthma") tend to have symptoms only intermittently either during the day or night and are treated with drugs when they develop symptoms. A variety of inhaled drugs open the airways (bronchodilators). Typical examples are albuterol and ipratropium. Older children and adolescents usually can take these drugs using a metered-dose inhaler. Children younger than 8 years or so often find it easier to use an inhaler with a spacer or holding chamber attached. Infants and very young children sometimes can use an inhaler and spacer if an infant-sized mask is attached. Those who cannot use inhalers may receive inhaled drugs at home through a mask connected to a nebulizer, a small device that creates a mist of drug using compressed air. Inhalers and nebulizers are equally effective at delivering the drug. Albuterol is best given in inhaled form, not by mouth. Sometimes severe asthma attacks are treated with corticosteroids by mouth.

Children with more severe "persistent asthma" may require daily preventive medications (inhaled or orally) to try to prevent asthma attacks from occurring. Different drugs are used depending on the frequency and severity of the child's attacks. Children with persistent asthma usually use inhaled drugs, such as cromolyn or nedocromil, or a low dose of an inhaled corticosteroid every day to help prevent attacks. These drugs block the release of the chemical substances that inflame the airways, and they reduce inflammation. Long-acting theophylline preparations are an alternative for prevention in some children but are now infrequently used. Children with even more frequent or more severe attacks may also receive one or more other drugs, including long-acting bronchodilators such as salmeterol, leukotriene modifiers such as zafirlukast or montelukast, and inhaled corticosteroids. If these drugs do not prevent severe attacks, children may need to take corticosteroids by mouth for short periods. Children who experience attacks mainly during exercise usually inhale a dose of bronchodilator just before exercising.

Children with very severe attacks are treated in the hospital with bronchodilators given in a nebulizer very frequently, sometimes even continuously. Sometimes doctors use injections of epinephrine, a bronchodilator, in children with very severe attacks if they are not able to breathe enough of the nebulized mist. Doctors usually give corticosteroids intravenously to children having a severe attack.

Because asthma is a long-term condition with a variety of treatments, doctors work with parents and children to make sure they understand the condition as well as possible. Parents and children should learn how to determine the severity of an attack, when to use drugs and a peak flow meter, when to call the doctor, and when to go to the hospital. Doctors may give families an "asthma action plan" which outlines steps to take when the child develops severe symptoms. It is extremely important for families to adhere to the drug plan. Often children will stop taking their daily preventive asthma drug if they haven't had an asthma attack in some time; unfortunately this may lead to an asthma attack. It is important to talk to the child's doctor about changes in asthma drugs.

Parents and doctors should inform school nurses, childcare providers, and others of the child's condition and drugs being used. Some children may be permitted to use inhalers in school as needed, and others must be supervised by the school nurse.

Bronchiolitis

Bronchiolitis is a contagious viral infection of the airways of infants and young children that causes difficulty in breathing, especially breathing out.

- Bronchiolitis causes airways to narrow in children younger than 18 months.
- Cold symptoms are followed by difficulty breathing and wheezing.
- Symptoms and results of a physical examination suggest the diagnosis.
- Most children recover at home in a few days, but those with severe symptoms should be hospitalized and sometimes require oxygen.

Bronchiolitis is most often caused by the respiratory syncytial virus, although other viruses, such as the parainfluenza and adenoviruses, are sometimes involved. Infection with these viruses causes inflammation of the airways. The inflammation causes the airways to narrow, obstructing the flow of air into and out of the lungs.

Bronchiolitis typically affects children younger than 18 months of age and is most common in infants younger than 6 months. During the first year of life, bronchiolitis affects about 11 of every 100 children, although during some epidemics a much higher proportion of infants is affected. Winter and early spring are the peak seasons for bronchiolitis. The disease may be more common in infants whose mothers smoke cigarettes, particularly those who smoked during pregnancy, and it appears to be less common among breastfed infants. Parents and older siblings can be infected with the same virus, but for them the virus usually causes only a mild cold.

Symptoms and Diagnosis

Bronchiolitis starts with symptoms of a cold—runny nose, sneezing, mild fever, and some coughing. After several days, the child develops difficulty breathing, with a worsened cough. Usually the child has a high-pitched sound on breathing out (wheezing). In most infants, the symptoms are mild; even though the infant may breathe somewhat rapidly and be very congested, he is alert, happy, and eating well. Other infants are more severely affected, breathing rapidly, shallowly, and with difficulty. Sometimes the child turns blue from a lack of oxygen. The rapid breathing creates a difficulty in drinking, which may result in dehydration.

A doctor bases the diagnosis on the symptoms and the physical examination. Sometimes the doctor swabs mucus from deep inside the nose to try to identify the virus in the laboratory.

DID YOU KNOW?

- The virus that usually causes bronchiolitis in young children usually causes only a mild cold in parents and older siblings.
- At birth, premature infants and infants at high risk of breathing problems may be given an antiviral drug to prevent bronchiolitis.

Prognosis and Treatment

Most children recover at home in 3 to 5 days. During the illness, frequent small feedings of clear fluids may be given. Increasing difficulty in breathing, bluish skin discoloration, fatigue, and dehydration indicate that the child should be hospitalized. Children with congenital heart or lung disease or an impaired immune system may be hospitalized sooner and are far more likely to become quite ill from bronchiolitis. With proper care, the chance of dying of bronchiolitis is low, even for children who need to be hospitalized.

In the hospital, oxygen levels are monitored with a sensor on a finger, toe, or an earlobe, and oxygen is given by an oxygen tent or face mask. A ventilator may be needed to assist breathing. Intravenous fluids are given if the child cannot drink adequately. Inhaled drugs that open the airways (bronchodilators) may be tried, although their effectiveness in bronchiolitis is questionable. The antiviral drug ribavirin may be given by nebulizer to infants who are premature or who have other conditions that put them at high risk for severe breathing problems, such as congenital heart or lung disease, cystic fibrosis, or AIDS. Antibiotics are not helpful.

Croup

Croup (laryngotracheobronchitis) is a contagious viral infection of the upper airways that causes cough and sometimes difficulty breathing, especially breathing in.

- Cold symptoms are followed by a barking cough and sometimes difficulty breathing, especially breathing in.
- Usually, giving children plenty of fluids and using a humidifier result in recovery in a few days.
- Children who do not respond to these measures should be hospitalized and are usually given drugs through a nebulizer, corticosteroids, and sometimes oxygen.

Croup is a viral infection that causes swelling of the lining of the airways, particularly the area just below the voice box (larynx). Parainfluenza virus is the most common cause, but croup can be caused by other viruses, such as the respiratory syncytial virus or an influenza virus. Although croup is most common in the fall and winter, it occurs throughout the year. Croup primarily affects children 6 months to 3 years of age, although it occasionally affects those younger or older. Croup caused by an influenza virus may be particularly severe and is more likely to occur in children between the ages of 3 and 7. The disease is usually spread by breathing in airborne droplets containing viruses or by having contact with objects contaminated by these droplets.

Symptoms and Diagnosis

Croup usually starts with symptoms of a cold—runny nose, sneezing, mild fever, and some coughing. Then the child develops a frequent, unusual-sounding cough, which is described as "brassy" or barking. Sometimes swelling of the airway causes difficulty breathing, which is most noticeable on breathing in (inspiration). In severe croup, there may be a loud squeaking noise (stridor) heard with each inspiration. All symptoms are typically much worse at night and may awaken the child from sleep. The child's condition often improves in the morning and worsens again the next night. A doctor distinguishes croup by its characteristic symptoms, especially the sound of the cough.

DID YOU KNOW?

- Taking a child with croup outside to breathe the cold night air may help him breathe more easily.

Treatment

A child who is mildly ill with croup may be cared for at home and usually recovers in 3 to 4 days. The child should be made comfortable, given plenty of fluids, and allowed to rest because fatigue and crying can worsen the condition. Home humidifying devices (for example, cool-mist vaporizers or humidifiers) may reduce drying of the upper airways and ease breathing. The humidity can be raised quickly by running a hot shower to steam up the bathroom. Carrying the child outside to breathe cold night air may also open the airways significantly—something parents often discover when the child's breathing returns to normal by the time they arrive at the hospital. Sometimes the doctor may prescribe an oral corticosteroid medication to the child for use for one night.

Children who do not respond to these measures need to be taken to the hospital. Children with increasing or continuing difficulty in breathing, rapid heart rate, fatigue, or bluish skin discoloration need to be hospitalized. In the hospital, oxygen is given when levels of oxygen in the blood are low. Doctors usually treat the child with epinephrine given in a nebulizer and corticosteroids given by mouth or injection. These drugs help shrink swollen tissue in the airways. Children who improve with these treatments may be sent home, although children with more severe cases should remain in the hospital. Antibiotics are used only in the rare situation when a child with croup also develops a bacterial infection. Rarely, a ventilator is needed. Fortunately, the vast majority of children with croup recover completely.

Cystic Fibrosis

Cystic fibrosis is a hereditary disease that causes certain glands to produce abnormal secretions, resulting in tissue and organ damage, especially in the lungs and the digestive tract.

- Children may cough, wheeze, and have difficulty breathing, frequent respiratory tract infections, and intestinal blockages.
- Weight gain and growth may be delayed.
- Cystic fibrosis has many serious complications and shortens life.

- The diagnosis is suggested by symptoms and confirmed by a sweat test or genetic tests.
- Ideally, a team of various practitioners provides treatment, which includes psychologic support, drugs and maneuvers to relieve respiratory symptoms, increased nutrition, and sometimes surgery.

Cystic fibrosis occurs in about 1 of 3,300 white infants and in 1 of 15,300 black infants. It is rare in Asians. Cystic fibrosis is equally common in boys and girls.

Cystic fibrosis results when a child inherits two defective copies (mutations) of a particular gene. This gene controls the production of a protein that regulates the transport of chloride and sodium (salt) across cell membranes. Worldwide, about 3 of 100 white people carry one defective copy of the gene; thus, they are carriers but they themselves do not get sick. About 3 of 10,000 white people inherit two defective copies of the gene; thus, they develop cystic fibrosis. In these people, chloride and sodium transport is disrupted and dehydration and increased stickiness of secretions occur.

Cystic fibrosis affects many organs throughout the body and nearly all the glands that secrete fluids into a duct (exocrine glands). The secretions are abnormal in different ways, and they affect gland function differently. In some glands, such as the pancreas, the secretions are thick or solid and may block the gland completely. Eventually, the pancreas can become scarred. The mucus-producing glands in the airways of the lungs produce abnormal secretions that clog the airways and allow bacteria to multiply. The sweat glands and small salivary glands in the cheek (parotid glands) secrete fluids containing more salt than normal.

Symptoms

The lungs are normal at birth, but breathing problems can develop at any time afterward. Thick secretions eventually block the small airways, which leads to inflammation and thickening of their walls. As larger airways fill with secretions, areas of the lung collapse and contract (a condition called atelectasis), and the lymph nodes enlarge. All these changes make breathing increasingly difficult and reduce the lungs' ability to transfer oxygen to the blood. Respiratory tract infections occur because of bacterial growth in the bronchial secretions and walls of the airways.

The blockage of pancreatic ducts and intestinal glands leads to digestive problems, including poor absorption of fats, proteins, and vitamins. This, in turn, can lead to nutritional deficiencies, and slower than expected growth. Some children have episodes of intestinal obstruction when abnormal stool contents block the bowel.

About 15 to 20% of newborns who have cystic fibrosis have meconium ileus, a serious obstruction of the small intestine. Meconium ileus is sometimes complicated by a twisting of the intestine on itself (volvulus—see page 99) or incomplete development of the intestine. Newborns who have meconium ileus almost always develop other symptoms of cystic fibrosis later. Meconium can also temporarily obstruct the large intestine in some newborns with cystic fibrosis, so that a bowel movement may not occur in these newborns until 1 to 2 days after birth.

The first symptom of cystic fibrosis in an infant who does not have meconium ileus is often a delay in regaining birth weight or poor weight gain at 4 to 6 weeks of age. Inadequate amounts of pancreatic enzymes, which are essential for proper digestion of fats and proteins, lead to poor digestion in most infants with cystic fibrosis. The infant has frequent, bulky, foul-smelling, oily stools and may have a distended abdomen and small muscles. Weight gain is slow despite a normal or large appetite.

About half the children with cystic fibrosis are first taken to the doctor because of frequent coughing, wheezing, and respiratory tract infections. Coughing, the most noticeable symptom, is often accompanied by gagging, vomiting, and disturbed sleep. As the disease progresses, the chest becomes barrel-shaped, and insufficient oxygen may make the fingers clubbed and the nail beds bluish. Polyps may form in the nose. The sinuses may fill with thick secretions, leading to chronic or recurrent sinus infections.

When a child with cystic fibrosis sweats excessively in hot weather or because of a fever, dehydration may result because of the increased loss of salt and water. A parent may notice the formation of salt crystals or even a salty taste on the child's skin.

Adolescents often have slowed growth, delayed puberty, and declining physical endurance. As the disease progresses, lung infection becomes a major problem. Recurrent bronchitis and pneumonia gradually destroy the lungs.

DID YOU KNOW?

- Cystic fibrosis is the most common life-shortening hereditary disease among white people in the United States.
- In the United States, about one half of children with cystic fibrosis live to age 33 or older.

Complications

Inadequate absorption of the fat-soluble vitamins—A, D, E, and K—may lead to night blindness, rickets, anemia, and bleeding disorders. In about 20% of untreated infants and toddlers, the lining of the rectum protrudes through the anus, a condition called rectal prolapse. Infants with cystic fibrosis who have been fed soy protein formula or breast milk may develop anemia and swelling of the extremities, because they are not absorbing enough protein.

Complications in adolescents with cystic fibrosis include a rupture of the small air sacs of the lung (alveoli) into the pleural space (the space between the lung and chest wall). This rupture can allow air to enter into this space (pneumothorax), which collapses the lung. Other complications include heart failure and massive or recurrent bleeding in the lungs.

Complications that develop mainly during adulthood can include diabetes mellitus, severe damage or cirrhosis of the liver, gallstones, infertility, and problems during pregnancy.

Diagnosis

The diagnosis of cystic fibrosis is usually confirmed in infancy or early childhood, but cystic fibrosis goes undetected until adolescence or early adulthood in about 10% of people with the disease.

The diagnosis is suggested by one or more of the typical symptoms and is confirmed by a sweat test. This test measures the amount of salt in sweat. The drug pilocarpine is placed on the skin to stimulate sweating, and filter paper or thin tubing is placed against the skin to collect the sweat. The concentration of salt in the sweat is then measured. A salt concentration higher than normal confirms the diagnosis in children who have symptoms of cystic fibrosis or who have a sibling with cystic fibrosis. Although the results of this test are valid any time after a newborn is 48 hours old, collecting a large enough sweat sample from a newborn younger than 3 or 4 weeks old may be difficult. The sweat test, which can be performed on an outpatient basis, can also confirm the diagnosis in older children and young adults.

In newborns with cystic fibrosis, the level of the digestive enzyme, trypsin, in the blood is high. This enzyme level can be measured in a small drop of blood collected on a piece of filter paper. Measurement of this enzyme in addition to sweat testing and genetic testing is the basis of cystic fibrosis newborn screening programs performed in many parts of the world. Many states in the USA are now testing for cystic fibrosis as part of their routine newborn screening.

The diagnosis of cystic fibrosis can also be confirmed by genetic testing in a child who exhibits one or more typical symptoms or has a history of cystic fibrosis in a sibling. Finding two abnormal cystic fibrosis genes (mutations) confirms the diagnosis. However, because genetic testing can confirm only a small percentage of the more than 1,000 different kinds of cystic fibrosis mutations, failure to detect two mutations does not exclude a diagnosis of cystic fibrosis. The disease can be diagnosed prenatally by performing genetic testing on the fetus using chorionic villus sampling or amniocentesis.

Because cystic fibrosis can affect several organs, other tests may be helpful. If pancreatic enzyme levels are reduced, an analysis of the child's stool may reveal low or undetectable levels of the digestive enzymes trypsin and chymotrypsin (both secreted by the pancreas) or high levels of fat. If insulin secretion is reduced, blood sugar levels are high. Pulmonary function tests may show that breathing is compromised and are good indicators of how well the lungs are functioning. Also, chest x-rays and computed tomography may be helpful to document lung infection and the extent of lung damage.

Carrier testing can be performed for prospective parents. In particular, relatives of a child with cystic fibrosis may want to know if they are likely to have children with the disease, and they should be offered genetic testing and counseling. A small blood sample is taken to help determine if a person has a defective cystic fibrosis gene. Unless both prospective parents have at least one such gene, their children will not have cystic fibrosis. If both parents carry a defective cystic fibrosis gene, each pregnancy has a 25% chance of producing a child with cystic fibrosis.

Treatment

A child with cystic fibrosis should have a comprehensive program of therapy directed by an experienced doctor—usually a pediatrician—along with a team of other doctors, nurses, a dietitian, social worker, genetics counselor, psychologist, and physical and respiratory therapists. The goals of therapy include long-term prevention and treatment of lung and digestive problems and other complications, maintenance of good nutrition, and encouragement of physical activity.

Children with cystic fibrosis need psychologic and social support because they may be unable to participate in normal childhood activities and may feel isolated. Much of the burden of treating a child with cystic fibrosis falls on the parents, who should receive adequate information and training so they can understand the condition and the reasons for the treatments.

The treatment of lung problems focuses on preventing airway blockage and controlling infection. Children should receive all routine vaccinations plus the pneumococcal vaccine and, because viral infections can further damage the lungs, the influenza vaccine.

Respiratory therapy—consisting of postural drainage, percussion, hand vibration over the chest wall, and encouragement of coughing—is started at the first sign of lung problems. Parents of a young child can learn these techniques and carry them out at home every day. Older children can carry out respiratory therapy independently, using special breathing devices or a compression vest.

Often, children are given drugs that help prevent their airways from narrowing (bronchodilators). Those with severe lung problems and a low level of oxygen in the blood may need supplemental oxygen therapy. In general, those with respiratory failure do not benefit from using a ventilator; however, occasional, short periods of mechanical ventilation in the hospital may help during an acute infection, after a surgical procedure, or while waiting for a lung transplant.

An aerosol drug, such as dornase alfa (recombinant human deoxyribonuclease I) is widely used to help thin the pus-filled mucus; such a drug makes it easier to cough up sputum, improves lung function, and may also decrease the frequency of serious respiratory tract infections. Mist tents have no proven benefit. Corticosteroids can relieve symptoms in infants with severe bronchial inflammation and in children who have narrowed airways that cannot be opened with bronchodilators. Sometimes, a nonsteroidal anti-inflammatory drug (NSAID) is used to slow the deterioration of lung function.

Respiratory tract infections must be treated as early as possible with antibiotics. At the first sign of a respiratory tract infection, a sample of coughed-up sputum or a throat culture is collected and tested, so that the infecting organism can be identified and the doctor can choose the drugs most likely to control it. *Staphylococcus aureus* and *Pseudomonas* species are commonly found. An antibiotic often can be given by mouth, or an antibiotic such as tobramycin can be given in an aerosol mist. However, if the infection is severe, intravenous antibiotics may be needed. This treatment often requires hospitalization but may be given at home. Taking oral or aerosol antibiotics intermittently or continuously may help prevent recurrences of infection and slow the decline in lung function.

Children who have pancreatic problems must take pancreatic enzyme replacements with each meal; a powder (for infants) and capsules are available. Special milk formulas containing protein and fats that are easy to digest may help infants who have pancreatic problems and poor growth.

The diet should provide enough calories and protein for normal growth. The proportion of fat should be normal to high. Because children with cystic fibrosis need more calories, they need to consume higher than normal amounts of fat to ensure adequate growth. Children with cystic fibrosis should take double the usual recommended daily amount of fat-soluble vitamins (A, D, E, and K) in a special formulation that is more easily absorbed. When they exercise, have a fever, or are exposed to hot weather, they should increase their salt intake. Children who cannot absorb enough nutrients from food may need supplementary feedings through a tube inserted into the stomach or small intestine.

At some time, surgery may be needed to treat a pneumothorax, chronic sinus infection, severe chronic infection restricted to one area of the lung, bleeding from blood vessels in the esophagus, gallbladder disease, or obstruction of the intestine. Massive or recurrent bleeding in the lung can be treated by a procedure called embolization, which blocks off the bleeding artery.

Liver transplantation has been successful for severe liver damage. Double lung transplantation for severe lung disease is becoming more routine and more successful with experience and improved techniques. One year after transplantation of both the right and the left lungs, about 75% of people are alive, and their condition is much improved.

Gene therapy, in which normal cystic fibrosis genes are delivered directly to the airways, holds great promise for treating cystic fibrosis. However, this therapy is only available in research trials. A number of new drugs, delivered by mouth or aerosol, are under investigation.

Prognosis

The severity of cystic fibrosis varies greatly from person to person regardless of age; the severity is determined largely by how much the lungs are affected. In the United States, half of the people with cystic fibrosis live about 33 years or longer. The outlook for longer survival has improved steadily over the past 50 years, mainly because treatments can now postpone some of the changes that occur in the lungs. Improved nutrition and comprehensive, coordinated medical care have helped immensely. Long-term survival is somewhat better in males and in people whose initial symptoms were restricted to the digestive tract; however, long-term survival is also significantly better in people who do not develop pancreatic problems.

However, deterioration is inevitable, leading to loss of lung function and eventually death. People with cystic fibrosis usually die of respiratory failure after many years of deteriorating lung function. A small number, however, die of heart failure, liver disease, bleeding into the airways, or complications of surgery. Despite their many problems, people with cystic fibrosis usually attend school or work until shortly before death.

CHAPTER 20

Digestive Disorders

Children can develop a variety of digestive disorders. All digestive disorders involve varying degrees of pain, vomiting, or changes in appetite and bowel function. The challenge for parents is to provide information that will help their doctors distinguish serious from nonserious disorders and, in some cases, to help their children adjust to chronic disorders that need medical attention over time.

DID YOU KNOW?

- Severe vomiting or diarrhea can cause dehydration requiring a doctor's attention.
- Parents should be alert for danger signs of severe dehydration:
  - ◆ Inability to keep down liquids
  - ◆ Lethargy
  - ◆ Dry mouth and lack of tears
  - ◆ No urine output for 6 hours or more.

Gastroenteritis

Gastroenteritis is inflammation of the digestive tract that results in vomiting and diarrhea, sometimes accompanied by fever or abdominal cramps.

- Gastroenteritis usually results from a viral, bacterial, or parasitic infection.
- If severe, the disorder can cause dehydration and an electrolyte imbalance.
- Diagnosis may include tests to identify any suspected bacteria or parasites.
- Encouraging children to wash their hands and teaching them to avoid improperly prepared or stored foods help prevent gastroenteritis.
- Fluids and sometimes electrolyte solutions are given at home, but sometimes children need to be taken to a doctor.

Gastroenteritis, sometimes called "stomach flu," is common in children. Severe gastroenteritis results in dehydration and an imbalance of blood chemicals (electrolytes) because of a loss of body fluids in the vomit and diarrhea. Although gastroenteritis is rarely serious when proper medical care is available, in developing countries it can be extremely serious; millions of children die each year from diarrhea caused by gastroenteritis.

Causes

A wide variety of viruses, bacteria, and parasites cause gastroenteritis. However, viruses (such as rotavirus) are a far more common cause than are bacteria (such as *Escherichia coli, Vibrio cholerae, Salmonella,* or *Shigella*) or parasites (such as *Giardia*).

Children usually contract viral gastroenteritis from other children who have had or who have been exposed to it, such as those in childcare centers, schools, and other crowded settings. Viral gastroenteritis is generally spread from hand to mouth but can also be spread by sneezing and spitting. It spreads particularly easily because of the way children play—putting hands and fingers in and near their mouths and then touching toys and each other.

Children can contract bacterial gastroenteritis from eating mayonnaise, dairy products, meat, and other foods that have not been refrigerated. Improper preparation of food, especially undercooking, can lead to gastroenteritis. Gastroenteritis contracted in this way is sometimes called "food poisoning." Children can also contract bacterial or parasitic gastroenteritis from swallowing contaminated water, such as from wells, streams, and swimming pools, and while traveling in developing countries.

Occasionally, gastroenteritis results when children eat things they are not supposed to, such as plants and vitamin pills. Rarely, gastroenteritis results because of an allergic condition (eosinophilic gastroenteritis) or from contact with animals at petting zoos.

DID YOU KNOW?

- Worldwide, millions of children die each year from diarrhea caused by gastroenteritis.
- Fluids given by mouth should be continued if children can keep the fluids down for at least 10 minutes before vomiting again.

Symptoms and Diagnosis

Symptoms are usually a combination of vomiting, diarrhea, abdominal cramps, fever, and poor appetite. Usually, vomiting predominates early in the illness, and diarrhea becomes more prominent later, but some children have both at the same time. The stools may be bloody if certain bacteria are a cause. These symptoms eventually improve in children who drink enough fluids. Children who are slightly dehydrated are thirsty, but seriously dehydrated children become listless, irritable, or lethargic, and may stop drinking. Infants are much more likely than older children to develop these serious side effects.

A doctor bases the diagnosis of gastroenteritis on the child's symptoms and on the parents' responses to questions about what the child has been exposed to. Diagnostic tests are not usually needed because most forms of gastroenteritis get better by themselves over a short time. Doctors who suspect a bacterial or parasitic infection may order additional tests, including stool and blood tests, and ones that measure white blood cells. Dehydrated children require blood tests to help doctors guide treatment.

Prevention and Treatment

The best way to prevent gastroenteritis is to encourage children to wash their hands and to teach them to avoid improperly prepared or stored foods. A vaccine to prevent rotavirus infection is now available in the United States.

Once a child has gastroenteritis, parents should encourage the child to take frequent sips of water and to try to take small amounts of juices and soups, which contain both fluids and electrolytes. If gastroenteritis persists longer than 12 to 24 hours, or the child cannot hold down juice, electrolytes usually should be replaced. Electrolyte replacement is done at home using nonprescription electrolyte solutions available as powders and liquids in pharmacies and some grocery stores.

For a vomiting child, the parents wait about 10 minutes and give the child a few sips of a liquid. If the liquid is not vomited, the sips are repeated every 10 or 15 minutes, increasing the amount given to an ounce or two after an hour or so. These larger amounts can be given less often, about every hour. Liquids are absorbed very quickly, so if the child vomits more than 10 minutes after drinking, most of the fluid was absorbed and fluids should be continued. The amount of liquid to give a child depends on the child's age, but generally should be about $1^{1}/_{2}$ to $2^{1}/_{2}$ ounces of solution for each pound the child weighs in a 24-hour period. If the child's vomiting or diarrhea improves while drinking electrolyte solutions, parents may try resuming a diet of juice, soups, and soft foods like bananas and applesauce the next day.

Children with diarrhea but little vomiting are fed their normal diet, with extra liquid given to make up for the fluid lost in the diarrhea.

Danger signs include inability to keep down even sips of liquid or signs of dehydration (such as lethargy, dry mouth, lack of tears, and no output of urine for 6 hours or more). Such children should see the doctor immediately. Children without such signs should see the doctor if symptoms last more than 1 or 2 days. If the dehydration is severe the doctor may give the child intravenous fluids.

Antidiarrheal drugs such as loperamide are not usually recommended for children; there is reason to think these may slow the resolution of infection by preventing the body from flushing the virus, bacteria, or parasites out with the stools. Antibiotics are of no value when a viral infection is the cause of gastroenteritis. Doctors give antibiotics only for certain bacteria that are known to respond to these drugs. Antiparasitic drugs may be given for a parasitic infection.

Gastroesophageal Reflux

Gastroesophageal reflux is the backward movement of food and acid from the stomach into the esophagus and sometimes into the mouth.

- Reflux may be caused by the infant's position during feeding, overfeeding, exposure to cigarette smoke or caffeine, or an abnormality of the digestive tract.
- Reflux may cause vomiting, excessive spitting up, damage to the esophagus, or breathing problems.
- If reflux is suspected, doctors may try treating it before diagnostic tests are done.
- Feeding and sleeping positions may be changed, and exposure to cigarette smoke and caffeine is eliminated.
- Antacids, proton pump inhibitors, or metoclopramide may be given.

Nearly all infants have episodes of gastroesophageal reflux; "burping up" that babies do after feeding is considered normal. Gastroesophageal reflux becomes a concern when it interferes with feeding and nutrition, causes poor weight gain, damages the esophagus, leads to breathing difficulties, or continues beyond infancy into childhood.

Causes

Healthy infants have reflux for many reasons. The circular band of muscle that normally keeps stomach contents from entering the esophagus (lower esophageal sphincter) is not fully developed in infants, allowing stomach contents to move backward into the esophagus. Being held flat during a feeding (instead of more upright) or lying down after a feeding promotes reflux. Overfeeding predisposes to reflux, as does exposure to cigarette smoke or caffeine in breast milk, both of which relax the lower esophageal sphincter and can cause the child to become irritable and eat poorly. Less commonly, children may have an anatomic abnormality, such as narrowing of the esophagus or abnormal position of the intestines (malrotation), which makes reflux even more likely. Immaturity of the nerves that control stomach emptying can also lead to gastroesophageal reflux. Milk allergy is a rare cause.

Symptoms

The most obvious symptoms of gastroesophageal reflux in infants are vomiting and excessive spitting up. Less obviously, the infant may be irritable, may not eat well, or may have "spells" of twisting and posturing that may be confused with seizures.

Reflux usually improves gradually until the age of 1 or 2 years, when the child starts eating solid foods and is able to eat on his own in an upright position. However, reflux occasionally leads to complications. Some infants lose weight. Some develop a low red blood cell count (anemia) because of bleeding from the esophagus, and some inhale (aspirate) stomach acid and food into their lungs. Aspiration of stomach contents can cause pneumonia, asthma, periods when breathing stops (apnea), a slow heart rate, and, extremely rarely, infant death.

Older children are usually able to describe chest pain or heartburn when they have gastroesophageal reflux. Chronic cough, hoarseness, hiccups, ear pain, and high-pitched breathing (stridor) may also be subtle signs of reflux in older children. In some children, reflux may be a cause of chronic ear infection (serous otitis media—see page 406).

Diagnosis and Treatment

Diagnosis of gastroesophageal reflux can be difficult when the symptoms are not obvious. Some doctors recommend simple measures to see if an infant's symptoms improve before ordering more extensive tests. For example, a doctor may recommend thicker, smaller, and more frequent feedings with more frequent burpings. Eliminating a child's exposure to cigarette smoke and caffeine also helps. Laying the child to sleep on the stomach or on an angle with the head elevated also reduces reflux. This is one of the few exceptions to the general recommendation that infants be put to sleep on their back and should be done only when a doctor specifically recommends it. Occasionally, doctors recommend a change of formula to determine if cow's milk or a formula ingredient is contributing to the infant's problem.

Some doctors recommend that infants whose symptoms do not improve with these measures and most older children try drug treatment for a short time before undergoing diagnostic testing. Drugs for reflux are generally safe and effective. Antacids neutralize stomach acid, and histamine-2 blockers and proton pump inhibitors suppress acid production by the stomach and improve reflux symptoms, at least temporarily. Promotility drugs, such as metoclopramide, stimulate the stomach to move its contents forward rather than backward and may tighten the lower esophageal sphincter.

Various tests can be used to diagnose reflux. X-rays taken after swallowing barium help doctors determine if the anatomy of the esophagus and stomach is normal. In addition, a diary can be kept to record the child's symptoms. Information from this diary, combined with monitoring of the level of acid in the esophagus through a small flexible tube that has been passed through the nose (called a "PH probe"), helps doctors determine if reflux episodes are the cause of the symptoms. A form of radionuclide imaging called a gastric emptying study can reveal to what degree stomach contents move forward appropriately or reflux backward. Examination of the esophagus using a flexible viewing tube (endoscopy) allows doctors to see if the esophagus is inflamed or bleeding. Rarely, examination of the voice box (larynx) and airways through a flexible viewing tube (bronchoscopy) gives information that helps doctors decide if reflux is a likely cause of lung or breathing problems.

Peptic Ulcer

A peptic ulcer is erosion of the lining of the stomach or duodenum due to excess stomach acid, breakdown of the stomach's protective lining, or both.

Peptic ulcers are much less common in children than in adults. As with adults, use of nonsteroidal anti-inflammatory drugs (NSAIDs) and infection with *Helicobacter pylori* bacteria can lead to the formation of peptic ulcers. Children whose parents have peptic ulcers are more likely to have ulcers, as are those whose parents smoke. Adolescents who drink alcohol or smoke are also more likely to develop ulcers. Children of any age can develop ulcers when they are extremely sick, such as after severe burns, injuries, and illnesses.

Infants with ulcers may be fussy and irritable around feedings. Ulcers in older children usually cause abdominal pain. At any age, peptic ulcers can perforate, bleed, or lead to obstruction. The diagnosis and treatment of peptic ulcers and their complications are the same in children as in adults.

Intussusception

Intussusception is the telescoping of one portion of the intestine into another, causing obstruction of the bowel and blockage of its blood flow.

- Abdominal pain comes and goes but eventually becomes constant and may be accompanied by vomiting or fever.
- A barium enema enables doctors to diagnose intussusception and may correct it.
- Sometimes surgery is needed.

Intussusception is an uncommon cause of abdominal pain that typically affects children between the ages of 6 months and 2 years. It can occasionally affect older children. In most cases, the cause is unknown. Rarely, thickening of the intestinal wall due to a diverticulum, polyp, or tumor may lead to intussusception.

Symptoms

Intussusception usually causes sudden pain in a child who is otherwise healthy. The pain initially comes and goes, and the child may pull his legs up to his trunk during pain spasms. The child may return to normal activities between episodes, but the pain eventually becomes constant. Some children simply become irritable or listless and apathetic between episodes of pain. After a time, the child may vomit, pass stools with blood and mucus ("currant jelly" stools), or develop a fever. If unrecognized and untreated, intussusception can cause death of bowel tissue, which spreads bacteria from the gut into the bloodstream.

Diagnosis and Treatment

A doctor may suspect intussusception based on the child's symptoms and a physical examination. X-rays may be useful, but results are normal about one third of the time. Ultrasound is better, but a barium enema can both diagnose and treat intussusception. With a barium enema, the doctor instills barium and air into the child's rectum and then takes x-rays. The pressure of the barium and air pushes the collapsed portion of the intestine back into place. Sometimes just air without barium is used. When this procedure is successful, the child can be sent home from the hospital after a short time. Parents are advised to watch for symptoms because intussusception can recur in the next 1 to 2 days.

Surgery is needed if the barium enema is not successful in correcting the intussusception, if the child is too ill to tolerate a barium enema, if the child has recurrences of the condition, or if complications occur. In the case of a recurrence, surgery is performed not only to correct the condition but also to look for a polyp, tumor, or other abnormality that could explain why the intussusception recurred.

Appendicitis

Appendicitis is inflammation and infection of the appendix.

- Pain—near the appendix or throughout the abdomen— may make children irritable or listless.
- If untreated, an infected appendix can rupture, causing a serious infection in the abdomen.
- Diagnosis in children may be difficult and may require blood tests, ultrasonography or computed tomography (CT), and repeated physical examinations.
- An infected appendix is surgically removed.

The appendix is a small finger-length portion of intestine that does not appear to have any essential bodily function. Appendicitis is a medical emergency that requires surgery. Appendicitis is rare in children younger than 1 year but becomes more common as children grow older and is most common in adolescents.

Appendicitis seems to develop when the appendix becomes blocked either as a result of infection in the digestive tract or elsewhere in the body or, less commonly, as a result of obstruction with hard feces. In either case, the appendix becomes infected. If an infected appendix is unrecognized or untreated, the appendix can rupture, creating a pocket of infection outside the intestine (abscess) or spilling contents of the intestines into the abdomen (peritonitis).

Symptoms and Diagnosis

Appendicitis almost always causes pain. The pain may start in the middle of the abdomen, near the navel, and gradually move to the lower right area of the abdomen. However, children younger than 2 years are often not able to complain of pain and are therefore more likely to be irritable or listless. They may lose consciousness partly or completely if a delay in diagnosis has led to rupture of the appendix with peritonitis. Older children sometimes develop diffuse abdominal pain rather than pain in the specific area of the appendix.

The diagnosis of appendicitis in children can be challenging for many reasons. The child can have gastroenteritis, Meckel's diverticulum, intussusception, or Crohn's disease, all of which may cause symptoms similar to those of appendicitis. The child may not have a fever or elevated white blood cell count, which are signs of infection. And the child may ask for food rather than avoid it in the way adults with appendicitis typically do.

Doctors who suspect appendicitis usually give intravenous fluids and antibiotics while waiting for results of blood tests. They may order ultrasound or computed tomography (CT) scans to see inside the abdomen. Repeated physical examinations help a doctor determine whether the condition is improving or getting worse and make a decision about treatment.

DID YOU KNOW?

- Appendicitis rarely occurs in children younger than 1 year but becomes more common as children grow older.
- Occasionally, doctors find a normal appendix during surgery for suspected appendicitis.

Treatment

The best treatment for appendicitis is surgical removal of the inflamed appendix (appendectomy). Appendectomy is fairly simple and safe, requiring a hospital stay of 2 to 3 days. If the appendix has ruptured, the doctor removes it and may wash out the abdomen with fluid, give antibiotics for several days, and watch for complications, such as infection and bowel blockage. About 10 to 20% of the time, surgeons discover a normal appendix while performing an appendectomy. This is not considered a medical error because the consequences of delaying surgery when appendicitis is suspected are serious. When the appendix is found to be normal, the surgeon looks within the abdomen for another cause of the pain. The doctor may remove the normal appendix so that the child will never develop appendicitis.

Meckel's Diverticulum

Meckel's diverticulum is a saclike outpouching of the wall of the small intestine present in some children at birth.

- Most children have no symptoms, but sometimes rectal bleeding occurs or the diverticulum becomes infected.
- Radionuclide scanning is the best way to diagnose the disorder.
- If the diverticulum causes symptoms, it is surgically removed.

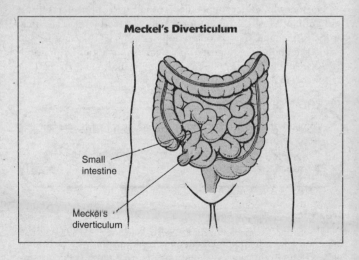

Meckel's Diverticulum

Small intestine

Meckel's diverticulum

About 3% of infants are born with Meckel's diverticulum. People can live their whole lives without ever knowing they have Meckel's diverticulum, but occasionally the abnormality can cause problems.

Symptoms and Diagnosis

Most children with Meckel's diverticulum have no symptoms, and many adults learn they have the condition only after surgeons discover it while performing surgery for another reason. The most common symptom in children younger than 2 years is painless rectal bleeding, which comes from ulcers in the small intestine caused by acid secreted by the diverticulum. Because of the bleeding, stools may appear bright red or brick- or currant jelly-colored because of a mixture of blood and mucus. Or they may appear black because of the breakdown of blood. Only rarely is the bleeding so severe that the child needs emergency attention.

DID YOU KNOW?

- Some people never find out that they have Meckel's diverticulum.

Sometimes, the diverticulum can become inflamed or infected, a condition called diverticulitis. Diverticulitis caused by a Meckel's diverticulum causes severe pain, abdominal tenderness, and sometimes vomiting and can easily be confused with appendicitis.

It is often difficult for doctors to diagnose Meckel's diverticulum. Blood tests, x-rays, computed tomography (CT), and barium enemas are not usually helpful. The best test is an imaging study called a Meckel radionuclide scan, in which a substance is given intravenously and is taken up by the diverticulum and detected by a camera.

Treatment

No treatment is needed for a diverticulum that does not cause symptoms. A bleeding diverticulum or one that causes symptoms must be surgically removed. If a Meckel's diverticulum is found in a child during an operation being performed for another reason, it is generally removed to prevent future complications.

Hemorrhagic Colitis

Hemorrhagic colitis is a type of gastroenteritis in which certain strains of the bacterium Escherichia coli (E. coli) *infect the large intestine and produce a toxin that causes bloody diarrhea and other serious complications.*

- Usually, this disorder results from eating undercooked beef or drinking unpasteurized milk or juice.
- Children have severe abdominal cramps and bloody diarrhea, and a few develop a life-threatening complication.
- Stool specimens are tested for strains of *E. coli*.
- Drinking plenty of fluids is usually all that is needed, but if complications develop, intensive care in a hospital is often required.

Hemorrhagic colitis is most common in children (and older people) but can occur in people of all ages.

In North America, the most common strain of *E. coli* that causes hemorrhagic colitis is found in the intestines of healthy cattle. Outbreaks can be caused by eating undercooked beef, especially ground beef, or by drinking unpasteurized milk. Unpasteurized juice can also be contaminated. The disease can be transmitted from child to child, particularly among children in diapers, and by touching cattle and other farm animals.

E. coli toxins damage the lining of the large intestine. If they are absorbed into the bloodstream, they can also affect other organs, such as the kidneys.

Symptoms

Severe abdominal cramps begin suddenly along with watery diarrhea, which typically becomes bloody within 24 hours. The diarrhea usually lasts 1 to 8 days. Fever is usually absent or mild but occasionally can exceed 102°F (38.9°C).

A few children with hemorrhagic colitis develop a severe complication called hemolytic-uremic syndrome. Symptoms include anemia (characterized by fatigue, weakness, and light-headedness) caused by the destruction of red blood cells (hemolytic anemia), a low platelet count (thrombocytopenia), and sudden kidney failure. Some children with hemolytic-uremic syndrome also develop complications of nerve or brain damage, such as seizures or strokes. These complications typically develop in the second week of illness and may be preceded by increasing fever.

Hemolytic-uremic syndrome is more likely to occur in children under age 5 (and in older people).

DID YOU KNOW?

- Antibiotics are not used to treat hemorrhagic colitis, an *E. coli* infection, because they increase the risk of serious complications.

Diagnosis and Treatment

A doctor usually suspects hemorrhagic colitis when a child has bloody diarrhea. To make the diagnosis, a doctor has stool specimens tested for strains of *E. coli*. Other tests, such as colonoscopy, may be performed if a doctor suspects that other diseases may be causing the bloody diarrhea.

The most important aspect of treatment is drinking enough fluids. Sometimes so much fluid is lost, however, that a doctor has to replace them intravenously. The diet is kept bland, with cooked cereals, bananas, rice, applesauce, and toast. Antibiotics are not given because they increase the risk of developing hemolytic-uremic syndrome. Children who develop complications are likely to require intensive care in the hospital and may need kidney dialysis.

Constipation

Constipation is the difficult and infrequent passing of hard, dry stools.

- Constipation is a functional problem that is often made worse by a lack of fiber in the diet.
- Children may feel intermittent abdominal discomfort or pain when stools are passed.
- Increased fiber in the diet, adequate intake of liquids, regular opportunities to defecate, and sometimes enemas and stool softeners can help.

Parents often worry about how often their children have bowel movements. However, constipation generally does not have any serious consequences and should be a concern only when passing stools becomes painful and leads to withholding of stools (encopresis), or when constipation causes other symptoms.

Causes and Symptoms

Constipation is extremely common in children. The most common cause is insufficient amounts of fruits, vegetables, whole grains (fiber), and fluids in the child's diet.

Children who are constipated often report intermittent abdominal discomfort. After a time, parents may notice soiling of the child's underwear because liquid stool from the intestine involuntarily leaks around hard stool in the rectum. Small amounts of blood may appear from small erosions (fissures) caused by the passage of hard stools. Occasionally, constipation can lead to difficulty with urination.

DID YOU KNOW?

- Soiled underwear is sometimes a sign of constipation.

Treatment

Minor cases of constipation can be treated by increasing the child's dietary fiber, either with whole grains and fruits or with a supplement such as psyllium. Good hydration is important. Sometimes, reducing the intake of milk helps constipation. Children become distracted and typically do not sit long enough on the toilet to pass constipated stools. They need to be guided to sit an adequate time on the toilet at regular intervals—at least twice a day—so they can establish a routine that gives them the opportunity to defecate fully. Parents can use enemas and stool softeners, such as mineral oil or milk of magnesia, to facilitate this process if necessary. A new medicine that contains polyethylene glycol is often prescribed for childhood constipation.

Children accustomed to withholding their stools may need several months of stool softeners to get them reconditioned to soft, comfortable stools.

Recurring Abdominal Pain

Recurring abdominal pain is abdominal pain that occurs 3 or more times over a period of at least 3 months.

- The cause is usually anxiety or other psychologic distress but may be a physical disorder.
- Pain due to a physical disorder, unlike pain due to psychologic distress, recurs at predictable times, in the same location, and sometimes at night and may be accompanied by other symptoms.
- Doctors ask the parent and child about the pain and other symptoms and examine the child to look for physical causes.
- Physical causes are treated, or measures to relieve psychologic distress (sometimes including antidepressants or anti-anxiety drugs) are taken.

About 1 in 10 school-aged children has recurring abdominal pain. It is most common in children between the ages of 8 and 10 and is rare in those younger than 4. Recurring abdominal pain is slightly more common among girls than boys and is fairly common among girls in early adolescence.

Causes

In most children, recurring abdominal pain is caused by anxiety and other psychologic distress that is a result of stress at school, with friends, between parents, or within a family. A significant number of children with the condition are depressed. About 1 in 10 have an identifiable physical cause, usually from a digestive or genitourinary tract disorder. The absence of a physical cause in most children is sometimes frustrating for parents.

DID YOU KNOW?

- About 1 in 10 school-aged children has recurring abdominal pain, usually due to psychologic distress.

When recurring abdominal pain has no physical cause, concerned responses from parents and teachers can make the pain better or worse to the extent that it favorably alters stressful situations to which the child is responding. For example, pain that distracts family members from arguing, garners attention for the child, or takes the child away from school or other stressful settings may be an effective way for a child to relieve anxieties he could otherwise not control. Importantly, most children do not intentionally use their symptoms to communicate distress to their parents or teachers. Rather, it is a symptom of true and significant emotional discomfort.

The most serious cause of recurring abdominal pain is sexual abuse. However, routine stresses at school or home are far more common causes of recurring abdominal pain than is sexual abuse.

SOME PHYSICAL CAUSES OF RECURRING ABDOMINAL PAIN

Intestinal disorders
- Hiatal hernia
- Esophagitis
- Peptic ulcer disease
- Hepatitis (inflammation of the liver)
- Cholecystitis (inflammation of the gallbladder) or cholelithiasis (gallstones)
- Irritable bowel syndrome
- Pancreatitis (inflammation of the pancreas)
- Inflammatory bowel disease (Crohn's disease, ulcerative colitis)
- Meckel's diverticulum
- Chronic appendicitis
- Intussusception
- Parasitic infection (for example, giardiasis)
- Tuberculosis of the intestine
- Celiac sprue
- Constipation
- Lactase deficiency

Genitourinary disorders
- Structural anomalies
- Urinary tract infection
- Normal monthly ovulation (in girls)
- Menstrual cramps (in girls)
- Pelvic inflammatory disease (in girls)

- Ovarian cysts (in girls)
- Endometriosis (in girls)

General illnesses

- Heavy metal poisoning (lead)
- Henoch-Schönlein purpura
- Sickle cell disease
- Food allergy
- Porphyria
- Familial Mediterranean fever
- Hereditary angioedema
- Abdominal migraine

Symptoms

Recurring abdominal pain caused by a physical condition generally recurs at predictable times or in the same location. It may be brought on by certain activities or foods and may worsen over days to months. Often, although not always, the pain may awaken the child from sleep. The child may also have other symptoms, such as loss of appetite, weight loss, changes in the form and color of bowel movements, constipation or diarrhea, vomiting of food or blood, swelling of the abdomen, recurring or persistent fever, jaundice, blood in the stools, or discomfort with urination.

Recurring abdominal pain without a clear physical cause is generally less likely to recur at predictable times and in the same location. It is often described in vague terms and occasionally disappears for weeks or months. It seldom disturbs a child during sleep but may wake him up early. The child can often be distracted from the pain by activities he enjoys; this is less likely to be the case when there are physical causes of the pain.

Diagnosis

The doctor asks the parent and child a series of questions about the character of the pain and about any symptoms that occur with it. The doctor also performs a physical examination, often including a rectal examination, looking for clues for a physical cause. The interview and examination give the doctor the information to decide what additional tests, if any, the child should undergo. Often, the doctor may strongly suspect a psychologic cause just from the child's answers to questions and from observing the child and parents in the interview.

Some possible tests for recurring abdominal pain range from urine and blood tests, which can detect infection, to more invasive procedures, such as colonoscopy, which can detect inflammation and other abnormalities within the large intestine. However, invasive tests are rarely needed. Given the frequency with which depression or anxiety accompanies symptoms of recurring abdominal pain, many doctors consider psychologic assessment to be the most important test.

Treatment

Physical causes of recurring abdominal pain are treated for the specific disorder responsible. When a physical cause for the child's symptoms cannot be found, a doctor may suspect a psychologic cause. Treatment then depends on good communication and a trusting relationship with the doctor as well as periodic monitoring of the child's symptoms.

The child should be supported in efforts to return to a full range of activities, including school. Teachers have a large role to play in limiting the child's withdrawal from activities with peers and in helping the child resolve conflicts related to school. A child who needs to leave class because of pain should be allowed to visit the school nurse for only a limited time. With the parents' permission, the nurse can give the child a mild pain reliever, such as ibuprofen or acetaminophen, if necessary. Typically, a child will request time in the nurse's office 1 or more times a day during the first week or two of treatment. Over time, the behavior becomes less frequent. Generally, when the parents stop treating the child as different or ill, pain with a psychologic cause initially worsens but then improves.

A child whose abdominal pain has no physical cause may be helped by seeing the doctor at regular intervals—weekly, monthly, or every other month—depending on the child's needs. In some cases, the doctor may prescribe antidepressants or antianxiety drugs, often in collaboration with a mental health professional. This treatment may result in a reduction or disappearance of the child's symptoms, but it is not always successful. Some children may develop new physical symptoms or emotional difficulties, or they may express unresolved emotional difficulties with new symptoms, such as a headache.

If the pain persists despite all efforts, especially if the child is severely depressed or if there are significant psychologic problems at home, the child may need to see a mental health professional.

Irritable Bowel Syndrome

Irritable bowel syndrome is a disorder of motility of the entire digestive tract that causes abdominal pain, constipation, or diarrhea.

- Symptoms may be triggered by stress, diet, drugs, hormones, or minor irritants.
- Doctors may do tests to exclude other more serious disorders.
- Eating small meals frequently, avoiding triggers, and, for some children, increasing dietary fiber may relieve symptoms.
- Eliminating foods that worsen symptoms can help, as can, for some children, limiting consumption of sorbitol (an artificial sweetener), fructose, or fat.

In irritable bowel syndrome, the digestive tract is especially sensitive to many stimuli. Stress, diet, drugs, hormones, or minor irritants may cause the digestive tract to contract abnormally, usually leading to diarrhea. Periods of constipation may occur between bouts of diarrhea.

The brain has enormous control over the digestive system. Stress, anxiety, depression, fear, virtually any strong emotion, or an emotional disorder can lead to diarrhea, constipation, and other changes in bowel function and can worsen a flare-up (bout or attack) of irritable bowel syndrome.

During a flare-up, the contractions of the digestive tract become stronger and more frequent, and the resulting rapid transit of food and stool through the large intestine often leads to diarrhea. Crampy pain seems to result from the strong contractions of the large intestine and the increased sensitivity of the receptors in the large intestine that sense stretching and pressure. Flare-ups almost always occur when a child is awake. They rarely wake a child from sleep.

For some children, high-calorie meals or a high-fat diet may be to blame. For other children, wheat, dairy products, coffee, tea, or citrus fruits appear to aggravate the symptoms, but it is not clear whether these foods are actually the cause. Others find that eating too quickly or eating after too long a period without food stimulates a flare-up of irritable bowel syndrome.

DID YOU KNOW?

- Irritable bowel syndrome usually causes diarrhea, sometimes alternating with constipation.
- Symptoms that wake a child from sleep are probably not due to irritable bowel syndrome.

Symptoms

Symptoms are commonly triggered by eating, often by eating too quickly or too much. A few minutes later, diarrhea with pain occurs. The diarrhea may begin very suddenly and with extreme urgency. Sometimes the urgency is so strong that the child loses control and cannot reach a bathroom in time. Diarrhea during the night is rare. Sometimes constipation and diarrhea alternate. Mucus often appears in the stool. The pain may come in bouts of continuous dull aching or cramps, usually over the lower abdomen. The child may experience bloating, gas, nausea, headaches, fatigue, depression, anxiety, and difficulty concentrating. Having a bowel movement often relieves the pain. Periods of stress may worsen symptoms.

Diagnosis

Most children with irritable bowel syndrome appear healthy. A physical examination generally does not reveal anything unusual except sometimes tenderness over the large intestine. Doctors generally perform some tests—for example, blood tests, a stool examination, and a sigmoidoscopy—to differentiate irritable bowel syndrome from Crohn's disease, ulcerative colitis, collagenous and lymphocytic colitis, and the many other diseases that can cause abdominal pain and changes in bowel habits. These test results are usually normal, although the stool may be watery. The results of a sigmoidoscopy, which may cause spasms and pain, are normal. Sometimes other tests—such as abdominal ultrasound, x-rays of the intestines, or a colonoscopy—are done.

Treatment

The treatment for irritable bowel syndrome differs from child to child. If particular foods or types of stress that trigger symptoms can be identified, these triggers should be avoided if possible. For most children, especially those who tend to be constipated, regular physical activity helps keep the digestive tract functioning normally.

In general, a normal diet is best. Many children do better eating frequent, smaller meals rather than less frequent, larger meals (for example, five or six small meals rather than three large meals a day). Children with bloating and increased gas (flatulence) should avoid beans, cabbage, and other foods that are difficult to digest. Sorbitol, an artificial sweetener used in dietetic foods and in some drugs and chewing gums, should not be consumed in large amounts. Fructose, a common constituent of fruits, berries, and some plants, should be eaten only in small amounts. A low fat diet helps some people. People who have both irritable bowel syndrome and lactase deficiency should not eat dairy products.

Some children benefit from eating more fiber. They can take a tablespoon of raw bran with plenty of water and other fluids at each meal, or they can take psyllium mucilloid supplements with two glasses of water. However, increasing the dietary fiber may aggravate some symptoms, such as flatulence and bloating.

Antispasmodic drugs, which slow the function of the digestive tract, are frequently prescribed but have not been proved effective in all children with irritable bowel syndrome. Antidiarrheal drugs help children with diarrhea. Aromatic oils, such as oil of peppermint, often relieve symptoms of flatulence and cramping.

If an emotional disorder is identified as the cause, treatment of the disorder may relieve irritable bowel syndrome symptoms. Such treatment may include the use of antidepressants, mild tranquilizers, psychotherapy, hypnosis, and behavior modification techniques.

Pinworm Infection

Pinworm infection (enterobiasis) is a disease caused by intestinal roundworms.

- Pinworm eggs are ingested, then hatch into roundworms in the intestine.
- Most children have no symptoms, but some feel an itching sensation around the anus or vagina.
- The diagnosis is made by finding the eggs or worms, which exit the anus to lay eggs.
- One dose of an antibiotic followed by a second dose 2 weeks later cures the infection.
- Reinfection is common because eggs can contaminate clothing and other objects.

Pinworms are the most common parasite in children in the United States.

Infection follows ingestion of pinworm eggs (ova). Eggs can be transferred from the area around the anus of an infected child to clothing, bedding, or toys. Eggs can survive outside the body for as long as 3 weeks at normal room temperature. These eggs can be transferred, often by the fingers, to the mouth of another child, who swallows them. Eggs sometimes are ingested in contaminated food. Children may reinfect themselves by transferring eggs from the area around the anus to their mouth. Children who suck their thumbs are at increased risk of infection.

After ingestion, the eggs hatch in the intestinal tract, and young worms migrate to the rectum and lower intestine. Pinworms mature in the lower intestine within 2 to 6 weeks. The female worm then moves to the area around the anus, usually at night, to deposit her eggs. The eggs are deposited in a sticky, gelatinous substance that adheres to the skin. The eggs and gelatinous material cause itching.

DID YOU KNOW?

- Pinworms are hair-thin but can be seen with the naked eye.
- Clothing, bedding, and toys should be washed and the environment should be vacuumed to try to eliminate any eggs.

Symptoms and Diagnosis

Most children who carry pinworms have no symptoms. Some, however, feel an itching sensation around the anus and scratch the area. The skin can become raw and superficially infected with bacteria. In girls, pinworms may cause vaginal itching and irritation.

The diagnosis of pinworm infection is made by finding the worms or eggs. The search for adult pinworms is best conducted by examining the child's anus about 1 to 2 hours after the child has been put to bed for the night. The worms are white and hair-thin, but they wiggle and are visible to the naked eye. Eggs can be obtained by patting the skin folds around the anus with the sticky side of a strip of transparent tape in the early morning before the child wakes up. The tape can be taken to the doctor for microscopic examination.

Treatment

A single dose of mebendazole, albendazole, or pyrantel, repeated after 2 weeks, effectively cures pinworm infection. Many doctors recommend treating the entire family. Despite drug therapy, reintroduction of the disease is common after treatment. Clothing, bedding, and toys should be washed and the environment vacuumed to try to eliminate any eggs. Anti-itching creams or ointments applied directly to the area around the anus may provide relief from itching.

CHAPTER 21

Ear, Nose, and Throat Disorders

Ear, nose, and throat disorders are extremely common in children. Ear infections occur almost as often as the common cold. They can occur behind the eardrum (in the middle ear, otitis media) or in front of the eardrum (in the outer ear, otitis externa). Throat infections are not usually serious, but they make children uncomfortable and can lead to missed school days and multiple doctor visits. Other disorders, such as hearing deficits and neck masses, affect fewer children but are potentially serious. In general, any abnormality of a child's ear, nose, or throat that does not improve within several days should be evaluated by a doctor.

Middle Ear Infections

- Viruses or bacteria from nasal secretions enter the middle ear through the eustachian tubes.
- Very young children are especially susceptible.
- Children may have a fever, cry, be irritable, sleep badly, or pull at their ears.
- To check the eardrum, doctors use a viewing tube (otoscope), often with a tube and rubber bulb that is used to squeeze air into the ear and thus see whether the eardrum can move.

- Acetaminophen or ibuprofen (to relieve fever and pain) and antibiotics may be given.
- If the infection persists or recurs despite antibiotics, tubes to ventilate the middle ear or surgery to repair the eardrum may be needed.

Middle ear infections are extremely common between the ages of 3 months and 3 years and often accompany the common cold. Young children are susceptible to middle ear infections for several reasons. The eustachian tube, which balances pressure within the ear, connects the middle ear with the nasal passages. In older children and adults, the tube is more vertical, wider, and fairly rigid, and secretions that pass into it from the nasal passages drain easily. But in younger children, the eustachian tube is more horizontal, narrower, and less rigid. The tube is more likely to become obstructed by secretions and to collapse, trapping those secretions in or close to the middle ear and impairing middle ear ventilation. Any viruses or bacteria in the secretions then multiply, causing infection. Viruses and bacteria can move back up the short eustachian tube of infants, causing middle ear infections.

DID YOU KNOW?

- Most middle ear infections are caused by the same viruses that cause the common cold, though many are caused by bacteria.
- Breastfeeding partially protects infants from ear infections because breast milk contains antibodies from the mother.
- Exposure to cigarette smoke increases the risk of middle ear infections.
- Many doctors recommend avoiding antibiotics at first, to see if the ear infection resolves on its own, and then prescribe antibiotics if not resolved.

Besides differences in anatomy of the ear, infants at about the age of 6 months become more susceptible to infection because they lose protection from their mother's antibodies, which they received through the placenta before birth. Breastfeeding appears to partially protect children from ear infections because the mother's antibodies are contained in breast milk. Children also become more sociable around this time and may develop viral infections by touching other children and objects and putting their fingers in their mouth and nose; these infections may in turn lead to middle ear infections. Exposure to cigarette smoke further increases the risk for middle ear infections, as does the use of a pacifier, both of which may impair the function of the eustachian tube and affect middle ear ventilation. Attendance at childcare centers increases the risk of exposure to the common cold and hence to ear infections.

Middle ear infections can resolve relatively quickly (acute), or they can recur or persist over a long time (chronic).

ACUTE MIDDLE EAR INFECTION

Acute middle ear infection (also called acute otitis media) is most often caused by the same viruses that cause the common cold. Acute infection may also be caused by bacteria found in the mouth and nose, such as *Streptococcus pneumoniae, Haemophilus influenzae*, and *Moraxella catarrhalis*. An infection initially caused by a virus sometimes leads to a bacterial infection.

Infants with acute middle ear infections have fever, crying or irritability that sometimes cannot be explained, and disturbances in sleep. They may also have a runny nose, cough, vomiting, and diarrhea. Infants and children who cannot fully communicate may pull at their ears. Older children are usually able to tell parents that their ear hurts or that they cannot hear well.

Commonly, fluid may accumulate behind the eardrum and persist after the acute infection has resolved (serous otitis media). Rarely, acute middle ear infection leads to more serious complications. Rupture of the eardrum can cause drainage of blood or fluid from the ear. Infection of the bone surrounding the ear (mastoiditis) is a rare disorder that can cause pain; infection of the inner ear (labyrinthitis) can cause dizziness and deafness; and infection of the tissues surrounding the brain (meningitis) or brain abscesses (collections of pus) can cause seizures and other neurologic problems. Recurring infections can promote growth of skinlike tissue through the eardrum (cholesteatoma). Cholesteatoma can damage the bones of the middle ear and cause hearing loss.

Doctors diagnose acute middle ear infections by looking for bulging and redness of the eardrum with an otoscope. They may need to clean wax from the ear first so they can see more clearly. Doctors may use a rubber bulb and tube attached to the otoscope to squeeze air into the ear to see if the eardrum moves. If the eardrum does not move or moves only slightly, then infection may be present.

Acetaminophen or ibuprofen is effective for fever and pain. Doctors used to give antibiotics to all children with acute middle ear infections. However, they now realize that many acute middle ear infections improve without antibiotics. Thus, many doctors use antibiotics (such as amoxicillin with or without clavulanate) only when the child does not improve after a brief period of time or if there are signs that the infection is not getting better.

Ventilating Tubes: Treating Recurring Ear Infections

Ventilating (tympanostomy) tubes are tiny, hollow plastic or metal tubes that are placed in the eardrum through a small slit. These tubes equalize the pressure between the environment and the middle ear. Doctors recommend ventilating tubes for children who have had recurring ear infections (acute otitis media) or chronic fluid collections in their middle ears (serous otitis media).

Placement of ventilating tubes is a common surgical procedure, performed in a hospital or doctor's office. After the procedure, children usually go home within a few hours. The tubes usually fall out on their own after a few months, although some types stay in for a year or more. Children with ventilating tubes may wash their hair and go swimming, but some doctors recommend that the children not submerge their head completely in water without using earplugs. Drainage of fluid from the ears indicates an infection and the doctor should be notified.

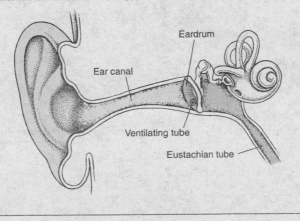

CHRONIC MIDDLE EAR INFECTION

Chronic middle ear infection occurs as a result of repeated acute infection or when recurring infections damage the eardrum or lead to formation of a cholesteatoma, which in turn promotes more infection. Chronic ear infections are more likely among children who are exposed to cigarette smoke, use pacifiers, and attend group day care centers. For children with chronic ear infections, doctors may recommend daily antibiotics for several months. If infection persists or recurs despite the use of antibiotics, or if chronic infections have led to eardrum damage or formation of cholesteatoma, doctors may recommend ventilating (tympanostomy) tubes, eardrum repair, or surgical removal of the cholesteatoma.

Serous Otitis Media

Serous otitis media is fluid accumulation behind the eardrum.

- Fluid may remain after a middle ear infection resolves or may accumulate because there is another blockage in the eustachian tube.
- The disorder usually causes no pain but can interfere with hearing and language development.
- Doctors examine the eardrum for changes in appearance.
- The disorder often heals on its own but may require surgery to drain the fluid.

Serous otitis media often occurs after acute otitis media. The fluid that has accumulated behind the eardrum during the acute infection remains after the infection resolves. Serous otitis media may also occur without preceding infection, and may be due to gastroesophageal reflux disease or a blockage of the eustachian tube by infection or enlarged adenoids. Serous otitis media is extremely common in children between the ages of 3 months and 3 years.

Although serous otitis media is painless, the fluid can impair hearing, understanding of speech, language development, learning, and behavior.

Doctors diagnose serous otitis media by looking for changes in the color and appearance of the eardrum and by squeezing air into the ear to see if the eardrum moves. If the eardrum does not move but there is no redness or bulging and the child has few symptoms, then serous otitis media is likely.

Serous otitis media does not improve more quickly when treated with antibiotics or other drugs, such as decongestants, antihistamines, or nasal sprays. The condition often resolves by itself after weeks or months.

If the condition persists without improvement after 3 months, surgery may help. In the United States, doctors perform myringotomy, in which they make a tiny slit in the eardrum, remove the fluid, and insert a small ventilating (tympanostomy) tube in the slit to provide drainage from the middle to the outer ear. Some doctors may perform a myringotomy to remove fluid but not to insert ventilating tubes; this procedure is called tympanocentesis.

Pharyngitis

Pharyngitis is infection of the throat (pharynx) and sometimes the tonsils.

- Viruses are usually responsible, but streptococcal bacteria can cause a more serious form (strep throat).
- Usually, the throat is sore and red, and swallowing is painful.
- Doctors examine the throat and lymph nodes in the neck and, if strep throat is suspected, may take a swab from the throat for testing or culture.
- Strep throat is usually treated with penicillin or another antibiotic.
- Ibuprofen or acetaminophen can relieve pain and fever, and fluids are useful.

Most pharyngitis is caused by the same viruses that cause the common cold. Like the common cold, viral pharyngitis gets better by itself and is a problem only because it makes children miserable and causes them to miss school. Streptococcus bacteria are a less common but more serious cause of pharyngitis ("strep throat"); strep throat is unusual in children younger than 2 years. Pharyngitis is also rarely caused by unusual infections, such as infectious mononucleosis or—in countries with low vaccination rates—diphtheria.

The tonsils (patches of lymphoid tissue at the back of the throat) also can become infected in children with pharyngitis. A doctor may use the term tonsillitis when the tonsils are particularly enlarged. Occasionally, the tonsils remain infected, inflamed, or enlarged (chronic tonsillitis) after an episode of pharyngitis.

Bacterial pharyngitis can cause persistent inflammation, infection, and enlargement of the tonsils (chronic tonsillitis); pus within folds of the tonsils (cryptic tonsillitis); and abscesses in the tissues to the side of the pharynx (lateral pharyngeal abscesses), behind the pharynx (retropharyngeal abscesses), or around the tonsils (peritonsillar abscesses). Some rare complications of streptococcal pharyngitis include rheumatic fever (see page 285), glomerulonephritis, or life-threatening infection of the tissues (necrotizing fasciitis) and bloodstream (toxic shock syndrome).

DID YOU KNOW?

- Most sore throats are caused by the same viruses that cause the common cold.

Symptoms

All children with pharyngitis have sore throats and some degree of pain when swallowing. Ear pain may occur because the throat and ears share the same nerves. The back of the throat and tonsils are typically red, and the tonsils may be enlarged or coated with white discharge.

Children with pharyngitis as part of a head cold have a runny nose, cough, and slight fever. Children with pharyngitis caused by strep throat may have tender, enlarged lymph nodes in the neck and a high fever. Occasionally, a child with strep throat has symptoms of scarlet fever, which include bright white or red changes of the tongue ("strawberry tongue") and a distinctive red skin rash (scarlatiniform rash).

Children with chronic tonsillitis may have a sore throat or discomfort or pain with swallowing.

Diagnosis and Treatment

Doctors suspect pharyngitis when they see redness and white discharge or pus in the back of the throat and when the lymph nodes in the neck are enlarged.

If doctors suspect strep throat, they may take a swab from the back of the throat and send it for two tests: rapid antigen testing and a bacterial culture. Rapid antigen testing can detect strep throat within minutes. If the result of a rapid test is positive, the bacterial culture is not needed. However, if the result of the rapid test is negative, most doctors perform a culture, which takes about 1 to 2 days for results.

Strep throat is usually treated with penicillin, either in a single injection or over 10 days by mouth. Often liquid amoxicillin is used for younger children who cannot swallow pills because liquid penicillin has poor taste. If the child is allergic to penicillin, the doctor may give erythromycin or another antibiotic. Treatment of strep throat and viral pharyngitis includes giving ibuprofen or acetaminophen for pain and fever and encouraging the child to drink fluids. Providing soup is a good way to keep the child well hydrated and nourished when swallowing is painful and before the appetite has returned. Gargling with saltwater or using an anesthetic throat spray may also help to temporarily relieve pain.

Enlarged Tonsils and Adenoids

- Tonsils and adenoids may become enlarged when they are infected, and they sometimes remain enlarged.
- Many children have no symptoms.
- Doctors check the tonsils for redness rather than for size and look for changes in breathing due to enlarged tonsils.
- Antibiotics may be given if a bacterial infection is suspected, and surgery to remove the tonsils and adenoids is recommended for some children.

Tonsils and adenoids are collections of lymphoid tissue that help the body fight infection. The tonsils are located on both sides of the back of the throat and are visible through the mouth. The adenoids are located higher and further back, where the nasal passages connect with the throat, and are not visible through the mouth. However, tonsils and adenoids can become enlarged—for example, when they become infected with bacteria that cause pharyngitis. When this happens, the tonsils become more prominent and the adenoids may block the nose. Usually, the tonsils and adenoids return to normal size once the infection is over. Sometimes they remain enlarged, particularly in children who have had

Locating the Tonsils and Adenoids

The tonsils are two areas of lymphoid tissue located on either side of the throat. The adenoids, also lymphoid tissue, are located higher and farther back, behind the palate, where the nasal passages connect with the throat. The adenoids are not visible through the mouth.

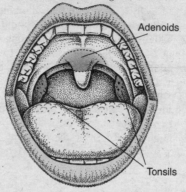

frequent or chronic infections. Extremely rarely, cancer can cause enlargement of lymph nodes, such as tonsils.

Symptoms

Most enlarged tonsils and adenoids cause no symptoms; some degree of tonsillar enlargement is even considered normal in preschool and adolescent children. However, children with enlarged tonsils or adenoids can experience sore throat and discomfort or pain with swallowing. Enlarged adenoids can give the voice a "pinched nose" quality and lead to changes in the shape of the child's palate and the position of the teeth.

Enlarged tonsils and adenoids are considered a problem when they cause more serious effects. They can cause chronic ear

DID YOU KNOW?

- Enlarged tonsils can interfere with breathing, sleeping, and eating.

infections and hearing loss due to obstruction of the eustachian tube and fluid accumulation in the middle ear. They can also cause recurring sinus infections and nosebleeds. Some children have obstructive sleep apnea, with snoring and brief periods without breathing; this can cause low oxygen levels in the blood, frequent waking, and daytime sleepiness. Rarely, obstructive sleep apnea caused by enlarged tonsils and adenoids can lead to serious complications, such as high blood pressure in the lungs (pulmonary hypertension) and changes in the heart that result from pulmonary hypertension (cor pulmonale).

Children with enlarged tonsils can also lose or fail to gain weight, either because of pain and difficulty eating or because of the constant physical effort it takes for them to breathe.

Diagnosis and Treatment

Doctors do not rely on the size of the tonsils alone to make the diagnosis. Very large tonsils may be normal, and chronically infected tonsils may be normal-sized. Instead, doctors look for redness of the tonsils, enlargement of lymph nodes at the jaw and in the neck, and the effect of the tonsils on breathing. The diagnosis of obstructive sleep apnea is suspected when parents report frequent periods without breathing. Doctors may also recommend a polysomnogram (also called a "sleep study"), in which oxygen in the blood is measured and the child is observed while sleeping.

Doctors may give antibiotics if they think a bacterial infection may be the cause of the enlarged tonsils. If antibiotics are not effective or if doctors think antibiotics will not be useful, they may recommend the surgical removal of the tonsils and adenoids (tonsillectomy and adenoidectomy).

Tonsillectomy and adenoidectomy used to be very common operations performed on children in the United States, but they are much less common now that doctors are more aware of which children will benefit from the operation. Children who benefit from surgery include those with obstructive sleep apnea and those whose talking and breathing are extremely uncomfortable. Doctors may also recommend surgery if they think cancer might be a cause of the enlargement, or if the child has had multiple throat or ear infections (defined by some as seven or more infections in 1 year, five or more infections a year over 2 years, or three or more a year over 3 years). A doctor may recommend adenoidectomy alone for ear infections, recurring nasal congestion, or sinus infections.

Tonsillectomy and adenoidectomy have not been shown to decrease the frequency or severity of colds, cough, and other symptoms. These procedures should be performed at least 3 weeks after any infection has cleared.

Tonsillectomy and adenoidectomy are usually performed on an outpatient basis. The surgical complication rate is low, but postoperative pain and difficulty swallowing may last up to a week. Bleeding is a less common complication but may occur anytime from the first day of surgery to the tenth day after surgery.

Hearing Deficits

- Hearing deficits are most often caused by genetic defects in newborns and by ear infections and earwax accumulation in older children.
- Children may not respond to sounds, may have difficulty talking, or may be slow learning to speak, but symptoms may be more subtle and hard to identify.
- Testing for hearing deficits before age 3 months is often recommended.
- A hearing aid is usually needed, but treatment of the cause can reverse some hearing deficits.

About 3 in every 1,000 children are born with severe hearing deficits. One in 10 may be born with deficits that are less severe, and many more who have normal hearing at birth develop hearing deficits before adulthood. Failure to recognize and treat a deficit can seriously impair a child's ability to speak and understand language. The impairment can lead to failure in school, teasing by peers, social isolation, and emotional difficulties.

Causes

Genetic defects are the most common cause of hearing deficits in newborns. Ear infections, including serous otitis media, are the most common cause of hearing deficits in older children. Another common cause is the accumulation of earwax. Other causes in older children are head trauma, loud noise (including loud music), prior use of aminoglycoside antibiotics (such as gentamicin) or thiazide diuretics, certain viral infections (for example, mumps), tumors or traumas that damage the auditory nerve, trauma from pencils or other foreign objects that get stuck deep in the ear, and rarely, autoimmune disease.

RISK FACTORS FOR HEARING DEFICITS IN CHILDREN

Newborns

- Low birth weight (especially less than 3.3 pounds)
- Low Apgar score (lower than 5 at 1 minute or lower than 7 at 5 minutes)
- Low blood oxygen or seizures resulting from a difficult delivery
- Infection with rubella, syphilis, herpes, cytomegalovirus, or toxoplasmosis before birth
- Cranial or facial abnormalities, especially those involving the outer ear and ear canal
- High level of bilirubin in the blood
- Bacterial meningitis
- Bloodstream infection (sepsis)
- Prolonged time spent on a ventilator
- Drugs (aminoglycoside antibiotics, some diuretics)
- History of early hearing loss in a parent or close relative

Older children

All the above, plus:
- Head trauma with skull fracture or loss of consciousness
- Chronic otitis media with cholesteatoma
- Some neurologic disorders, such as neurofibromatosis and neurodegenerative disorders
- Exposure to noise
- Perforation of the eardrum from infection or trauma

Symptoms

Parents may suspect a severe hearing deficit if the child does not respond to sounds or if the child has difficulty talking or delayed speech. Less severe hearing deficits can be more subtle and lead to symptoms that are misinterpreted by parents and doctors. Children who ignore their parents or other people who are talking to them some, but not all of the time, may be doing so because of modest hearing deficits. Children who talk and hear well at home but not in school may have a mild or moderate hearing deficit that is a problem only in the midst of the background noise of a classroom. In general, children who are developing well in one setting but who have significant social, behavioral, language, or learning difficulties in a different setting should be screened for hearing deficits.

DID YOU KNOW?

- Hearing aids are available for children as young as 2 months.

Screening and Diagnosis

Because hearing plays such an important role in a child's development, many doctors recommend that all newborns be tested for hearing deficits by the age of 3 months. This testing is required by law in many states.

Screening is usually done in two parts. First, the child is tested for echoes produced by healthy ears in response to soft clicks made by a handheld device (evoked otoacoustic emissions testing). If this test raises questions about a child's hearing, a second test measures electrical signals from the brain in response to sounds (the auditory brain stem response test [ABR]). The ABR is painless and usually performed while the child is sleeping; it can be performed on children of any age. If results of the ABR are abnormal, the test is repeated in 1 month. If hearing loss is still detected, the child may be fitted with hearing aids and may benefit from placement in an educational setting responsive to children with hearing deficits.

Several different tools are used to diagnose hearing deficits in older children. One involves asking a series of questions to detect delays in a child's normal development or to assess a parent's concern about language and speech development. The child's ears may also be examined for abnormalities. Children between the ages of 6 months and 2 years may be tested for their response to various sounds. Additionally, the response of the eardrum to a range of sound frequencies (tympanometry) may indicate if there is fluid in the middle ear. After the age of 2 years, children can usually demonstrate that they hear and understand speech by following simple commands, and they can be tested for responses to sounds using earphones.

Treatment

Some causes of hearing loss can be treated so that a child can regain hearing. For example, ear infections can be treated with antibiotics or surgery, earwax can be manually removed or dissolved with ear drops, and cholesteatomas can be surgically removed.

In other cases, however, the cause of a child's hearing loss cannot be reversed, and treatment involves use of a hearing aid to compensate for the deficit as much as possible.

Hearing aids are available for children as young as 2 months. Children with a mild or moderate hearing deficit that occurs only in the classroom may also respond well to radio systems that transmit a teacher's voice directly to a set of speakers, hearing aids, or earphones. Cochlear implants (devices placed in the inner ear to stimulate the auditory nerve with an electrical current in response to sounds) are used for children with severe hearing deficits.

A sense of pride has grown in recent years among people in deaf communities concerning their rich culture and alternative forms of communication. Many people oppose the aggressive treatment of hearing deficits on the grounds that it denies children the opportunities available in those communities. Families who wish to consider this approach should discuss it with their doctor.

Objects in the Ears and Nose

- Children may put various objects in their ears or nose, sometimes resulting in pain or infection.

Cotton, pieces of pencils, paper, pebbles, and beans are just a few of the many objects children put in their ears and nose. Insects sometimes crawl into ears and cause significant pain.

Objects in the ear can be removed by flushing with sterile water or saline, using suction, or with forceps or other tools. A doctor may remove an insect by putting a topical anesthetic or mineral oil in the ear, which kills the insect, stops pain, and makes removal easier. Younger, more frightened children may need sedation or general anesthesia for these procedures.

> **DID YOU KNOW?**
>
> • Before objects inserted into an ear or the nose are removed, children may need general anesthesia.

Sharp objects, such as pencils, can perforate the child's eardrum. Perforations require evaluation by an ear specialist, but most heal by themselves over time without loss of hearing.

Objects stuck up the nose are of greater concern because they can obstruct the child's airway, cause infection, and be difficult to remove. Children are often scared to admit they put an object in their nose; many parents become aware of the problem only after the child develops persistent bleeding, a runny nose, a foul-smelling discharge, or difficulty breathing on one side of the nose only.

Doctors use a topical anesthetic and attempt to remove the object using suction or forceps. If these measures do not work, the doctor may need to sedate the child or give general anesthesia to remove the object.

Neck Masses

Neck masses are swellings that change the shape of the neck.

- The neck may swell because of enlarged lymph nodes, infected cysts, injury, or tumors.
- Most masses cause no symptoms, but infected lymph nodes or cysts may be painful.
- Tests may be done to look for the cause.
- Treatment may involve antibiotics, surgery, or no treatment, depending on the cause.

Neck masses are extremely common in children. The most common cause of a neck mass is one or more enlarged lymph nodes. A lymph node may enlarge if it is infected (lymphadenitis) or if there is an infection nearby, such as the throat. Some neck masses are the result of a cyst (a fluid-filled sac) present from birth that is noticed only after it becomes inflamed or infected.

Other causes include swelling due to trauma to the neck, inflammation of the salivary glands, or noncancerous (benign) tumors. Rarely, lymphoma and thyroid tumors or other cancerous (malignant) tumors are causes.

Most neck masses cause no symptoms and are of greater concern to parents than to the children who have them. However, infected lymph nodes or cysts are tender and painful.

DID YOU KNOW?

- Usually, tests are not needed unless a neck mass persists for several weeks.

Because many neck masses are caused by viral infections and disappear without treatment, tests are usually not needed unless a mass persists for several weeks. However, doctors may take a swab from the back of the throat to test for a bacterial infection, or they may perform blood tests to look for such conditions as infectious mononucleosis, leukemia, hyperthyroidism, or bleeding problems. Doctors may also perform x-rays and computed tomography (CT) to determine if the mass is a tumor or a cyst and to determine more precisely how big it is and where it extends. A skin test may determine if tuberculosis is a likely cause, and a biopsy gives the doctor information about whether a cancerous tumor is present.

Treatment of a neck mass depends on the cause. Antibiotics are useful for lymphadenitis and other bacterial infections. Masses caused by viral infections and swelling from trauma gradually disappear with time. Tumors and cysts generally require surgery.

Laryngeal Papillomas

Laryngeal papillomas are rare noncancerous (benign) tumors of the voice box (larynx).

Laryngeal papillomas are caused by human papillomavirus. Although they can occur at any age, papillomas mostly affect children between the ages of 1 and 4 years. Papillomas are suspected when parents notice hoarseness, a weak cry, or other changes in the child's voice. Papillomas recur often and occasionally spread into the windpipe and lungs, obstructing the airway. Rarely, they become cancerous.

Laryngeal papillomas are detected using a laryngoscope to view the voice box. Doctors perform a biopsy in which they take a sample of the papilloma to confirm the diagnosis. Surgery is the usual treatment. Drug treatment is available for papillomas that rapidly recur or spread beyond the larynx. Many children require numerous procedures through childhood to remove the tumors as they reappear. At puberty, some papillomas may disappear on their own.

CHAPTER 22

Eye Disorders

Congenital glaucoma and congenital cataracts (see page 78) are rare disorders that can affect a newborn. Although disorders that most often blur vision, such as nearsightedness, farsightedness, and astigmatism (refractive errors), do develop in children, they more often require treatment among adults. Certain disorders, including misalignment between the two eyes (strabismus), occur more often among children. Refractive errors and strabismus can cause a loss of vision (amblyopia)

DID YOU KNOW?

- Teachers and school nurses are sometimes the first to notice eye disorders in children.
- Vision can be tested in children as young as 3 or 4 years by having them read charts with pictures, figures, or letters.

Amblyopia

Amblyopia is loss of vision that occurs because the brain ignores the image from the eye.

- Amblyopia often results from an eye disorder that causes the eyes to provide different images to the brain, which the brain cannot fuse.
- Depth perception is lost.

419

- Doctors check infants and young children for eye disorders that can cause amblyopia.
- Amblyopia is more likely to be permanent when it begins at an early age or persists for a long time.
- Usually, putting a patch over the normal eye or eye drops to blur vision in the normal eye helps by forcing the brain to use images from the other eye.

In amblyopia, vision loss is usually caused by the abnormal functioning of the brain, not of the eye. It develops only during childhood. Amblyopia is the most common cause of vision loss in children.

People have depth perception because the two images—one from each eye—are recorded from slightly different angles. The brain combines, or fuses, the separate images into one, three-dimensional picture. The brain develops the ability to fuse images only during childhood. When the input to the brain from one eye is of poor quality, such as a relatively blurred image or a double image, the brain suppresses the images, actually ignoring the input from that eye. The person is unaware of the image from one eye even though the eye itself is normal.

Causes

One of the most common causes of amblyopia is misalignment between the two eyes (strabismus). With strabismus, the eyes do not point to the same object, so the brain sees two very different images. These images are too different to be fused. In adults, seeing two different images results in double vision (diplopia). However, in children, if the ability to fuse images has not yet developed, the brain learns to ignore the image from the misaligned eye.

Similarly, poor vision in one eye (due to severe nearsightedness, farsightedness, or even congenital cataract) can impair a child's ability to fuse images. If the images the brain receives from the eyes are vastly different from each other, the brain learns to ignore the image that is more blurred.

Symptoms and Diagnosis

Children with amblyopia may be too young to describe symptoms. Or, a child may not realize that there is a problem, such as

REFRACTIVE ERRORS IN CHILDREN

Refractive errors, such as nearsightedness, farsightedness, and astigmatism, are conditions that result in blurring of vision because the eye cannot focus images precisely on the retina. If only one eye is affected, loss of vision (amblyopia) may develop.

The symptoms of refractive errors are the same in children as adults, although young children are often not able to make their vision problems known. Sometimes a teacher or school nurse may be the first to notice a child is having a problem seeing correctly.

All children need to be checked for refractive errors. Diagnosis is generally similar in children and adults. Children as young as 3 or 4 years can read charts with pictures, figures, or letters used to test vision. Vision is tested in each eye separately to detect loss of vision that affects only one eye. The eye not being tested is covered with a patch or other object.

Refractive errors are generally treated with eyeglasses in children and adults. However, contact lenses are not used often in children prior to adolescence. Many children are not able to care for and clean their contact lenses; inadequate cleaning or sterilization of contact lenses can lead to eye infections. In addition, some children tend to lose contact lenses.

not being able to see out of one eye. Because only one image is perceived, the child lacks depth perception, although the child may not realize it.

In addition to performing a routine eye examination, doctors examine children at the earliest possible age for strabismus and refractive errors, which can cause amblyopia.

Prognosis and Treatment

Sometimes amblyopia is mild and temporary. Amblyopia is more likely to be permanent when it begins at an early age or persists for a long time. Amblyopia from any cause that has not been treated by the age of 10 usually cannot be fully reversed.

The sooner treatment is begun, the more likely amblyopia can be prevented or corrected. Treatment entails forcing the brain to use the visual images from the problem eye. Sometimes this is accomplished by correcting the vision in the problem eye with eyeglasses. The most effective way is to "handicap" the normal, stronger eye by putting a patch over it or giving eye drops that blur vision, such as atropine.

Strabismus

Strabismus (squint, cross-eyes, wandering eye) is a misalignment or wandering of one eye so that its line of vision is not pointed at the same object as the other eye.

- Vision may be double, or the brain may ignore the image from one eye.
- Children should be checked periodically for strabismus, starting when they are only a few months old.
- Strabismus sometimes resolves on its own, but in some cases, eyeglasses, eye drops, or surgery is needed.

The causes of strabismus are varied and include an imbalance in the pull of muscles that control the position of the eyes or poor vision in one eye.

Strabismus: A Misaligned Eye

There are several types of strabismus. In the most common types, an eye turns inward (esotropia or cross-eye) or outward (exotropia or walleye). In this illustration, the child's right eye is affected.

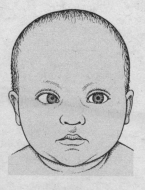

Esotropia

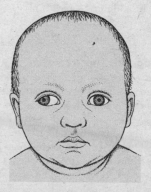

Exotropia

There are several different types of strabismus, each developing in different ways. Some types of strabismus are characterized by inward turning of the eye (esotropia) and some by outward turning (exotropia). Others are characterized by upward turning (hypertropia) or downward turning (hypotropia).

Parents sometimes notice strabismus because the child's eyes appear to be positioned abnormally. Strabismus may cause double vision (diplopia) in the older child or amblyopia in the younger child.

The child should be examined periodically to detect strabismus, beginning at the age of a few months. To examine an infant, a doctor shines a light into the eyes to see if the light reflects back from the same location on each pupil. Older children can be examined more thoroughly; they may be asked to stare at objects, sometimes with one eye covered. The more thorough examination may reveal mild strabismus that would otherwise be impossible to detect. Children with strabismus need frequent examinations by an eye doctor.

If strabismus is mild, treatment may not be needed. However, if strabismus is severe or worsening, treatment is usually required. Treatment depends on the particular characteristics of the strabismus.

Phoria is a tendency for misalignment of the eyes. The tendency is so minor that, for most of the day, the eye muscle and brain can completely correct any misalignment and maintain fusion. Phoria usually does not cause symptoms, but if sufficiently severe, it can lead to strabismus and double vision. Eye doctors can perform tests to diagnose phoria. Usually, no treatment is needed for phorias without symptoms.

Infantile Esotropia: Infantile esotropia is inward turning of the eyes that develops before 6 months of age; it often runs in families and tends to be severe. The eyes often begin to turn in by 3 months of age. The inward turning tends to be constant and is easily noticeable.

Surgery, which is accomplished by changing the pull of the eye muscles, is usually needed to realign the eyes. Repeated operations may be necessary. Rarely, even the best possible treatment may not fully correct strabismus. Occasionally, amblyopia can develop by the age of 2, even with treatment.

Accommodative Esotropia: Accommodative esotropia is inward turning of the eyes that develops between the ages of 6 months and

7 years, most often in 2- to 3-year-olds and is related to optical focusing (accommodation) of the eyes.

The misalignment is the result of how the eyes move when focusing on nearby or distant objects. Children with accommodative esotropia are often farsighted. Although everyone's eyes turn inward when focusing on very close objects, eyes that are farsighted also turn inward when looking at distant objects. In mild cases, the eyes may turn too far inward only when looking at nearby objects. In more severe cases, the eyes turn too far inward all the time. With treatment, accommodative esotropia can usually be corrected. The first treatment tried is usually eyeglasses, which can help the child focus on objects, reducing the tendency for the eyes to turn inward when viewing those objects. Many children outgrow farsightedness and eventually do not need eyeglasses.

Occasionally, drugs (such as echothiophate eye drops) are used to help the eyes to focus on nearby objects. If eyeglasses and eye drops fail to properly align the eyes, surgery may help. Permanent amblyopia develops less often in children with accommodative esotropia than in children with infantile esotropia.

Paralytic Strabismus: In paralytic strabismus, one or more of the eye muscles that move the eye in a different direction become paralyzed. As a result, the muscles no longer work in balance. The eye muscle paralysis is usually caused by a disorder affecting the nerves to the eye muscles. For example, brain injuries or tumors can increase pressure within the skull, compressing nerves to the eye muscles.

In children with paralytic strabismus, movement of the affected eye is impaired only when the eye tries to move in a specific direction, not in all directions. Amblyopia or double vision may develop. The double vision is made worse by looking in directions normally controlled by the paralyzed eye muscles.

Paralytic strabismus may be treated with eyeglasses that contain prism lenses, which bend the light so that both eyes receive nearly the same image. It may heal by itself over time. Alternatively, surgery may be needed. If paralytic strabismus results from another condition affecting the nerves, such as a brain tumor, the other condition also needs to be treated.

Intermittent Exotropia: Exotropia is outward turning of the eyes. The eyes turn out only sometimes (intermittently), usually when the child is looking at distant objects. Intermittent exotropia is detectable after the age of 6 months.

Intermittent exotropia that does not cause troublesome symptoms, such as double vision, may not need treatment. Amblyopia rarely develops. If symptoms are occasionally troublesome, eyeglasses may help. Rarely, a doctor may recommend exercises for the eye muscles. If symptoms worsen despite the use of eyeglasses, surgery may be effective.

Conjunctivitis

Infectious conjunctivitis is inflammation of the conjunctiva caused by viruses, bacteria, or fungi.

- Typically, the eye itches, is red, and produces a discharge.
- Good hygiene, particularly hand washing, can help prevent transmission.
- Symptoms usually resolve on their own.
- Antibiotics or antiviral drugs, usually applied to eyes, may be needed.

The conjunctiva is the thin, transparent lining that covers the back of the eyelid and loops back to cover the white of the eye (sclera), right up to the edge of the cornea, the transparent part of the eye that covers the pupil and iris. The conjunctiva helps protect the eye by keeping small foreign objects and microorganisms out and by helping keep the eye covered with moisture (the tear film).

The most common disorder of the conjunctiva is inflammation (conjunctivitis). There are many causes of inflammation, including infections by bacteria, viruses (such as adenoviruses and occasionally herpesvirus), or fungi. Allergic reactions, chemicals or foreign bodies in the eye, and overexposure to sunlight can also cause inflammation. Conjunctivitis tends to be relatively short-lived, but it sometimes lasts for months or years. Symptoms of conjunctivitis are typically the same, regardless of the cause. They include itching, redness, a discharge, and, occasionally, pain or blurred vision.

DID YOU KNOW?

- Conjunctivitis caused by certain adenoviruses is particularly severe and contagious.

A variety of microorganisms may infect the conjunctiva. The most common organisms are viruses, particularly those from the group known as adenoviruses. Bacterial infections are less-frequent. The term pinkeye, when used by doctors, usually means conjunctivitis caused by viruses or bacteria. Both viral and bacterial conjunctivitis are quite contagious, easily passing from one child to another or from a child's infected eye to the uninfected eye. Fungal infections are rare.

Newborns are particularly susceptible to eye infections, which they acquire from microorganisms in the mother's birth canal. *Neisseria gonorrhoeae*, which causes gonorrhea (a sexually transmitted disease), can spread from mother to newborn during birth and cause conjunctivitis. Another common cause of conjunctivitis in newborns is the bacteria *Chlamydia trachomatis*. Conjunctivitis due to either of these bacteria spreads through contact with genital secretions. Rarely, such spreads occur during child abuse or adolescent sexual encounters. Certain strains of *Chlamydia* cause a particularly long-lasting form of conjunctivitis called inclusion conjunctivitis.

Severe infections may scar the conjunctiva, causing abnormalities in the tear film. Sometimes severe conjunctival infections spread to the cornea.

Symptoms and Diagnosis

When infected, the eye sometimes feels irritated, and bright light may cause discomfort. The conjunctiva becomes pink because blood vessels dilate, and a discharge appears in the eye. The discharge tends to be watery in viral conjunctivitis and thicker and white or yellow in bacterial conjunctivitis, but this distinction is not absolute. Often, the discharge causes the eyes to stick shut, particularly overnight. This discharge may also cause vision to blur. Vision improves when the discharge is washed away. If the cornea is infected, vision also blurs but does not improve with washing. Very rarely, severe infections that have scarred the conjunctiva lead to long-term vision difficulties.

Children and adolescents with inclusion conjunctivitis or with conjunctivitis due to *N. gonorrhoeae* often have symptoms of a genital infection, such as a discharge from the penis or vagina and burning during urination.

Doctors diagnose infectious conjunctivitis by its symptoms and appearance. The eye is often examined with a slit lamp, an instrument that magnifies the surface of the eye. The slit lamp allows the doctor to see inflammation of the conjunctiva or infection of the cornea and front part of the eye (anterior chamber).

It is difficult to distinguish viral from bacterial conjunctivitis by appearance, although the presence of an upper respiratory infection increases the likelihood of a viral cause. Upper respiratory infections often accompany conjunctivitis caused by viruses, but they are rare in bacterial conjunctivitis. Samples of infected secretions may be sent to a laboratory to identify the infecting organism by a culture. However, a culture is usually done when the symptoms are severe or recurrent or when chlamydia or *N. gonorrhoeae* is thought to be the cause.

WHAT IS EPIDEMIC KERATOCONJUNCTIVITIS?

One of the most severe forms of infectious conjunctivitis results from infection with several particular strains of adenovirus. This infection, epidemic keratoconjunctivitis, is extremely contagious and often results in large outbreaks within a community or school. The infection is spread through contact with infected secretions—from person to person or through contaminated objects, including doctors' instruments.

The symptoms of this infection are similar to other types of viral conjunctivitis—redness, irritation, light sensitivity, and a thin, watery discharge. The lymph node in front of the ear on the affected side often becomes swollen. Symptoms typically last from 1 to 3 weeks. Some children have blurred vision, which may last for weeks or months before resolving.

Epidemic keratoconjunctivitis resolves completely without specific treatment. Doctors sometimes give corticosteroid drops to children with blurred vision or severe light sensitivity. Good hygiene, particularly hand washing, is needed to minimize the spread of the infection. Children generally stay home from school for several days.

Prognosis and Treatment

Most children with infectious conjunctivitis eventually get better on their own. However, some infections, particularly those caused by some bacteria, may last a long time if not treated. Inclusion conjunctivitis persists for months.

The eyelid should be gently washed with tap water and wiped with a clean washcloth to keep the eyelid clean and free of discharge. Cool compresses sometimes soothe the feeling of irritation. Because infectious (bacterial or viral) conjunctivitis is highly contagious, hand washing before and after cleaning the eye or applying drugs is essential. Also, the child should be warned against touching the infected eye and then touching the other eye. Towels and washcloths used to clean the eye should be kept separate from other towels and washcloths. Children with infectious conjunctivitis generally stay home from school for a few days, just as they would with a cold.

Antibiotics are helpful only in bacterial conjunctivitis. However, because it is difficult to distinguish between bacterial and viral infection, doctors often prescribe antibiotics for everyone with conjunctivitis. Antibiotic eye drops or ointments (such as sulfacetamide or trimethoprim-polymyxin) that are effective against many types of bacteria are used for 7 to 10 days. Eye drops must be applied every 2 to 3 hours because the drug is washed away by tears. Ointments last longer and are applied every 6 hours but blur vision.

Inclusion conjunctivitis requires antibiotics, such as erythromycin, azithromycin, or doxycycline, which are taken by mouth. Conjunctivitis due to *N. gonorrhoeae* may be treated with an injection of ceftriaxone. Corticosteroid eye drops may be needed by some children with severe adenoviral conjunctivitis, particularly if conjunctivitis is interfering with important daily activities. If viral conjunctivitis is caused by herpesvirus, antiviral drugs may be applied to the eyes (trifluridine or idoxuridine eye drops or vidarabine ointment) or given by mouth (acyclovir). Antiviral drugs are not useful for infections caused by other viruses

CHAPTER 23

Bone Disorders

- If the growth plate is damaged, bones may not grow normally, and joints may be distorted or permanently damaged, causing arthritis.
- Many bone disorders cause pain, interfere with walking, or both.
- Common bone disorders such as injuries are usually treated the same in children as in adults, but if the growth plate is damaged, surgery may be needed.

Although most bone disorders affecting children are similar to those affecting adults, there are some differences. Children's bones are continually growing and extensively reshaping themselves (remodeling). Growth proceeds from a vulnerable part of the bone called the growth plate. In remodeling, old bone tissue is gradually replaced by new bone tissue. Children's bones can remodel more extensively than adults' can. Also, in children, bones heal more rapidly, and scarring and stiffening develop less often. Most childhood bone disorders are minor and do not cause permanent problems.

Causes

Bone disorders in children can develop from any of the causes that affect adults, such as injuries and infections. Causes that affect mainly children include gradually developing misalignment of bones. In children, the bones in the legs can be very curved, which usually results from the way the legs were positioned in the uterus before birth.

COMMON FOOT, KNEE, AND LEG DISORDERS IN INFANTS AND YOUNG CHILDREN

Many knee and foot problems that parents notice in their infants and young children eventually resolve on their own without treatment. Some problems develop because of the way the legs were positioned in the uterus before birth. Rarely, treatment may be needed.

In **flat feet,** the middle of the feet, which are normally arched, appear sunken. An infant with normal feet may appear flat-footed because a fat pad appears in the arch of the foot. Flat feet may result when the arch of the foot is unusually flexible **(flexible flatfeet).** Another cause of flat feet is stiffening of the foot joints that fixes the foot in a position with a flattened arch **(tarsal coalition).** Tarsal coalition may be a birth defect or result from conditions such as injuries or prolonged swelling.

Usually fat pads and flexible flatfeet cause no symptoms. Sometimes flexible flatfeet cause pain or cramps in the feet. Tarsal coalition may cause pain or cramping. Feet with tarsal coalition are stiff, which can interfere with walking or running.

Fat pads do not require treatment. Flexible flatfeet usually do not require treatment. However, if an older child has pains or cramps in the feet, corrective shoes may be needed. Treatment for tarsal coalition often includes a cast. Sometimes surgically separating the attached internal structures restores mobility to the foot.

In **bowlegs** (physiological genu varum), the knees appear rotated away from each other. Bowlegs develop because of the way the legs bend to fit in the uterus before birth. Bowlegs develop in toddlers and are considered normal. Usually the only symptom is the appearance of the knees. Usually the condition corrects itself within about a year after the child begins to walk.

In **knock knees** (genu valgum), the knees point inward. Knock knees most often affect children aged 3 to 5 years. Usually the condition corrects itself by the age of 10 without treatment.

Femoral torsion is curving of the thighbone (femur). With internal femoral torsion, the thighs curve inward. The knees, and usually the toes, point toward each other. With external femoral torsion, the thighs curve outward. The knees and toes point away from each other. Internal femoral torsion develops much more often than external femoral torsion. Children with internal femoral torsion sometimes have abnormally flexible joints and ligaments.

Internal and external femoral torsion usually correct themselves when the child is older and begins to walk. Sometimes, internal femoral torsion is corrected by making sure that the child sits straight. Maintaining a straight sitting position may not be possible until the child reaches school age. In the rare circumstance when internal femoral torsion persists past the age of 10, surgically straightening the bone may be necessary. It can take years for internal or external femoral torsion to improve. Tibial torsion is curving of the shinbone (tibia).

Tibial torsion develops before birth and is very common. In internal tibial torsion, the tibia curves inward, pointing the toes toward each other. In external tibial torsion, the shinbone curves outward, pointing the toes away from each other. Tibial torsion is often noticed during the second year of life when the child begins to walk. The shinbone appears curved but gradually straightens after the child begins walking.

Poor blood supply can also damage the growth plate, as can separation from the rest of the bone or even minor misalignment. Damage to the growth plate suppresses the growth of bones, distorts the joint, and can cause long-standing joint damage (arthritis).

Certain rare hereditary disorders of connective tissue (see page 443) affect the bones, such as Marfan syndrome, mucopolysaccharidoses, osteogenesis imperfecta, chondrodysplasias, and osteopetroses.

DID YOU KNOW?

- Bowlegs usually corrects itself within about 1 year after children start walking.
- Children's bones heal more quickly and with less scarring than adults' bones.

Symptoms and Diagnosis

Children usually experience the same symptoms as adults. Pain is common and may develop slowly, over weeks or longer.

Infants and very young children may be unable to communicate their pain. Bone disorders sometimes cause painless deformities. Some deformities may affect a child's ability to walk or use the limbs. Diagnosis of bone disorders is similar in children and adults.

Treatment

Treatment of most bone disorders, such as fractures and infections, is usually similar in children and adults.

If the growth plate becomes damaged, surgery may help. Accurately realigning separated or misaligned ends of the growth plate surgically may restore normal bone growth. By decreasing the irritation caused by misalignment, surgery may prevent the development of arthritis in the joint.

If a bone disorder causes a physical deformity, the child may become anxious or depressed. Some treatments for bone disorders may also be psychologically difficult to accept. For example, adolescents may be reluctant to wear a back brace for treatment of scoliosis, because doing so makes them appear different from peers. Professional counseling may relieve anxiety or depression. Counseling may also help a child go through with difficult treatments.

Scoliosis

Scoliosis is abnormal curvature of the spine.

- Doctors can detect scoliosis more easily when the child bends forward.
- The progression of scoliosis is monitored to determine whether and when treatment is needed.
- Children may have to wear a brace or device (orthosis) to keep the spine straight and prevent worsening.

Scoliosis is very common, especially among girls. Scoliosis may result from a birth defect or develop later in life, most often in adolescence. Usually, the cause cannot be found. The spine usually bulges toward the right when the curvature is in the upper back and to the left when it is in the lower back. The result is that the right shoulder is usually higher than the left. One hip may be higher than the other. Scoliosis often develops in children with kyphosis (kyphoscoliosis).

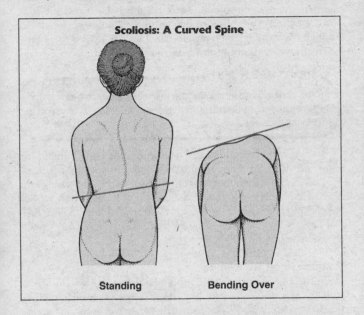

Scoliosis: A Curved Spine

Standing   Bending Over

Symptoms and Diagnosis

Mild scoliosis usually produces no symptoms. With more severe scoliosis, the back may sometimes becomes sore or stiff after the child sits or stands for a long period of time.

Mild scoliosis may be discovered during a routine physical examination. A parent, teacher, or doctor may suspect scoliosis when one of the child's shoulders seems higher than the other or when the child's clothes do not hang straight.

In about half of affected children, scoliosis is likely to worsen. The more severe the curve, the greater the likelihood of it worsening. Likewise, the more symptoms that develop, the greater the likelihood that scoliosis will worsen.

Because scoliosis tends to worsen when the child reaches puberty, the earlier it develops, the longer it has to worsen. Thus, a small curve in a 10-year-old is of much greater concern than that same curve in a 16-year-old. Worsening scoliosis may eventually cause permanent problems, such as noticeable deformities or chronic pain. Severe scoliosis may even affect internal organs, for example, deforming and damaging the lungs. Sometimes, scoliosis can worsen even if symptoms have not developed.

DID YOU KNOW?

- The earlier scoliosis begins, the worse it is likely to be.
- Scoliosis should be treated if it causes symptoms, is worsening, or is severe.

To diagnose the condition, a doctor asks the child to bend forward and views the spine from behind, because the abnormal spinal curve can be seen more easily in this position. X-rays show the precise angles of curvature. If doctors think scoliosis may worsen significantly, they may examine the child several times a year. Special devices may be used to more precisely measure the curve of the spine.

Prognosis and Treatment

In the vast majority of children who have scoliosis, the curvature will not progress more but rather remain small. However, it needs to be followed by a doctor regularly. Scoliosis that causes symptoms, is worsening, or is severe may need to be treated. The earlier treatment is begun, the better the chance of preventing a severe deformity.

A brace or object fashioned to hold the spine (orthosis) may be worn to keep the spine straight. In the most severe cases, the vertebrae need to be bonded together surgically; a metal rod may be inserted during surgery to keep the spine straight until the vertebrae have bonded permanently.

Kyphosis

In kyphosis (Scheuermann disease), changes in the cartilages of the vertebrae (osteochondritis) cause a humpback.

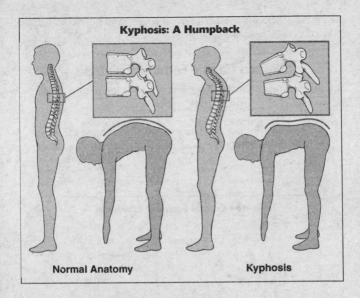

Kyphosis: A Humpback

Normal Anatomy　　　**Kyphosis**

Some amount of kyphosis is common and begins in adolescence, affecting boys more often than girls. The cause is unknown. The vertebrae curve forward on each other, usually in the upper back. As a result, the back develops a hump. Scoliosis also often develops in children with kyphosis (kyphoscoliosis).

Kyphosis often produces no symptoms. Sometimes, mild, persistent back pain develops. Kyphosis may be noticed only because it alters the body's appearance. The shoulders may appear rounded. The upper spine may appear more curved than normal, or a hump may be visible. Mild kyphosis that does not produce symptoms is sometimes detected only during a routine physical examination. A doctor confirms the diagnosis by taking x-rays of the spine, which show the curve and the deformity of the vertebrae.

Treatment most often consists of wearing a spinal brace or sleeping on a rigid bed. In mild kyphosis, the spine may straighten slightly with treatment, although symptoms may not improve. It is unclear whether treating mild kyphosis prevents the curve from worsening. When kyphosis is more severe, treatment may improve symptoms and prevent the curve from worsening. Rarely, despite treatment, kyphosis worsens to such an extent that surgery is needed to straighten the spine.

Slipped Capital Femoral Epiphysis

Slipped capital femoral epiphysis is a separation within the thigh-bone (femur) at its growth plate in the hip joint.

- This disorder usually causes pain and a limp.
- This disorder occurs most frequently among boys who are obese.

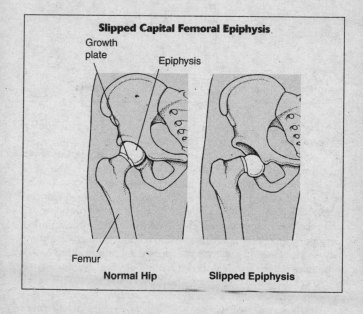

Slipped Capital Femoral Epiphysis

Growth plate

Epiphysis

Femur

Normal Hip　　　**Slipped Epiphysis**

Slipped capital femoral epiphysis usually develops in over-weight adolescents, most commonly boys. The cause is not known. However, the disorder may result from a thickening in the part of a bone where growth occurs or from changes in levels of hormones in the blood, which normally occur around puberty.

The separation causes the top part of the thighbone to eventually lose its blood supply, decay, and collapse.

DID YOU KNOW?

- Pain due to a slipped capital femoral epiphysis originates in the hip but may seem to come from the knee.

The first symptom may be stiffness or mild pain in the hip. However, the pain may seem to come from the knee. The pain improves with rest and worsens with walking or moving the hip. Later, a limp develops, followed by hip pain that extends down the inner thigh to the knee. The affected leg is usually twisted outward.

X-rays of the affected hip show a slippage or separation of the head of the thighbone from the rest of the bone. Early diagnosis is important because treatment becomes more difficult and gives less satisfactory results later.

Surgery is usually needed to align the separated ends of the thighbone and to fasten them together with metal pins. The hip is immobilized in a cast for several weeks to 2 months.

Legg-Calvé-Perthes Disease

Legg-Calvé-Perthes disease is destruction of the growth plate of the thighbone, causing pain and a limp.

Legg-Calvé-Perthes disease develops most commonly in boys between the ages of 5 and 10. It is caused by a poor blood supply to the upper growth plate of the thighbone. The reason for the poor blood supply is not known.

Legg-Calvé-Perthes disease can cause severe hip damage without causing severe symptoms at first. The severe damage may, however, lead to permanent arthritis of the hip. The first symptom is often hip or thigh pain. Pain begins gradually and progresses slowly. The pain tends to worsen when moving the hip or walking. A limp can develop, sometimes before the child experiences much pain. Eventually, joint movement becomes restricted, and the thigh muscles may become wasted (atrophied) from lack of use. X-rays may show changes around the growth plate, such as a fracture or destruction of the bone.

DID YOU KNOW?

- Legg-Calvé-Perthes disease usually takes at least 2 years to heal, no matter how it is treated.

Treatment includes prolonged immobilization of the hip. Sometimes the partial immobilization provided by bed rest is sufficient. Sometimes nearly total immobilization for 12 to 18 months is necessary, requiring traction, slings, plaster casts, or splints. Such treatments keep the legs rotated outward. Physical therapy is also given to keep the muscles from contracting and wasting away. If a child is older than 6 and has moderate or severe bone destruction, surgery may be helpful. Regardless of how it is treated, Legg-Calvé-Perthes disease usually takes at least 2 years to heal.

Osgood-Schlatter Disease

Osgood-Schlatter disease is painful inflammation of the bone and cartilage at the top of the shinbone (tibia).

Osgood-Schlatter disease develops between the ages of 10 and 15, usually in boys. The cause is thought to be repetitive, excessive pulling by the tendon of the kneecap (patellar tendon) on its point of attachment at the top of the shinbone (tibia). This point of attachment is called the tibial tubercle.

The major symptom is pain at the tibial tubercle. The pain worsens with activity and is relieved with rest. Swelling and tenderness eventually develop at the site. X-rays of the knee may show enlargement or fragmentation of the tibial tubercle.

Avoiding sports and excessive exercise helps reduce pain. Avoiding deep knee bending is particularly helpful. Use of nonsteroidal anti-inflammatory drugs (NSAIDs) may help the pain. Several weeks or months may be required for healing. Occasionally, the entire leg, from the ankle to the upper thigh, must be immobilized in a plaster cast for several weeks.

Chondromalacia Patellae

Chondromalacia patellae is damage to the cartilage under the knee-cap (patella), usually causing dull, aching pain around the knee.

Chondromalacia patellae typically develops in adolescents. Joggers are especially susceptible. The cause is probably a minor, repetitive injury resulting from misalignment of the kneecap. The misalignment causes the cartilage on the underside of the kneecap to grate against other bones when the knee bends.

Dull, aching pain is felt all around and behind the knee. Climbing, especially going up or down stairs, and running usually worsen the pain. Prolonged sitting may also worsen the pain. A doctor makes the diagnosis based on the symptoms and physical examination and may recommend exercises to strengthen the quadriceps muscles, which straighten, or extend, the knee joint. Increasing knee flexibility with stretching exercises helps. Activities that worsen the pain should be avoided. Analgesic or nonsteroidal anti-inflammatory drugs (NSAIDs), such as ibuprofen or naproxen, can help relieve symptoms.

Tumors

- Bone tumors may be noncancerous (benign) or cancerous (malignant).
- Tumors may cause bone pain or a lump or may weaken bones, making them easy to fracture.
- Diagnosis involves x-rays, computed tomography (CT) or magnetic resonance imaging (MRI), and biopsy.

Noncancerous bone tumors are relatively common, but cancerous ones are rare. Also, bone tumors may be primary—noncancerous or cancerous tumors that originate in the bone itself—or metastatic—cancerous tumors that originate elsewhere in the body and then spread to bone. In children, most cancerous bone tumors are primary.

Bone pain is the most common symptom of bone tumors. The pain can be severe (somewhat like a toothache, which is also a form of bone pain). In addition, a lump may be noticeable. Sometimes a tumor, especially if cancerous, weakens a bone, causing it to fracture with little or no stress (pathologic fracture).

A persistently painful joint or limb should be x-rayed. However, x-rays tend to show only that there is an abnormality suggestive of an abnormal growth, usually without indicating whether a tumor is noncancerous or cancerous. Computed tomography (CT) and magnetic resonance imaging (MRI) often help determine the exact location and size of the tumor and give additional information as to the nature of the tumor, but these tests rarely provide a specific diagnosis.

DID YOU KNOW?

- Some noncancerous bone tumors do not require treatment.

Usually, removing a tissue sample of the tumor for examination under a microscope (biopsy) is necessary for diagnosis. For many tumors, a sample may be taken by inserting a needle into the tumor and withdrawing some cells (aspiration biopsy); however, because the needle used is very small, sometimes normal cells may be sampled and cancer cells missed, even when cancer cells are lying right beside the normal cells. Sometimes, a surgical procedure called open biopsy is necessary to obtain an adequate sample for diagnosis.

NONCANCEROUS TUMORS

Osteochondromas (osteocartilaginous exostoses), the most common type of noncancerous bone tumors, usually occur in people aged 10 to 20 years. These tumors are growths on the surface of a bone, which protrude as hard lumps. A person may have one or several tumors. The tendency to develop several tumors may run in families.

At some point in their lives, about 10% of children who have more than one osteochondroma develop a cancerous bone tumor called a chondrosarcoma (presumably formed from an existing osteochondroma); surgical removal is generally appropriate if one of the tumors enlarges or causes new symptoms. Such children should also visit their doctor for regular examinations. However, children who have only one osteochondroma are unlikely to develop a chondrosarcoma; therefore, a single osteochondroma usually does not need to be removed unless it causes problems, such as increased swelling.

Chondromas, which usually occur in people aged 10 to 30 years, develop in the central part of a bone. These tumors often are discovered when x-rays are taken for other reasons and often can be diagnosed by their appearance on the x-ray. Some chondromas cause pain. If a chondroma does not cause pain, it does not have to be removed or treated. However, follow-up x-rays may be taken to monitor its size. If the tumor cannot be diagnosed with certainty on x-rays or if it causes pain, a biopsy may be needed, usually consisting of the entire tumor (excisional biopsy), to determine whether it is noncancerous or cancerous.

Chondroblastomas are rare tumors that grow in the ends of bones. They usually occur in people aged 10 to 20 years. These tumors may cause pain, leading to their discovery. If untreated, these tumors may continue to grow and destroy bone; therefore, treatment consists of surgical removal. Occasionally, these tumors recur after surgery.

PRIMARY CANCEROUS TUMORS

Osteosarcoma (osteogenic sarcoma) is the second most common type of primary cancerous bone tumor. Although most common in people aged 10 to 20 years, osteosarcomas can occur at any age. About half these tumors occur in or around the knee, but they can originate in any bone. They tend to spread (metastasize) to the lungs. Usually, these tumors cause pain and swelling. A biopsy is needed for diagnosis.

Osteosarcomas are usually treated with a combination of chemotherapy and surgery. Usually, chemotherapy is given first; pain often subsides during this phase of treatment. Then the tumor is surgically removed. About 75% of people who have this type of tumor survive for at least 5 years after diagnosis. Because surgical procedures have improved, the affected arm or leg can usually be saved; in the past, the affected limb often had to be amputated.

Chondrosarcomas are tumors composed of cancerous cartilage cells. Many chondrosarcomas are slow-growing or low-grade tumors, meaning that they are less likely to spread than some other tumors; they often can be cured with surgery. However, some chondrosarcomas are high-grade tumors, which tend to spread. A biopsy is needed for diagnosis. During treatment, a chondrosarcoma must be completely removed surgically, because it does not respond to chemotherapy or radiation therapy. Amputation of the arm or leg is rarely necessary. More than 75% of people who have a chondrosarcoma survive if the entire tumor is removed.

Ewing's tumor (Ewing's sarcoma) is a cancerous tumor that affects males more often than females and appears most commonly in people aged 10 to 20 years. Most of these tumors develop in the arms or legs, but they may develop in any bone. Pain and swelling are the most common symptoms. Tumors may become quite large, sometimes affecting the entire length of a bone. Although CT and MRI can help determine the exact size of the tumor, a biopsy is needed for diagnosis. Treatment consists of a combination of surgery, chemotherapy, and radiation therapy, which can cure more than 60% of people who have Ewing's tumor.

CHAPTER 24

Hereditary Connective Tissue Disorders

- Hereditary connective tissue disorders develop in childhood but last throughout life.
- Some hereditary connective tissue disorders can be diagnosed before birth.

Muscles, bones, cartilage, ligaments, and tendons are built mostly of connective tissue. Connective tissue is also found in other parts of the body, such as the skin and internal organs. Connective tissue is strong and thus able to support weight and tension.

Certain hereditary disorders cause connective tissue throughout the body to form abnormally. In general, the hereditary connective tissue disorders develop in childhood but last throughout life. Muscular dystrophies are a group of hereditary muscle disorders that lead to muscle weakness.

Most hereditary connective tissue disorders are diagnosed by their symptoms and findings on a physical examination. Analysis of genes, usually from a blood test, may help doctors diagnose some hereditary disorders. Biopsy (removal of a tissue sample for examination under a microscope) can also help; the tissue is usually removed using local anesthesia. X-rays can reveal bone abnormalities.

Ehlers-Danlos Syndrome

Ehlers-Danlos syndrome is a rare disorder of connective tissue that results in unusually flexible joints, very elastic skin, and fragile tissues.

- Ehlers-Danlos syndrome causes children to develop small hard lumps under the skin and a humpback with an abnormal curve of the spine.
- The body's response to injuries may be altered.
- There is no way to cure Ehlers-Danlos syndrome or to correct the connective tissue abnormalities.
- Special protective clothing should be worn to prevent injuries.

Ehlers-Danlos syndrome is caused by an abnormality in one of the genes that controls the production of connective tissue. There are several variations (with widely varying severity), each affecting a different gene and producing slightly different changes. The result is abnormally fragile connective tissue, which causes problems in joints and bones and may weaken internal organs.

Children with Ehlers-Danlos syndrome usually have very flexible joints. Some develop small, hard, round lumps under the skin; a humpback with an abnormal curve of the spine (kyphoscoliosis); or flat feet. The skin can be stretched several inches but returns to its normal position when released.

DID YOU KNOW?

- Children with Ehlers-Danlos syndrome usually have a normal iife span.

Ehlers-Danlos syndrome may alter the body's response to injuries. Minor injuries may result in wide gaping wounds. Although these wounds usually do not bleed excessively, they leave wide scars. Sprains and dislocations develop easily.

In a small number of children with Ehlers-Danlos syndrome, the blood clots poorly. Bleeding from minor wounds may be difficult to stop.

The intestines can bulge through the abdominal wall (hernias), and abnormal outpouchings (diverticula) can develop in the intestine. Rarely, a fragile intestine bleeds or ruptures (perforates).

If a pregnant woman has Ehlers-Danlos syndrome, delivery may be premature. If the fetus has Ehlers-Danlos syndrome, its surrounding membranes may rupture early (premature rupture of membranes). A mother or baby who has Ehlers-Danlos syndrome can bleed excessively around the time of delivery.

A doctor makes the diagnosis based on the symptoms and results of a physical examination. The doctor can confirm the diagnosis of some types of Ehlers-Danlos syndrome by taking a sample of skin to examine under a microscope.

Treatment and Prognosis

There is no way to cure Ehlers-Danlos syndrome or correct the abnormalities in the connective tissue. Injuries can be treated, but it may be difficult for a doctor to stitch cuts because stitches tend to tear out of the fragile tissue. Usually, using an adhesive tape or medical skin glue closes cuts more easily and leaves less scarring.

Special precautions should be taken to prevent injuries. For example, protective clothing and padding may be worn in children with severe forms; surgery requires special techniques that minimize injury and ensure that a large supply of blood is available for transfusion.

Despite the many and varied complications people with Ehlers-Danlos syndrome may have, their life span is usually normal. However, in a few people with one specific type of Ehlers-Danlos syndrome, complications (usually bleeding) are fatal.

Marfan Syndrome

Marfan syndrome is a rare disorder of connective tissue, resulting in abnormalities of the eyes, bones, heart, and blood vessels.

- Affected people are unusually tall, have an arm span that is greater than their height, and have long, thin fingers and flexible joints.
- Marfan syndrome may be suspected in a tall, thin person who has characteristic symptoms.
- Doctors monitor people with Marfan syndrome to detect heart and lung complications.

- There is no cure for Marfan syndrome.
- Treatment is directed toward identifying and managing complications as soon as they occur.

In Marfan syndrome, which is caused by a dominant gene, some fibers and other parts of connective tissue undergo changes that ultimately weaken the tissue. The weakening affects bones and joints as well as internal structures, such as the heart, blood vessels, eyes, and intestines. Weakened tissues stretch, distort, and can even tear. For example, the aorta may weaken, bulge, or tear. Connective tissues that join structures may weaken or break, separating formerly attached structures. For example, the eye's lens or retina may separate from its normal attachments.

Symptoms can range from mild to severe. Many people with Marfan syndrome never notice symptoms. In some people, symptoms may not become apparent until adulthood. People with Marfan syndrome are taller than expected for their age and family. Their arm span (the distance between fingertips when the arms are outstretched) is greater than their height. Their fingers are long and thin. Often, the breastbone (sternum) is deformed and pushed either outward or inward. The joints may be very flexible. Flat feet and a humpback with an abnormal curve of the spine (kyphoscoliosis) are common; so are hernias. Usually, the person has little fat under the skin. The roof of the mouth is often high.

The most dangerous complications develop in the heart and lungs. Weakness may develop in the connective tissue of the wall of the body's main artery, the aorta. The weakened wall may result in blood seeping between the layers of the aorta's wall (aortic dissection) or a bulge (aneurysm), which can rupture. Pregnancy in a woman with Marfan syndrome increases the risk of dissection. Delivery by caesarean section is often recommended to minimize the risk.

DID YOU KNOW?

- Marfan syndrome may be so mild that people never notice symptoms.
- The most dangerous complications affect the heart and lungs.
- Most people with Marfan syndrome live until their 60s.

If the aorta gradually widens, the aortic valve, which leads from the heart into the aorta, may begin to leak (aortic regurgitation). The mitral valve, which is located between the left atrium and ventricle, may leak or become prolapsed (bulge backward into the left atrium). These heart valve abnormalities can impair the heart's ability to pump blood. Abnormal heart valves can also develop serious infections (infective endocarditis). Air-filled sacs (cysts) may develop in the lungs. The cysts may rupture, bringing air into the space that surrounds the lungs (pneumothorax).

The lens of one or both eyes may be displaced in Marfan syndrome. The light-sensitive area at the back of the eye (retina) may detach from the rest of the eye. Displacement of the lens and detachment of the retina may cause permanent loss of vision.

Doctors may suspect the diagnosis if an unusually tall, thin person has any of the characteristic symptoms, or if Marfan syndrome has been recognized in other family members.

It is most important for doctors to monitor for complications that can cause serious symptoms. Echocardiography is used to evaluate the heart and aorta and is usually repeated yearly. The eyes are usually examined yearly. Echocardiography and eye examinations are also performed whenever symptoms develop.

Treatment and Prognosis

There is no cure for Marfan syndrome nor any way to correct the abnormalities in the connective tissue. Treatment is aimed at fixing abnormalities before dangerous complications develop. Some doctors prescribe drugs, such as beta-blockers, that make blood flow more gently through the aorta. However, whether these drugs help is controversial. If the aorta has widened or developed an aneurysm, the affected section can be repaired or replaced surgically. A displaced lens or retina can usually be reattached surgically.

Years ago, most people with Marfan syndrome died in their 40s. Now, most people with Marfan syndrome live until their 60s. Prevention of aortic dissection and rupture probably explains why the life span has been lengthened.

Pseudoxanthoma Elasticum

Pseudoxanthoma elasticum is a disorder of connective tissue that causes abnormalities in the skin, eyes, and blood vessels.

- Pseudoxanthoma elasticum causes the elastic fibers of the body to stiffen.
- The skin of the neck, underarms, and groin becomes thick, grooved, inflexible, and loose.
- Yellowish pebbly bumps appear in the skin, giving an appearance similar to a plucked chicken.
- Blood vessels become stiff, which may lead to high blood pressure, nosebleeds, or internal bleeding.
- There is no cure, so treatment is aimed at preventing complications.

Pseudoxanthoma elasticum stiffens the fibers that enable tissue to stretch and then spring back into place (elastic fibers). Elastic fibers are in the skin and various other tissues throughout the body, including blood vessels. The blood vessels may stiffen, losing their normal ability to expand and allow more blood to flow as needed; stiffness also prevents the blood vessels from contracting.

The skin of the neck, underarms, groin, and around the navel eventually becomes thick, grooved, inflexible, and loose. Yellowish, pebbly bumps give the skin an appearance similar to an orange or a plucked chicken. The change in appearance may be mild and overlooked during early childhood but becomes more noticeable as the child ages.

Stiff blood vessels lead to high blood pressure. Nosebleeds and bleeding in the brain, uterus, and intestine may occur. Too little blood flow may result in chest pain (angina) and leg pain while walking (intermittent claudication). Bleeding may continue for prolonged periods. Damage to the back of the eye (retina) can cause severe loss of vision or blindness.

Treatment and Prognosis

There is no cure for pseudoxanthoma elasticum nor any way to correct the abnormalities in the connective tissue. Treatment is aimed at preventing complications. People should avoid drugs that may cause stomach or intestinal bleeding, such as aspirin, other nonsteroidal anti-inflammatory drugs (NSAIDs), and anticoagulants. People with pseudoxanthoma elasticum should avoid contact sports because of the risk of injury to the eye. Complications often limit life span.

Cutis Laxa

Cutis laxa is a rare disorder of connective tissue that causes the skin to stretch easily and hang in loose folds.

- The disease may be mild, or it may be more severe and affect internal organs.
- Symptoms may become noticeable shortly after birth or may develop suddenly in older children or adolescents.
- Plastic surgery may improve the appearance of the skin.

In cutis laxa, the elastic fibers contained in the connective tissue become loose. Sometimes only the skin is affected, but connective tissues throughout the body can be affected. Cutis laxa is usually hereditary. In some kinds of cutis laxa, the abnormal genes cause problems unrelated to connective tissues—for example, mental retardation.

Cutis laxa can be mild, affecting only a person's appearance, or severe, affecting the internal organs. The skin may be very loose at birth, or it may become loose later. The loose skin is often most noticeable on the face, resulting in a prematurely aged appearance. The lungs, heart, intestines, or arteries may be affected with a variety of severe impairments.

DID YOU KNOW?

- In some kinds of cutis laxa, other problems that are not related to connective tissue occur.

Although symptoms often become noticeable shortly after birth, they may begin suddenly in children and adolescents, sometimes with a fever and rash. In some people, symptoms develop gradually in adulthood.

A doctor can usually diagnose cutis laxa by examining the skin. Sometimes, a skin biopsy is necessary.

Treatment and Prognosis

Plastic surgery can often improve the appearance of the skin, although the improvement may be only temporary. Severe impairments of the heart, lungs, arteries, or intestines can be fatal.

Mucopolysaccharidoses

The mucopolysaccharidoses are a group of hereditary disorders affecting the connective tissue that result in a characteristic facial appearance and abnormalities of the bones, eyes, liver, and spleen, sometimes accompanied by mental retardation.

- Short stature, hairiness, and abnormal development are noticeable symptoms.
- Other symptoms may include mental retardation, vision or hearing impairments, heart and blood vessel problems, and stiff finger joints.

Mucopolysaccharides are essential parts of connective tissue. In the mucopolysaccharidoses, the body lacks enzymes needed to break down and store mucopolysaccharides. As a result, excess mucopolysaccharides enter the blood and are deposited in abnormal locations throughout the body.

During infancy and childhood, short stature, hairiness, and abnormal development become noticeable. The face may appear coarse. Some types of mucopolysaccharidoses cause mental retardation to develop over several years. In some types, vision or hearing may become impaired. The arteries or heart valves can be affected. Finger joints are often stiff.

A doctor usually bases the diagnosis on the symptoms and findings on a physical examination. The presence of a mucopolysaccharidosis in other family members also suggests the diagnosis. Urine tests may help but are sometimes inaccurate. X-rays may show characteristic bone abnormalities. Mucopolysaccharidoses can be diagnosed before birth using amniocentesis or chorionic villus sampling.

Treatment and Prognosis

In one type of mucopolysaccharidosis, attempts at replacing the abnormal enzyme have had limited, temporary success. Bone marrow transplantation may help some people. However, death or disability often results, and this treatment remains controversial.

The prognosis depends on the type of mucopolysaccharidosis. A normal life span is possible. Some types, usually those that affect the heart, cause premature death.

Osteogenesis Imperfecta

Osteogenesis imperfecta is a group of disorders of bone formation that make the bones abnormally fragile.

- Bones fracture easily, even with minor injuries, such as those that occur when a child learns to walk.
- Hearing loss is common.
- X-rays show the abnormal bone structure, and a bone biopsy is used to confirm the diagnosis.
- Treatment is with drugs that strengthen bones and measures to avoid injury.
- Doctors may have to insert metal rods to stabilize fractured bones.

Osteogenesis imperfecta is the best known of a group of disorders that disturb bone growth; these disorders are called osteodysplasias. In osteogenesis imperfecta, synthesis of collagen, one of the normal components of bone, is impaired. The bones become weak and fracture easily. There are several types of osteogenesis imperfecta.

Osteogenesis imperfecta can range from mild to severe. Most people with osteogenesis imperfecta have fragile bones and hearing loss. Infants with severe osteogenesis imperfecta are usually born with many broken bones; the skull may be so soft that the brain is not protected from pressure applied to the head during childbirth. With moderate osteogenesis imperfecta, bones often break after very minor injuries, usually when the child begins to walk. Children with mild osteogenesis imperfecta may sustain few broken bones during childhood and even fewer after puberty, when bones strengthen. Sometimes heart or lung diseases develop in children with osteogenesis imperfecta.

DID YOU KNOW?

- Osteogenesis imperfecta is one of a group of disorders that disturb bone growth (osteodysplasias).
- Infants with severe disease may be born with many broken bones.

X-rays may show abnormal bone structure that suggests osteogenesis imperfecta. A bone biopsy is used to confirm the diagnosis. A test called audiometry is performed often throughout childhood to monitor hearing.

Treatment

Bisphosphonate drugs (such as pamidronate, alendronate, etidronate, and risedronate) may strengthen bones. Treatment of broken bones is similar for children with osteogenesis imperfecta as for children without the disorder. However, broken bones can become deformed or fail to grow. As a result, body growth can become permanently stunted in children with many broken bones, and deformities are common. Bones may require stabilization with metal rods (intramedullary rods). Taking measures to avoid even minor injuries can help prevent fractures.

Chondrodysplasias

The chondrodysplasias are a group of rare disorders of cartilage that cause the skeleton to develop abnormally.

- Chondrodysplasias usually cause short stature and sometimes short limbs, bowlegs, a bulky forehead, an unusually shaped nose, and an arched back.
- Diagnosis is made by physical examination and x-rays of the bones.
- Sometimes surgery is needed if a person's joints do not have their full range of motion.

In chondrodysplasias, the growth plate, which contains cartilage, does not make new bone cells. Thus, growth of bone is impaired.

Each type of chondrodysplasia produces different symptoms. Chondrodysplasias usually cause short stature (dwarfism). Some cause more shortening of the limbs than the trunk (short-limbed dwarfism); others cause more shortening of the trunk than the limbs. Some children and adults have short limbs, bowlegs, a bulky forehead, an unusually shaped nose (saddle nose), and an arched back. Sometimes, joints do not develop the capacities for their full range of motion.

A doctor usually makes the diagnosis based on the symptoms, physical examination, and x-rays of the bones. Sometimes the abnormal genes responsible for chondrodysplasias can be detected, usually by a blood test. Analyzing the genes is most helpful for predicting the disease before birth. Diagnosis of severe types before birth is also possible using other methods; in some cases, the fetus can be directly viewed with a flexible scope (fetoscopy), or an ultrasound is performed. Surgery may be needed to replace joints that have severely restricted movement with artificial ones.

Osteopetroses

The osteopetroses are a group of rare disorders that increase the density of bones.

- Symptoms, which may begin in infancy, include impaired bone growth, easy bone breakage, anemia, infection, and bleeding.
- X-rays can show the appearance of the very dense bones.
- Corticosteroids may strengthen bones by decreasing formation of new bone cells.

In osteopetroses (sometimes called marble bone diseases), the body fails to recycle old bone cells. The result is increased density of the bones. The increased density makes bones weaker than normal. The dense bone tissue also crowds out the bone marrow.

The osteopetroses range from mild to severe and can even be life threatening. Symptoms may begin in infancy (early onset) or later in life (delayed onset).

Although the osteopetroses are different disorders, many of the same symptoms develop in most of them. Bone growth is usually impaired. Bones thicken and break easily. Formation of blood cells may be impaired because of a lack of bone marrow, leading to anemia, infection, or bleeding. Bone overgrowth in the skull can compress nerves, causing facial paralysis or loss of vision or hearing, and can distort the face and teeth.

DID YOU KNOW?

- Bone marrow transplantation may help some children whose symptoms began in infancy.

Doctors usually establish the diagnosis based on the symptoms and the appearance of very dense bone on x-rays. When the person has no symptoms, osteopetrosis is sometimes detected only by chance, after a doctor sees very dense bones on x-rays taken for an unrelated purpose.

Treatment and Prognosis

There is no cure. Corticosteroids, such as prednisone, decrease formation of new bone cells and may increase the rate of removal of old bone cells, strengthening bones. Bone marrow transplantation appears to have cured some infants with early-onset disease. However, the long-term prognosis after transplantation is unknown.

Fractures, anemia, bleeding, and infection require treatment. If nerves leaving the skull are compressed, surgery may be required to release the nerve. Orthodontic treatment may be needed.

Early-onset osteopetrosis that is not treated with bone marrow transplantation usually causes death during infancy or early childhood. Death usually results from anemia, infection, or bleeding. Late-onset osteopetrosis is often very mild.

CHAPTER 25

Juvenile Rheumatoid Arthritis

Juvenile rheumatoid arthritis is persistent or recurring inflammation of the joints similar to rheumatoid arthritis but beginning before age 16.

- Juvenile rheumatoid arthritis may cause fever, rash, and lymph node swelling and affect the heart or kidneys.
- Diagnosis is based on the child's symptoms and a physical examination because there is no single definitive laboratory test to diagnose juvenile rheumatoid arthritis.
- Children receive drugs to treat pain and inflammation.
- Flexibility exercises help enhance joint movement.

Juvenile rheumatoid arthritis is an uncommon disease characterized by inflammation of joints or connective tissue. The cause is unknown. Although juvenile rheumatoid arthritis is not considered a hereditary disorder, hereditary factors may increase a child's chance of developing it.

Symptoms and Complications

There are several types of juvenile rheumatoid arthritis, each with different characteristics. The type of juvenile rheumatoid arthritis is determined by which symptoms develop during the first months of the disease and how many joints are affected.

In pauciarticular juvenile rheumatoid arthritis, four or fewer joints, usually those of the leg, are affected. The knee is usually the first joint affected. The hip and shoulder are usually spared. Occasionally, a single toe, a finger, a wrist, or the jaw becomes stiff and swollen. The back may also be involved. The joint pain and swelling may persist or come and go.

In polyarthritis, five or more (sometimes as many as 20 to 40) joints are affected. The inflammation usually affects the same joint on both sides of the body—for example, both knees or both hips. The jaw, neck joints, and wrists may be affected. Symptoms may develop slowly; fever and enlargement of the spleen or lymph glands can occur. Inflammation may develop in the tendons and connective tissues around joints (tenosynovitis), causing pain, swelling, and warmth.

In systemic disease (Still's disease), any number of joints can be involved. Inflammation also occurs at sites other than the joints. The liver, spleen, and lymph nodes may enlarge, and sometimes inflammation develops in the membrane surrounding the heart (pericarditis). Rarely, the kidneys become inflamed. A high fever and rash may appear before joint pain and swelling. The fever comes and goes, usually for at least 2 weeks. Temperature is usually highest in the afternoon or evening (often 103°F or higher), then returns rapidly to normal. A child with fever may feel tired and less energetic. A rash made up of flat, pink or salmon-colored patches—mainly on the trunk and the upper part of the legs or arms—appears for hours (often in the evening). The rash can reappear days later on a different part of the body.

With any type of juvenile rheumatoid arthritis, the joints may be stiff when the child awakens. Joints often become swollen and warm. Later, joints may become painful, but the pain may be milder than expected from the amount of swelling. Pain may become worse when the joint is moved. A child may be reluctant to walk. Joint pain tends to persist for weeks or months.

Any type of juvenile rheumatoid arthritis can interfere with physical growth. Joint deformities often develop. When juvenile rheumatoid arthritis interferes with growth of the jaw, a small chin (micrognathia) can result. Long-standing (chronic) joint inflammation can eventually cause deformities or permanent damage of the affected joint.

Inflammation of the iris in the eye (iridocyclitis) can develop with any kind of juvenile rheumatoid arthritis, but most often iridocyclitis develops with pauciarticular juvenile rheumatoid arthritis or polyarthritis. Iridocyclitis may cause eye redness, eye pain, or loss of vision, but it can develop without any symptoms. If untreated, iridocyclitis can lead to permanent eye damage.

DID YOU KNOW?

- There are several types of juvenile rheumatoid arthritis, each with different characteristics.
- Eye damage can occur, sometimes without producing symptoms.
- Symptoms of juvenile rheumatoid arthritis eventually disappear in a high proportion of affected children.

Diagnosis

A doctor diagnoses juvenile rheumatoid arthritis based on the child's symptoms and the results of a physical examination. There is no single, definitive laboratory test for juvenile rheumatoid arthritis. Blood is tested for rheumatoid factor and antinuclear antibodies, which are present in some people with rheumatoid arthritis and related diseases (for example, autoimmune diseases, such as lupus, polymyositis, or scleroderma). However, many children with juvenile rheumatoid arthritis do not have rheumatoid factor or antinuclear antibodies in their blood. Also, children with many other conditions can have rheumatoid factor or antinuclear antibodies in their blood. X-rays eventually may show characteristic changes in the bones or joints. The child must be examined regularly by an ophthalmologist for iridocyclitis regardless of whether symptoms are present.

Treatment and Prognosis

The types of juvenile rheumatoid arthritis are treated similarly, and the drugs used to reduce pain and inflammation are the same as for rheumatoid arthritis, including, for example, nonsteroidal anti-inflammatory drugs (NSAIDs) such as ibuprofen and naproxen, corticosteroids, and methotrexate or other immunosuppressive drugs. However, children with juvenile rheumatoid arthritis often also need treatment for iridocyclitis. Iridocyclitis is treated with corticosteroid eye drops or ointments, which suppress inflammation. Eye drops that widen (dilate) the pupil can decrease eye pain from iridocyclitis. Both types of drugs can prevent glaucoma and blindness. For unusually severe iridocyclitis, eye surgery may be needed.

As in rheumatoid arthritis in adults, non-drug therapies are also used in children; for example, splinting and flexibility exercises, to prevent permanent stiffening of joints.

Symptoms of juvenile rheumatoid arthritis completely disappear in a high proportion of affected children. Up to half of the children with pauciarticular juvenile rheumatoid arthritis and about one quarter or more of children with polyarthritis or systemic disease have a complete remission.

CHAPTER 26

Muscular Dystrophy and Related Disorders

Muscular dystrophies are a group of inherited muscle disorders that lead to muscle weakness of varying severity. Other inherited muscle disorders include myotonic myopathies, periodic paralysis, Charcot-Marie-Tooth disease, spinal muscular atrophies, and glycogen storage diseases. Glycogen storage diseases are a group of rare inherited disorders in which muscles cannot metabolize sugars normally (see page 476), so they build up large stores of glycogen (a starch that is formed from sugars).

Duchenne and Becker Muscular Dystrophies

Duchenne and Becker muscular dystrophies cause weakness in the muscles closest to the torso.

- These dystrophies are the most common muscular dystrophies and nearly always occur in boys.
- The diagnosis is confirmed by genetic testing, a muscle biopsy, or both.
- Genetic counseling is recommended.

On average, 1 of 3,300 boys born has Duchenne muscular dystrophy, whereas on average 1 of 18,000 boys born has Becker muscular dystrophy.

The gene defect that causes Duchenne muscular dystrophy is different from the gene defect that causes Becker muscular dystrophy, but both defects involve the same gene. The gene for either of these traits is recessive and is carried on the X chromosome. Therefore, although a female can carry the defective gene, she will not develop the disease because the normal gene on one X chromosome compensates for the gene defect on the other X chromosome. However, any male who receives the defective gene will have the disease, because he has only one X chromosome.

Boys with Duchenne muscular dystrophy lack almost totally the muscle protein, dystrophin, which is important for maintaining the structure of muscle cells. Boys with Becker muscular dystrophy produce dystrophin, but because the protein structure is altered, the dystrophin does not function properly.

Symptoms

In boys with Duchenne muscular dystrophy, the first symptoms are developmental delay (particularly a delay in starting to walk), difficulty walking or climbing stairs, and falling. Starting between the ages of 3 and 7, the gait becomes waddling, and the child has difficulty rising from a sitting position.

Weakness in the shoulder muscles usually follows and gets steadily worse. As the muscles weaken they also enlarge, but the abnormal muscle tissue is not strong. In over 80% of boys with Duchenne muscular dystrophy, the heart muscle also enlarges and weakens, causing problems with the heartbeat, which show up on an electrocardiogram.

In boys with Duchenne muscular dystrophy, the arm and leg muscles usually contract around the joints, so that the elbows and knees cannot fully extend. Eventually, an abnormally curved spine (scoliosis) develops. By age 10 or 12, most children with the disease are confined to a wheelchair. The increasing weakness also makes them susceptible to pneumonia and other illnesses, and most die by the age of 20.

In boys with Becker muscular dystrophy, weakness is less severe and first appears a little later, at about age 12. The pattern of weakness resembles that of Duchenne muscular dystrophy.

However, very few adolescents become confined to a wheelchair. The average age of death is 42 years.

Diagnosis

Doctors suspect muscular dystrophy when a young boy becomes weak and grows weaker. An enzyme (creatine kinase) leaks out of muscle cells, causing levels of creatine kinase in the blood to be abnormally high. However, high blood levels of creatine kinase do not necessarily mean that a person has muscular dystrophy; other muscle diseases may also cause elevated levels of this enzyme. Duchenne muscular dystrophy is diagnosed when blood tests show the gene for the protein dystrophin to be absent or abnormal and a muscle biopsy shows extremely low levels of dystrophin in the muscle. Under the microscope, the muscle generally shows dead tissue and abnormally large muscle fibers. In the late stages of muscular dystrophy, fat and other tissues replace the dead muscle tissue. Similarly, Becker muscular dystrophy is diagnosed when blood tests show the gene for the protein dystrophin to be abnormal and a muscle biopsy shows low levels of dystrophin in the muscle, but not as low as in Duchenne muscular dystrophy.

Other tests to support the diagnosis include electrical studies of muscle function (electromyography) and nerve conduction studies.

Families with members who have either Duchenne or Becker muscular dystrophy are advised to consult a genetic counselor for help in evaluating the risk of passing the muscular dystrophy trait on to their children. In families with a history of these disorders, doctors can perform prenatal tests on the fetus to determine whether the child is likely to be affected.

Treatment

Neither Duchenne nor Becker muscular dystrophy can be cured. Physical therapy and exercise help prevent the muscles from contracting permanently around joints. Sometimes surgery is needed to release tight, painful muscles.

Taking either of the corticosteroids prednisone or deflazacort by mouth daily, can improve the boy's strength. However, long-term use causes many side effects, so it is not given to every child with muscular dystrophy. Use of prednisone is generally reserved for people whose muscle weakness has severely interfered with the normal activities of daily living. Thus, whether to give these drugs depends on the boy's degree of incapacitation as well as the severity of the drug's side effects. Creatine, a supplement taken by mouth, improves strength, but usually not very much. Gene therapy that would enable muscles to produce dystrophin and thereby relieve the weakness is under investigation but has so far not proved successful.

Other Muscular Dystrophies

- Several much less common forms of muscular dystrophy, all inherited, also cause progressive muscle weakness.
- The diagnosis is confirmed by a muscle biopsy.
- Gene therapy holds promise for the future.

Facioscapulohumeral (Landouzy-Dejerine) muscular dystrophy is transmitted by an autosomal dominant gene; therefore, a single abnormal gene is sufficient to cause the disorder, and the disorder can appear in either males or females. Symptoms usually begin between the ages of 7 and 20. The facial and shoulder muscles are always affected, so that a child has difficulty whistling, closing the eyes tightly, or raising the arms. Some people with the disease also develop a footdrop (the foot flops down). The weakness is rarely severe, and people who have Landouzy-Dejerine muscular dystrophy have a normal life expectancy.

Mitochondrial myopathies are muscle disorders inherited through faulty genes in mitochondria (the energy factories of cells; they carry their own genes). Because sperm do not contribute mitochondria during fertilization, all mitochondrial genes come from the mother. Therefore, although they are equally likely in males and females, these disorders can never be inherited from the father. These rare disorders sometimes cause increasing weakness in one or a few muscle groups, such as the eye muscles (ophthalmoplegia). Symptoms usually develop before 20 years of age. One mitochondrial myopathy is called the Kearns-Sayre syndrome.

Diagnosis and Treatment

Diagnosis requires taking a sample of the weak muscle tissue for biopsy and either examining it under a microscope or performing chemical tests on it. Specific treatments are not available, but gene therapy holds promise for the future.

Myotonic Myopathies

Myotonic myopathies are inherited disorders in which the muscles are not able to relax normally after contraction; muscle weakness and spasms may also occur.

- Drug treatment can relieve stiffness and cramping but has side effects.

Myotonia congenita (Thomsen's disease) is a rare autosomal dominant disorder that affects males and females. Symptoms usually start in infancy. The hands, legs, and eyelids become very stiff because of an inability to relax the muscles. Muscle weakness, however, is usually minimal. The diagnosis is made from the child's characteristic appearance, inability to relax the grip of the hand rapidly after closing the hand, and prolonged contraction after the doctor taps a muscle. An electromyogram (a test in which electrical impulses from muscles are recorded is needed to confirm the diagnosis. Myotonic congenita is treated with phenytoin, quinine, procainamide, or mexiletine to relieve muscle stiffness and cramping; however, each of these drugs has undesirable side effects. Regular exercise may be beneficial. People with myotonic congenita have a normal life expectancy.

Myotonic dystrophy (Steinert's disease) is an autosomal dominant disorder affecting males and females. The disorder produces weakness and stiff muscles, especially in the hands. Drooping eyelids are also common. Symptoms can appear at any age and can range from mild to severe. Only about half of affected people develop symptoms before age 20. People with the most severe form of the disorder have extreme muscle weakness, mental retardation, diabetes, and many other symptoms. They usually die by age 50. Treatment with quinine, phenytoin, procainamide, and other drugs has been used, but these drugs do not improve the weakness, which is the most bothersome symptom to the person. Also, each of these drugs has undesirable side effects. The only treatment for muscle weakness is supportive measures, such as ankle braces and other devices.

Periodic Paralysis

Periodic paralysis is an autosomal dominant inherited disorder that causes sudden attacks of weakness and paralysis; there are several variants.

- During an attack of weakness, blood levels of potassium are often abnormally high or abnormally low.
- Drug treatment and sometimes other measures can help prevent sudden attacks.

During an attack of periodic paralysis, muscles do not respond to normal nerve impulses or even to artificial stimulation with an electronic instrument. The person remains completely awake and alert. The precise form that the disorder takes varies in different families. In some families, the paralysis is related to high levels of potassium in the blood (hyperkalemia); in others, the paralysis is related to low levels of potassium in the blood (hypokalemia) or, rarely, to normal levels.

Symptoms and Diagnosis

In the hyperkalemic form of the disorder, attacks often begin by age 10. The attacks last 15 minutes to 1 hour. In the hypokalemic form, attacks usually, but not always, first appear before age 16. The attacks last longer (occasionally for 2 to 3 days) and are more severe. Fasting, strenuous work, and exposure to cold may precipitate attacks in people who have the hyperkalemic form. Some people with the hypokalemic form are prone to attacks of paralysis after eating meals rich in carbohydrates (sometimes hours or even the day after), but exercise also precipitates attacks. Eating carbohydrates and exercising vigorously drive sugar into cells; potassium moves with the sugar and the result is lowered potassium levels in the blood. On awakening the day after engaging in vigorous exercise, a person with either the hyperkalemic form or the hypokalemic form may feel some weakness or even paralysis in certain muscle groups or in the arms and legs. The weakness generally lasts 1 or 2 days.

A doctor's best clue to the diagnosis is a person's description of a typical attack. If possible, the doctor draws blood while an attack is in progress to check the level of potassium. Doctors usually perform additional tests to be sure abnormal potassium levels in the blood are not from other causes.

Prevention and Treatment

Acetazolamide, a drug that alters the blood's acidity, may prevent attacks in all types of periodic paralysis. People with the hypokalemic form can take potassium chloride in an unsweetened solution while the attack is in progress. Usually symptoms improve considerably within an hour. People with the hypokalemic form should also avoid meals rich in carbohydrates and strenuous exercise. People with the hyperkalemic form can prevent attacks by eating frequent meals rich in carbohydrates and low in potassium.

Charcot-Marie-Tooth Disease

Charcot-Marie-Tooth disease (peroneal muscular atrophy) is a hereditary neuropathy in which the muscles of the lower legs become weak and waste away (atrophy).

Charcot-Marie-Tooth disease affects 1 of 2,500 children. There are 3 types and several subtypes of the disease. In some types, axons (the part of the nerve that sends messages) die because the myelin sheath surrounding them is damaged or destroyed (demyelinated). In other types, axons die even though the sheath is not damaged. Most types of the disease are inherited as an autosomal (not sex-linked) dominant trait: only one gene from one parent is required for the disease to develop.

DID YOU KNOW?

- Charcot-Marie-Tooth disease is the most common hereditary neuropathy.

Symptoms vary by type of the disease. In type 1, symptoms begin in middle childhood, adolescence, or later. Weakness begins in the lower legs, which causes an inability to flex the foot (footdrop) and wasting away of the calf muscles (stork leg deformity). Later, hand muscles begin to waste away. There is little loss of sensation. In milder subtypes of type 1, high arches and hammer toes may be the only symptoms. In one subtype of type 1, boys have severe symptoms, and girls have mild symptoms or may be unaffected. The disease progresses slowly and does not affect life span.

Children with type 2 disease, which progresses more slowly, develop somewhat similar symptoms, often beginning in their teens.

Type 3 disease starts in infancy. Walking and running are delayed, and the peripheral nerves become enlarged. Muscle weakness in the legs progresses at a faster rate than in type 1. Sensation in the legs is lost.

Diagnosis and Treatment

The distribution of weakness, the age at which the disease began, the family history, the presence of foot deformities (high arches and hammer toes), and the results of nerve conduction studies help doctors identify the different types of Charcot-Marie-Tooth disease and distinguish them from other causes of neuropathy. Genetic testing and counseling for Charcot-Marie-Tooth disease is available.

No treatment can stop the progression of the disease. Wearing braces helps correct footdrop, and sometimes orthopedic surgery is needed.

Spinal Muscular Atrophies

Spinal muscular atrophies are hereditary disorders in which nerve cells in the spinal cord and brain stem degenerate, causing progressive muscle weakness and wasting.

The disorders are usually inherited as a recessive autosomal (not sex-linked) trait: two genes are required, one from each parent. There are three main types of spinal muscular atrophy.

Symptoms

Symptoms first appear during infancy and childhood. In acute (type I) spinal muscular atrophy (Werdnig-Hoffmann disease), muscle weakness is apparent at or within a few days of birth. Death occurs in 95% of children by age 1 1/2 years and in all by age 4 years, usually due to respiratory failure.

In children with intermediate (type II) spinal muscular atrophy, weakness develops by age 6 months. Most children are confined to a wheelchair by age 2 to 3 years. The disorder is often fatal in early life, usually because of respiratory problems, but some children survive with permanent weakness that does not continue to worsen.

Chronic (type III) spinal muscular atrophy (Wohlfart-Kugelberg-Welander disease) begins in children between the ages of 5 and 15 years and worsens slowly. Consequently, people with this disorder usually live longer than those with type I or II spinal muscular atrophy. Weakness and wasting of muscles begin in the legs and later spread to the arms.

Diagnosis and Treatment

Doctors test for these rare disorders when unexplained weakness and muscle wasting occur in young children. Because these disorders are inherited, a family history may help doctors make the diagnosis. Electromyography also helps. The specific defective gene has been identified for some of the types and can be detected by blood tests. If there is a family history of one of the disorders, amniocentesis can be performed to help determine whether an unborn child has the defective gene.

No specific treatments are available. Physical therapy and wearing braces can sometimes help.

CHAPTER 27

Diabetes Mellitus

Diabetes mellitus is a disorder in which blood sugar (glucose) levels are abnormally high because the body does not produce enough insulin.

- Symptoms of type 1 diabetes tend to occur rapidly and include excessive thirst and urination and dehydration, which lead to fatigue and lethargy.
- Increases in thirst and urination are milder and develop more gradually in type 2 diabetes.
- Diagnosis is by determining the level of sugar in the blood.
- Damage to the heart, kidneys, arteries, and eyes is less likely to develop if blood sugar is kept close to normal levels.
- Treatment includes diet and exercise plus insulin or drugs taken by mouth.

The symptoms, diagnosis, and treatment of diabetes are similar in children and adults. However, treatment of diabetes in children may be more complex and must be tailored to the child's physical and emotional maturity level.

Insulin is a hormone released by the pancreas that controls the amount of sugar in the blood. A child with diabetes has high blood sugar levels either because the pancreas produces little or no insulin (type 1 diabetes, formerly called juvenile-onset diabetes) or because the body is insensitive to the amount of insulin that is produced (type 2 diabetes). In either case, the amount of insulin available is insufficient for the body's needs.

Type 1 diabetes occurs throughout childhood, even in infancy, with a usual age of onset between 6 and 13 years. Type 2 diabetes occurs mainly in adolescents and is almost always associated with obesity.

Up until the 1990s, more than 95% of children who developed diabetes had type 1, usually as a result of an attack by the immune system on the cells in the pancreas that make insulin (islet cells). Recently, the number of children, especially adolescents, with type 2 diabetes has been steadily increasing. Today, 10 to 40% of children newly diagnosed with diabetes have type 2. The increase in childhood type 2 diabetes has been particularly prominent among Native Americans, blacks, and Hispanics. Obesity and a family history of type 2 diabetes are major factors in the development of type 2 diabetes (but not type 1).

WHICH CHILDREN ARE AT RISK FOR TYPE 2 DIABETES?

Children and adolescents meeting these criteria should be tested with a fasting blood sugar test every 2 years beginning at about age 10:

- Being overweight (weighing more than 85% of children of similar age, sex, and height or weighing more than 120% of the ideal weight for height)

Plus any two of the following factors:

- Having a close relative with type 2 diabetes
- Being Native American, black, Hispanic, Asian/Pacific Islander
- Having high blood pressure, high blood levels of lipids (fats), or polycystic ovary syndrome.

Symptoms

High blood sugar levels are responsible for a variety of immediate symptoms and long-term complications.

Symptoms develop quickly in type 1 diabetes, usually over 2 to 3 weeks or less, and tend to be quite obvious. High blood sugar levels cause the child to urinate excessively. This fluid loss causes an increase in thirst and the consumption of fluids. Some children become dehydrated, resulting in weakness, lethargy, and a rapid pulse. Vision may become blurred.

Diabetic ketoacidosis occurs at the beginning of the disease in about one third of children with type 1 diabetes. Without insulin, cells cannot use the sugar that is in the blood. Cells switch to a back-up mechanism to obtain energy and break down fat, producing compounds called ketones as byproducts. Ketones make the blood too acidic (ketoacidosis), causing nausea, vomiting, fatigue, and abdominal pain. The ketones make the child's breath smell like nail polish remover. Breathing becomes deep and rapid as the body attempts to correct the blood's acidity. The increase of ketones in the blood leads to diabetic ketoacidosis. Diabetic ketoacidosis can progress to coma and death, sometimes within a few hours. Children with ketoacidosis often have other chemical imbalances in the blood, such as an abnormal level of potassium and high levels of lipids (fats).

Symptoms in children with type 2 diabetes are milder than those in type 1 and develop more slowly—over weeks or even a few months. Parents may notice an increase in the child's thirst and urination or only vague symptoms, such as fatigue. Typically, children with type 2 diabetes do not develop ketoacidosis or severe dehydration.

DID YOU KNOW?

- The number of children with type 2 diabetes has been steadily increasing and is due to childhood obesity.
- A few children who have type 2 diabetes might be able to stop taking drugs that treat diabetes if they lose weight, improve their diet, and exercise regularly.
- Ideally, blood sugar is measured 4 times per day in children who have diabetes.
- Because low blood sugar is so harmful in children younger than 5 years of age, their target blood sugar level is higher than that of older children.

Diagnosis

Doctors suspect diabetes when children have typical symptoms or when a urine test done during a routine physical examination reveals sugar. The diagnosis is confirmed by measurement of the blood sugar level. Preferably, the blood test is done after fasting overnight. A child is considered to have diabetes if the fasting blood sugar level is 126 milligrams per deciliter (mg/dL) or higher. Rarely, doctors order a blood test that detects antibodies to islet cells to help distinguish type 1 diabetes from type 2; however, this information is rarely useful.

Because prompt measures (such as dietary changes, an increase in physical activity, and weight loss) may help prevent or delay the onset of type 2 diabetes, children at risk should be screened with a blood test. Nothing can be done to prevent type 1 diabetes.

In an increasing number of adolescents, type 2 diabetes is part of a constellation of disorders called the metabolic syndrome. This syndrome includes obesity (particularly abdominal obesity), insulin resistance, high blood pressure, and high triglyceride levels. This cluster of medical problems markedly raises the likelihood of future heart disease.

Treatment

The main goal of treatment is to keep blood sugar levels as close to the normal range as can be done safely. To control blood sugar, children with diabetes take drugs (such as insulin usually given by injection or drugs given by mouth) and change their lifestyle. Changes include adjustments in diet, regular exercise, and, for overweight children, weight loss.

When type 1 diabetes is first diagnosed, children are usually hospitalized. Children with diabetic ketoacidosis are treated in an intensive care unit. Children with type 1 diabetes always require insulin because nothing else is effective. They typically receive two or more daily injections of insulin, although a few may receive insulin continuously delivered under the skin by a pump. Insulin treatment is usually begun in the hospital so that blood sugar levels can be tested often and doctors can change insulin dosage in response. Rarely, treatment is started at home.

Children with type 2 diabetes do not usually need to receive treatment in the hospital. They do require treatment with diabetic drugs taken by mouth. The drugs used for adults with type 2 diabetes (such as metformin, sulfonylureas, meglitinides, thiazolidinediones, and glucosidase inhibitors) are safe for children, although some of the side effects—particularly diarrhea—cause more problems in children. Some children with type 2 diabetes need insulin. A major part of treatment is weight loss. Some children who lose weight, improve their diet, and exercise regularly may be able to stop taking the drugs.

Nutritional management and education are particularly important for all children with diabetes. Because carbohydrates in food are turned into glucose by the body, variations in carbohydrate intake cause variations in blood sugar levels. Thus, children with diabetes need to eat meals on a regular schedule; long periods between eating should be avoided because blood sugar may fall too low. Large amounts of sugar, such as soda, candy, and pastries, are discouraged because blood sugar may rise too high. Parents and older children are taught how to gauge the carbohydrate content of food and adjust what children eat as needed to maintain a consistent daily intake of carbohydrates. Children of all ages find it difficult to consistently follow a properly balanced meal plan (consumed at regular intervals) and avoid the temptations of sugary snacks. Infants and preschool-aged children present a particular challenge to parents because of the concern arising from the dangers of frequent and severe low blood sugar (hypoglycemia).

Emotional issues affect children with diabetes and their families. The realization that they have a lifelong condition may cause some children to become sad, angry, and sometimes even deny that they have an illness. A doctor needs to address these emotions to secure the child's cooperation in complying with the required regimen of meal plan, physical activity, blood glucose testing, and drugs. Failure to resolve these issues can lead to difficulties with glucose control.

Summer camps for children with diabetes allow these children to share their experiences with one another while learning how to become personally more responsible for their condition.

If treating the diabetes is difficult, the doctor may enlist the aid of a team of other professionals, possibly including a pediatric endocrinologist, dietitian, diabetes educator, social worker, or psychologist. Family support groups may also help. The doctor may provide parents with information to bring to school so that school personnel understand their roles.

Monitoring Treatment: Children and parents are taught to monitor the blood sugar level at least 4 times a day using a blood sample obtained by pricking a fingertip or the forearm with a small implement called a lancet. Once experience is gained, parents and many children can adjust the insulin dose as needed to achieve the best control. In general, by 10 years of age, children start to become interested in testing their blood sugar levels and injecting insulin themselves. Parents should encourage this independence but make sure the child is being responsible. Doctors teach most children how to adjust their insulin dosage in accordance with the patterns of their home blood glucose records.

Children with diabetes typically should see their doctor at least 4 times a year. The doctor evaluates their growth and development, reviews blood sugar records that the family member keeps, provides guidance and counseling about nutrition, and measures glycosylated hemoglobin (hemoglobin A_{1c})—a substance in the blood that reflects blood glucose levels over the long term. The doctor screens for long-term complications once a year by measuring protein in the urine, assessing function of the thyroid gland, and performing neurologic and eye examinations.

Some children with diabetes do very well and control their diabetes without undue effort or conflict. In others, diabetes becomes a constant source of stress within the family, and control of the condition deteriorates. Adolescents in particular often find it difficult to follow the proper treatment routine given the demands on their schedule and the limitations on their freedom that arise from diabetes. An adolescent benefits if the doctor considers the adolescent's desired schedule and activities and takes a flexible approach to problem solving—working with the adolescent rather than imposing solutions. The ultimate goals are tight control of blood glucose levels to prevent long-term complications and a healthy and normal lifestyle.

Complications of Treatment and Illness: No treatment completely maintains blood sugar at normal levels. The goal of treatment is to avoid blood sugar levels that are too high and too low. The complications of diabetes include heart disease, kidney failure, blindness, peripheral vascular disease, and other serious disorders. Although these events take years to develop, the better the control of diabetes, the less likely that complications will ever occur.

Low blood sugar (hypoglycemia) occurs when too much insulin or diabetic drugs are taken or when the child does not eat regularly. Hypoglycemia produces weakness, confusion, seizures and even coma. In adolescents and older children, episodes of hypoglycemia rarely cause long-term problems. However, frequent episodes of hypoglycemia in children younger than 5 may permanently impair intellectual development. Young children also may not be aware of the warning symptoms of hypoglycemia. To minimize the possibility of hypoglycemia, doctors and parents monitor young children with diabetes particularly closely and also use a slightly higher target range for their blood sugar level.

Children and adolescents with type 1 diabetes who miss insulin injections may develop diabetic ketoacidosis within days. The long-term insufficient or inadequate use of insulin can lead to a syndrome of stunted growth, delayed puberty, and an enlarged liver (Mauriac syndrome).

CHAPTER 28

Hereditary Disorders of Metabolism

- The process of converting ingested substances into material the body can use is called metabolism.
- Metabolic disorders result from the body's inability to break down some substance that should be broken down.
- A toxic intermediate substance builds up, or the body is unable to produce some essential substance.

Most of the foods and drinks people ingest are complex materials that the body must break down into simpler substances. This process may involve several steps. The simpler substances are then used as building blocks, which are assembled into the materials the body needs to sustain life. The process of creating these materials may also require several steps. The major building blocks are carbohydrates, amino acids, and fats (lipids). This complicated process of breaking down and converting the substances ingested is called metabolism.

DID YOU KNOW?

- Some hereditary disorders of metabolism can be detected before birth.

Metabolism is carried out by chemical substances called enzymes, which are made by the body. If a genetic abnormality affects the function of an enzyme or causes it to be deficient or missing altogether, various disorders can occur. The disorders usually result from an inability to break down some substance that should be broken down—so that some intermediate substance that is toxic builds up—or from an inability to produce some essential substance. Metabolic disorders are classified by the particular building block that is affected.

Some hereditary disorders of metabolism (such as phenylketonuria and the lipidoses) can be diagnosed in the fetus using amniocentesis or chorionic villus sampling. Usually, the diagnosis of a hereditary disorder of metabolism is made using a blood test or an examination of a tissue sample to determine whether a specific enzyme is deficient or missing.

Carbohydrate Metabolism

- Carbohydrates are sugars that the body uses for energy.
- The body must break down complex sugars into simpler forms in order to use them.

Carbohydrates are sugars. Some sugars are simple, and others are more complex. Sucrose (table sugar) is made of two simpler sugars called glucose and fructose. Lactose (milk sugar) is made of glucose and galactose. Both sucrose and lactose must be broken down into their component sugars by enzymes before the body can absorb and make use of them. The carbohydrates in bread, pasta, rice, and other carbohydrate-containing foods are long chains of simple sugar molecules. These longer molecules must also be broken down by the body. If an enzyme needed to process a certain sugar is missing, the sugar can accumulate in the body, causing problems.

GLYCOGEN STORAGE DISEASES

- Sugar that is not needed for the body's immediate needs is stored in the liver, muscles, and kidneys.
- People who have glycogen storage diseases lack an enzyme needed to change glucose into glycogen for storage or to break down glycogen into glucose again.

- Some of these diseases cause few symptoms, whereas others are fatal.
- Treatment usually involves regulating the intake of carbohydrates.

Glycogen is made of many glucose molecules linked together. The sugar glucose is the body's main source of energy for the muscles (including the heart) and brain. Any glucose that is not immediately used for energy is held in reserve in the liver, muscles, and kidneys in the form of glycogen and released when needed by the body.

There are many different glycogen storage diseases (also called glycogenoses), each identified by a roman numeral. These diseases are caused by a hereditary lack of one of the enzymes that is essential to the process of forming glucose into glycogen and breaking down glycogen into glucose. About 1 in 20,000 infants has some form of glycogen storage disease.

Some of these diseases cause few symptoms; others are fatal. The specific symptoms, age at which symptoms start, and their severity vary considerably among these diseases. For types II, V, and VII, the main symptom is usually weakness. For types I, III, and VI, symptoms are low levels of sugar in the blood and protrusion of the abdomen (because excess or abnormal glycogen may enlarge the liver). Low levels of sugar in the blood cause weakness, sweating, confusion, and sometimes seizures and coma. Other consequences for children may include stunted growth, frequent infections, or sores in the mouth and intestines. Glycogen storage diseases tend to cause uric acid, a waste product, to accumulate in the joints (which can cause gout) and in the kidneys (which can cause kidney stones). In type I glycogen storage disease, kidney failure is common in the second decade of life or later.

The specific diagnosis is made when a chemical examination of a sample of tissue, usually muscle or liver, determines that a specific enzyme is missing.

Treatment depends on the type of glycogen storage disease. For many people, eating many small carbohydrate-rich meals every day helps prevent blood sugar levels from dropping. For people who have glycogen storage diseases that produce low blood sugar, glucose levels are maintained by giving uncooked cornstarch every 4 to 6 hours around the clock. Sometimes carbohydrate solutions are given through a stomach tube all night to prevent low blood sugar levels from occurring atnight.

Types and Characteristics of Glycogen Storage Diseases

NAME	AFFECTED ORGANS	SYMPTOMS
Type O	Liver, muscle	Enlarged liver with accumulation of fat inside the liver cells (fatty liver); episodes of low blood sugar levels (hypoglycemia) when fasting
von Gierke's disease (Type IA)	Liver, kidney	Enlarged liver and kidney; slowed growth; very low blood sugar levels; abnormally high levels of acid, fats, and uric acid in blood
Type IB	Liver, white blood cells	Same as in von Gierke's disease but may be less severe; low white blood cell count; recurring mouth and intestinal infections or Crohn's disease
Pompe's disease (Type II)	All organs	Enlarged liver and heart, muscle weakness
Forbes' disease (Type III)	Liver, muscle, heart, white blood cells	Enlarged liver or cirrhosis; low blood sugar levels; muscle damage and heart damage in some people
Andersen's disease (Type IV)	Liver, muscle, most tissues	Cirrhosis in juvenile type; muscle damage and heart failure in adult (late-onset) type
McArdle's disease (Type V)	Muscle	Muscle cramps or weakness during physical activity
Hers' disease (Type VI)	Liver	Enlarged liver; episodes of low blood sugar when fasting; often no symptoms
Tarui's disease (Type VII)	Skeletal muscle, red blood cells	Muscle cramps during physical activity; red blood cell destruction (hemolysis)

GALACTOSEMIA

- Children with galactosemia are missing one of the enzymes needed to metabolize a sugar in milk.
- The liver, kidneys, and lenses of the eyes are damaged.
- A blood test is performed on newborns to detect this disorder.
- Treatment involves completely eliminating milk and milk products from the diet.

Galactosemia (a high blood level of galactose) is caused by lack of one of the enzymes necessary for metabolizing galactose, a sugar present in lactose (milk sugar). A metabolite builds up that is toxic to the liver and kidneys and also damages the lens of the eye, causing cataracts.

A newborn with galactosemia seems normal at first but within a few days or weeks loses his appetite, vomits, becomes jaundiced, has diarrhea, and stops growing normally. White blood cell function is affected, and serious infections can develop. If treatment is delayed, affected children remain short and become mentally retarded or may die.

Galactosemia is detectable with a blood test. This test is performed as a routine screening test on newborns in nearly all states in the United States and particularly in those with a family member known to have the disorder.

Galactosemia is treated by completely eliminating milk and milk products—the source of galactose—from an affected child's diet. Galactose is also present in some fruits, vegetables, and sea products, such as seaweed. Doctors are not sure whether the small amounts in these foods cause problems in the long term. People who have the disorder must restrict galactose intake throughout life.

If galactosemia is recognized at birth and adequately treated, the liver and kidney problems do not develop, and initial mental development is normal. However, even with proper treatment, children with galactosemia often have a lower intelligence quotient (IQ) than their siblings, and they often have speech problems. Girls often have ovaries that do not function, and only a few are able to conceive naturally. Boys, however, have normal testicular function.

HEREDITARY FRUCTOSE INTOLERANCE

- Children who have hereditary fructose intolerance are missing an enzyme needed to break down fructose (a sugar in table sugar and some fruits).
- Ingesting fructose, even in tiny amounts, results in low blood sugar levels and can lead to kidney and liver damage.

In this disorder, the body is missing an enzyme that allows it to use fructose, a sugar present in table sugar (sucrose) and many fruits. As a result, a by-product of fructose accumulates in the body, blocking the formation of glycogen and its conversion to glucose for use as energy. Ingesting more than tiny amounts of fructose or sucrose causes low blood sugar levels (hypoglycemia), with sweating, confusion, and sometimes seizures and coma. Children who continue to eat foods containing fructose develop kidney and liver damage, resulting in jaundice, vomiting, mental deterioration, seizures, and death. Chronic symptoms include poor eating, failure to thrive, digestive symptoms, liver failure, and kidney damage.

The diagnosis is made when a chemical examination of a sample of liver tissue determines that the enzyme is missing. Treatment involves excluding fructose (generally found in sweet fruits), sucrose, and sorbitol (a sugar substitute) from the diet. Acute attacks respond to glucose given intravenously; milder attacks of hypoglycemia are treated with glucose tablets, which should be carried by anyone who has hereditary fructose intolerance.

Amino Acid Metabolism

Amino acids are the building blocks of proteins and have many functions in the body. Hereditary disorders of amino acid processing can be the result of defects either in the breakdown of amino acids or in the body's ability to get the amino acids into cells. Because these disorders produce symptoms early in life, newborns are routinely screened for several common ones. In the United States, newborns are commonly screened for phenylketonuria, maple syrup urine disease, homocystinuria, tyrosinemia, and a number of other inherited disorders, although screening varies from state to state.

DID YOU KNOW?

- Newborns are usually screened for the most common disorders of amino acid metabolism.

PHENYLKETONURIA

- In phenylketonuria, the body is not able to rid itself of excess phenylalanine (an essential amino acid present in food).
- Phenylalanine builds up in the blood and eventually causes mental retardation.
- An infant may be sleepy, eat poorly, and have seizures, nausea, vomiting, an eczema-like rash, and a "mousy" body odor.
- Treatment is a diet that restricts intake of foods that contain phenylalanine.

Phenylketonuria (PKU) is a disorder that causes a buildup of the amino acid phenylalanine, which is an essential amino acid that cannot be synthesized in the body but is present in food. Excess phenylalanine is normally converted to tyrosine, another amino acid, and eliminated from the body. Without the enzyme that converts it to tyrosine, phenylalanine builds up in the blood and is toxic to the brain, causing mental retardation.

PKU occurs in most ethnic groups. If PKU runs in the family and DNA is available from an affected family member, amniocentesis or chorionic villus sampling with DNA analysis can be performed to determine whether a fetus has the disorder.

Most affected newborns are detected during routine screening tests. Newborns with PKU rarely have symptoms right away, although sometimes an infant is sleepy or eats poorly. If not treated, affected infants progressively develop mental retardation over the first few years of life, which eventually becomes severe. Other symptoms include seizures, nausea and vomiting, an eczema-like rash, lighter skin and hair than their family members, aggressive or self-injurious behavior, hyperactivity, and sometimes psychiatric symptoms. Untreated children often give off a "mousy" body and urine odor as a result of a by-product of phenylalanine (phenylacetic acid) in their urine and sweat.

To prevent mental retardation, phenylalanine intake must be restricted (but not eliminated altogether as people need some phenylalanine to live) beginning in the first few weeks of life. Because all natural sources of protein contain too much phenylalanine for children with PKU, affected children cannot have meat, milk, or other common foods that contain protein. Instead, they must eat a variety of phenylalanine-free processed foods, which are specially manufactured. Low-protein natural foods, such as fruits, vegetables, and restricted amounts of certain grain cereals, can be eaten.

A restricted diet, if started early and maintained well, allows for normal development. However, if very strict control of the diet is not maintained, affected children may begin to have difficulties in school. Dietary restrictions started after 2 to 3 years of age may control extreme hyperactivity and seizures and raise the child's eventual IQ but do not reverse mental retardation. Recent evidence suggests that functioning of some mentally retarded adults with PKU (born before newborn screening tests were available) may improve when they follow the PKU diet.

A phenylalanine-restricted diet should continue for life or intelligence may decrease and neurologic and psychiatric problems may ensue.

MAPLE SYRUP URINE DISEASE

- Children can develop vomiting, confusion, coma, and the odor of maple syrup.
- Treatment is a diet that restricts the intake of certain foods.

Children with maple syrup urine disease are unable to metabolize certain amino acids. By-products of these amino acids build up, causing neurologic changes, including seizures and mental retardation. These by-products also cause body fluids, such as urine and sweat, to smell like maple syrup. This disease is most common among Mennonite families.

There are many forms of maple syrup urine disease; symptoms vary in severity. In the most severe form, infants develop neurologic abnormalities, including seizures and coma, during the first week of life and can die within days to weeks. In the milder forms, children initially appear normal but develop vomiting, staggering, confusion, coma, and the odor of maple syrup particularly during physical stress, such as infection or surgery.

In some states, newborns are routinely screened for this disease with a blood test.

Infants with severe disease are treated with dialysis. Some children with mild disease benefit from injections of the vitamin B_1 (thiamin). After the disease has been brought under control, children must always consume a special artificial diet that is low in the particular amino acids that are affected by the missing enzyme.

HOMOCYSTINURIA

- Symptoms, including decreased vision and skeletal abnormalities, develop after 3 years of age.
- Vitamin B_6 or vitamin B_{12} may be given.

Children with homocystinuria are unable to metabolize the amino acid homocysteine, which, along with certain toxic by-products, builds up to cause a variety of symptoms. Symptoms may be mild or severe, depending on the particular enzyme defect.

Infants with this disorder are normal at birth. The first symptoms, including dislocation of the lens of the eye, causing severely decreased vision, usually begin after 3 years of age. Most children have skeletal abnormalities, including osteoporosis; the child is usually tall and thin with a curved spine, elongated limbs, and long, spiderlike fingers. Psychiatric and behavioral disorders and mental retardation are common. Homocystinuria makes the blood more likely to spontaneously clot, resulting in strokes, high blood pressure, and many other serious problems.

In a few states, children are screened for homocystinuria at birth with a blood test. The diagnosis is confirmed by a test measuring enzyme function in liver or skin cells.

Some children with homocystinuria improve when given vitamin B_6 (pyridoxine) or vitamin B_{12} (cobalamin).

TYROSINEMIA

- Children who have type I tyrosinemia usually become ill within the first year of life.
- Treatment is with a diet that restricts certain foods and a drug that blocks the production of toxic metabolites.

Children with tyrosinemia are unable to completely metabolize the amino acid tyrosine. By-products of this amino acid build up, causing a variety of symptoms. In some states, the disorder is detected on the newborn screening tests.

There are two main types of tyrosinemia: I and II. Type I tyrosinemia is most common in children of French-Canadian or Scandinavian descent. Children with this disorder typically become ill sometime within the first year of life with dysfunction of the liver, kidneys, and nerves, resulting in irritability, rickets, or even liver failure and death. Children are treated by taking a drug, that blocks the production of toxic metabolites and by restricting tyrosine and phenylalanine from their diet. Sometimes, children with type I tyrosinemia require a liver transplant.

Type II tyrosinemia is less common. Affected children sometimes have mental retardation and frequently develop sores on the skin and eyes. Restriction of tyrosine in the diet can prevent problems from developing.

Lipid Metabolism

- Lipidoses are disorders caused by excess fatty substances.
- Fatty acid oxygenation disorders result when the body cannot convert fat into energy.

Fats (lipids) are an important source of energy for the body. The body's store of fat is constantly broken down and reassembled to balance the body's energy needs with the food available. Groups of specific enzymes help the body break down and process fats. Certain abnormalities in these enzymes can lead to the buildup of specific fatty substances that normally would have been broken down by the enzymes. Over time, accumulations of these substances can be harmful to many organs of the body. Disorders caused by the accumulation of lipids are called lipidoses. Other enzyme abnormalities result in the body being unable to properly convert fats into energy. These abnormalities are called fatty acid oxidation disorders.

OTHER RARE HEREDITARY DISORDERS OF LIPID METABOLISM

Wolman's disease is a disorder that results when specific types of cholesterol and glycerides accumulate in tissues. This disease causes enlargement of the spleen and liver. Calcium deposits in the adrenal glands cause them to harden, and fatty diarrhea (steatorrhea) also occurs. Infants with Wolman's disease usually die by 6 months of age.

Cerebrotendinous xanthomatosis occurs when cholestanol, a product of cholesterol metabolism, accumulates in tissues. This disease eventually leads to uncoordinated movements, dementia, cataracts, and fatty growths (xanthomas) on tendons. The disabling symptoms often appear after age 30. If started early, the drug chenodiol helps prevent progression of the disease, but it cannot undo any damage already done.

In **sitosterolemia,** fats from fruits and vegetables accumulate in blood and tissues. The buildup of fats leads to atherosclerosis, abnormal red blood cells, and fatty deposits on tendons (xanthomas). Treatment consists of reducing the intake of foods that are rich in plant fats, such as vegetable oils, and taking cholestyramine resin.

In **Refsum's disease,** phytanic acid, which is a product of fat metabolism, accumulates in tissues. A buildup of phytanic acid leads to nerve and retinal damage, spastic movements, and changes in the bone and skin. Treatment involves avoiding eating green fruits and vegetables that contain chlorophyll. Plasmapheresis, in which phytanic acid is removed from the blood, may be helpful.

GAUCHER'S DISEASE

- Children have an enlarged liver and spleen, brownish skin pigmentation, and yellow spots on the eyes.
- Children who have the infantile form usually die within a year, but children and adults who develop the disease later in life may survive for many years.
- Treatment is enzyme replacement therapy.

In Gaucher's disease, glucocerebrosides, which are a product of fat metabolism, accumulate in tissues. Gaucher's disease is the most common lipidosis. The disease is most common in Ashkenazi (Eastern European) Jews. Gaucher's disease leads to an enlarged liver and spleen and a brownish pigmentation of the skin. Accumulations of glucocerebrosides in the eyes cause yellow spots called pinguec-ulae to appear. Accumulations in the bone marrow can cause pain and destroy bone.

Most people who have Gaucher's disease develop type 1, the chronic form, which results in an enlarged liver and spleen and bone abnormalities. Most are adults, but children also may have type 1. Type 2, the infantile form, develops in infancy; infants with the disease have an enlarged spleen and severe nervous system abnormalities and usually die within a year. Type 3, the juvenile form, can begin at any time during childhood. Children with the disease have an enlarged liver and spleen, bone abnormalities, and slowly progressive nervous system abnormalities. Children who survive to adolescence may live for many years.

Many people with Gaucher's disease can be treated with enzyme replacement therapy, in which enzymes are given intrave-nously, usually every 2 weeks. Enzyme replacement therapy is most effective for people who do not have nervous system complications.

TAY-SACHS DISEASE

In Tay-Sachs disease, gangliosides, which are products of fat metabolism, accumulate in tissues. The disease is most common in families of Eastern European Jewish origin. At a very early age, children with this disease become progressively retarded and appear to have floppy muscle tone. Spasticity develops and is fol-lowed by paralysis, dementia, and blindness. These children usu-ally die by age 3 or 4. Tay-Sachs disease can be identified in the fetus by chorionic villus sampling or amniocentesis. The disease cannot be treated or cured.

NIEMANN-PICK DISEASE

In Niemann-Pick disease, the deficiency of a specific enzyme results in the accumulation of sphingomyelin (a product of fat metabolism) or cholesterol. Niemann-Pick disease has several forms, depending on the severity of the enzyme deficiency and thus accumulation of sphingomyelin or cholesterol. The most severe forms tend to occur in Jewish people. The milder forms occur in all ethnic groups.

In the most severe form (type A), children fail to grow properly and have multiple neurologic problems. These children usually die by age 3. Children with type B disease develop fatty growths in the skin, areas of dark pigmentation, and an enlarged liver, spleen, and lymph nodes; they may be mentally retarded. Children with type C disease develop symptoms in childhood, with seizures and neurologic deterioration.

Some forms of Niemann-Pick disease can be diagnosed in the fetus by chorionic villus sampling or amniocentesis. After birth, the diagnosis can be made by a liver biopsy (removal of a tissue specimen for examination under a microscope). None of the types of Niemann-Pick disease can be cured, and children tend to die of infection or progressive dysfunction of the central nervous system.

FABRY'S DISEASE

In Fabry's disease, glycolipid, which is a product of fat metabolism, accumulates in tissues. Because the defective gene for this rare disorder is carried on the X chromosome, the full-blown disease occurs only in males. The accumulation of glycolipid causes noncancerous skin growths (angiokeratomas) to form over the lower part of the trunk. The corneas become cloudy, resulting in poor vision. A burning pain may develop in the arms and legs, and the person may have episodes of fever. People with Fabry's disease eventually develop kidney failure and heart disease, although most often they live into adulthood. Kidney failure may lead to high blood pressure, which may result in stroke.

DID YOU KNOW?

• Only boys can develop Fabry's disease.

Fabry's disease can be diagnosed in the fetus by chorionic villus sampling or amniocentesis. Fabry's disease is usually treated by replacing the deficient enzyme and taking analgesics to help relieve pain and fever. People with kidney failure may need a kidney transplant.

FATTY ACID OXIDATION DISORDERS

- In fatty acid oxidation disorders, the enzymes needed to break down fats are missing or deficient.
- Mental and physical development may be delayed.
- Some states screen newborns for the most common enzyme deficiencies.

Several enzymes help break fats down so that they may be turned into energy. An inherited defect or deficiency of one of these enzymes leaves the body short of energy and allows breakdown products, such as acyl-CoA, to accumulate. The enzyme most commonly deficient is medium chain acyl-CoA dehydrogenase (MCAD). MCAD deficiency is one of the most common inherited disorders of metabolism, particularly in people of Northern European descent.

Symptoms usually develop between birth and age 3. Children are most likely to develop symptoms if they go without food for a period of time (which depletes other sources of energy) or have an increased need for calories because of exercise or illness. The level of sugar in the blood drops significantly, causing confusion or coma. The child becomes weak and may have vomiting or seizures. Over the long term, children have delayed mental and physical development, an enlarged liver, heart muscle weakness, and an irregular heartbeat. Sudden death may occur.

Some states screen newborns for MCAD deficiency with a blood test. Immediate treatment is with intravenous glucose. For long-term treatment, the child must eat often, never skipping meals, and consume a diet high in carbohydrates and low in fats. Supplements of the amino acid carnitine may be helpful. The long-term outcome is generally good.

Pyruvate Metabolism Disorders

- Pyruvate is an energy source for cells.
- A deficiency in any one of the enzymes involved in pyruvate metabolism leads to a disorder.

Pyruvate is a substance formed in the processing of carbohydrates and proteins that serves as an energy source for cells. Problems with pyruvate metabolism can limit a cell's ability to produce energy and allow a buildup of lactic acid, a waste product. Many enzymes are involved in pyruvate metabolism. A hereditary deficiency in any one of these enzymes results in one of a variety of disorders, depending on which enzyme is missing. Symptoms may develop any time between early infancy and late adulthood. Exercise and infections can worsen symptoms, leading to severe lactic acidosis. These disorders are diagnosed by measuring enzyme activity in cells from the liver or skin.

Pyruvate dehydrogenase complex deficiency is a lack of a group of enzymes needed to process pyruvate. This deficiency results in a variety of symptoms, ranging from mild to severe. Some newborns with this deficiency have brain malformations. Other children appear normal at birth but develop symptoms, including weak muscles, seizures, poor coordination, and a severe balance problem, later in infancy or childhood. Mental retardation is common. This disorder cannot be cured, but some children are helped by a diet that is high in fat and low in carbohydrates.

Absence of pyruvate carboxylase, an enzyme, is a very rare condition that interferes with or blocks the production of glucose from pyruvate in the body. Lactic acid and ketones build up in the blood. Often this disease is fatal. Children who survive have seizures and severe mental retardation, although there are recent reports of children with milder symptoms. There is no cure, but some children are helped by eating frequent carbohydrate-rich meals and restricting dietary protein.

CHAPTER 29

Childhood Cancers

- The most common childhood cancers are leukemia, lymphoma, and brain tumors, which also occur in adults.
- Because children are still growing, treatment may cause side effects in children that do not occur in adults.
- Treatment is complex and can cause long-term consequences, so children are best treated in centers with expertise in childhood cancers.

Cancer is a rare disease among children, occurring in only 1 of 5,000 children every year. Although the most common childhood cancers are leukemia, lymphoma, and brain tumors, these cancers also occur in adults, and the diagnosis and treatment are similar in adults and children. Several of the more common cancers that occur mainly in children are Wilms' tumor, neuroblastoma, and retinoblastoma. Bone cancers also affect children (see page 441).

In contrast to many adult cancers, cancers in children tend to be much more curable. About 75% of children with cancer survive at least 5 years. Nonetheless, cancer kills over 2,000 children each year.

As in adults, doctors use a combination of treatments, including surgery, chemotherapy, and radiation therapy. However, because children are still growing, these treatments may have side effects that do not occur in adults. For example, in a child, an arm or leg that received radiation may not grow to full size. Children who receive radiation to the brain may not have normal intellectual development.

Children who survive cancer have more years than adults to develop long-term consequences of chemotherapy and radiation therapy, such as infertility, poor growth, damage to the heart, and even development of second cancers (which occurs in 3 to 12% of children who survive cancer). Because of these significant possible consequences and the complexity of treatment, children with cancer are best treated in centers with expertise in childhood cancers.

DID YOU KNOW?

- Cancers in children tend to be more curable than cancers in adults.
- Children who survive cancer have an increased risk of developing a second cancer.

The impact of being diagnosed with cancer and the intensity of the treatment are overwhelming to the child and family. It is difficult for the health care team and the family to maintain a sense of normalcy for the child, especially considering the child's frequent hospitalizations and office visits for treatment of the cancer and its complications. Overwhelming stress is typical, as parents struggle to continue to work, be attentive to siblings, and still attend to the many needs of the child with cancer (see page 540). The situation is even more difficult when the child is being treated at a specialty center far from home. The treatment team should include pediatric cancer specialists, other needed specialists, and the primary care doctor. Other essential personnel are a social worker (who can provide emotional support and advice regarding financial aspects of care), a teacher (who can work with the child, the school, and the health care team to ensure that the child's education continues), and a psychologist (who can help the child, siblings, and parents throughout treatment). Many centers also include a parent advocate—a parent who had a child with cancer who can offer guidance to family members.

Wilms' Tumor

Wilms' tumor (nephroblastoma) is a specific kind of cancer of the kidneys.

- Symptoms include a large abdomen, abdominal pain, fever, a poor appetite, nausea, and vomiting.
- Treatment involves surgical removal of the kidney that has the tumor, taking chemotherapy drugs after surgery, and sometimes receiving radiation therapy.

Wilms' tumor usually develops in children younger than 5 years of age, although it occasionally occurs in older children and rarely in adults. Very rarely, it develops before birth and appears in the newborn. In about 4% of cases, Wilms' tumor occurs simultaneously in both kidneys.

The cause of Wilms' tumor is not known, although a genetic abnormality may be involved in some cases. Children with certain birth defects, such as absence of the irises or excessive growth of one side of the body, both of which may be caused by a genetic abnormality, have an increased risk of developing Wilms' tumor. However, most children with Wilms' tumor have no such recognizable abnormalities.

Symptoms and Diagnosis

Symptoms include a large abdomen (for example, a rapid change to a larger diaper size), abdominal pain, fever, poor appetite, nausea, and vomiting. Blood appears in the urine in 15 to 20% of cases. Because the kidneys are involved in controlling blood pressure, Wilms' tumor may cause high blood pressure. This cancer can spread to other parts of the body, especially the lungs. Involvement of the lungs can lead to a cough and shortness of breath.

The first sign of Wilms' tumor, a painless mass in their child's abdomen, is most often noticed by the parents. A doctor is usually able to feel a lump (mass) in the child's abdomen. If the doctor suspects Wilms' tumor, ultrasound, computed tomography (CT), or magnetic resonance imaging (MRI) is performed to determine the nature and size of the lump.

DID YOU KNOW?

- Wilms' tumor may develop before birth.
- Typically, the first symptom, a lump in the abdomen, is noticed by the child's parents.
- Most children with Wilms' tumor survive.

Prognosis and Treatment

Younger children, children with smaller tumors, and children whose tumor has not spread tend to fare better. In general, Wilms' tumor is very curable; about 70 to 95% of children with Wilms' tumor survive, depending on how widespread the disease is. Even older children and children with widespread tumors have a very good prognosis. However, one particular type of Wilms' tumor (present in less than 5% of cases) is more resistant to treatment. Children with this type of tumor, which is recognized by its microscopic appearance, have a poorer prognosis.

Doctors treat Wilms' tumor by removing the kidney that contains the tumor. During the operation, the other kidney is examined to determine whether it also has a tumor. After surgery, doctors give the child chemotherapy drugs—most commonly actinomycin D, vincristine, and doxorubicin. Children with larger or widespread tumors also receive radiation therapy. Sometimes the tumor cannot be removed initially; in that case, the child is first treated with chemotherapy and radiation, and the tumor is removed when it is smaller.

Neuroblastoma

Neuroblastoma is a common childhood cancer that grows in parts of the nervous system.

- Symptoms can vary greatly, depending on where the cancer originated and where it has spread.
- Usually, surgery is performed to remove the cancer, and then the child is given chemotherapy drugs.

A neuroblastoma develops in a certain kind of nerve tissue located in many places of the body. It usually originates in nerves in the abdomen or chest, most commonly in the adrenal glands (located above each kidney). Very rarely, a neuroblastoma originates in the brain.

Neuroblastoma is the most common cancer in infants and one of the most common tumors in children of any age. About 80% of all neuroblastomas occur in children younger than 5 years. Although its cause is not known, this cancer sometimes runs in families.

Symptoms and Diagnosis

The symptoms depend on where the neuroblastoma originated and whether it has spread. For cancers originating in the abdomen, the first symptoms include a large abdomen, a sensation of fullness, and abdominal pain. Cancers in the chest may cause cough or difficulty breathing. In over half of the children, the cancer has spread beyond the original location by the time the child sees a doctor. Symptoms in these children relate to spread of the cancer. For example, cancer that has invaded the bones causes pain. Cancer that has reached the bone marrow may reduce the number of various types of blood cells. A reduced number of red blood cells (anemia) causes a weak and tired feeling; a reduced number of platelets causes bruising; and a reduced number of white blood cells lowers the resistance to infection. The cancer can spread to the skin, where it produces lumps, or to the spinal cord, where it may cause weakness of the arms or legs. About 90% of neuroblastomas produce hormones, such as epinephrine, which can increase heart rate and cause anxiety.

Early diagnosis of a neuroblastoma is not easy. If the cancer grows large enough, the doctor may be able to feel a lump (mass) in the abdomen. A doctor who suspects a neuroblastoma may suggest an ultrasound examination, computed tomography (CT), or magnetic resonance imaging (MRI) of the chest and abdomen. A urine sample can be tested for excessive production of epinephrine-like hormones. To see if the cancer has spread, the doctor may obtain a bone scan, take x-rays of bones, or examine tissue samples from the liver, lung, skin, bone marrow, or bone.

Prognosis and Treatment

Children younger than 1 year and children with small cancers have a very good prognosis. If the cancer has not spread, it usually can be removed by surgery. Nearly all children receive chemotherapy drugs such as vincristine, cyclophosphamide, doxorubicin, etoposide, and cisplatin. Also, radiation therapy may be used. In children older than 1 year, the cure rate is low for cancer that has spread.

Retinoblastoma

Retinoblastoma is a cancer of the retina, the light-sensing area at the back of the eye.

- Symptoms may include a white pupil or cross-eyes, and some retinoblastomas may affect vision.
- With treatment, most children with retinoblastoma are cured.
- Treatment is usually surgery or chemotherapy, but sometimes both are needed.

Retinoblastomas represent about 2% of childhood cancers and almost always occur before age 4. They occur in both eyes at the same time in 20 to 30% of children. This cancer is the result of damage to specific, known genes that control eye development. Sometimes a damaged gene is inherited from a parent or becomes damaged very early during embryonic development. Children with this type of damage may pass the defective gene on to their offspring, who may also develop retinoblastoma. Other times, genes are damaged later in embryonic development only in the embryo's eye cells. This damage cannot be passed on to offspring. Retinoblastoma is hereditary in all of the children with cancer in both eyes and in 15 to 20% of children with cancer in one eye.

Retinoblastoma usually spreads to the brain along the optic nerve (the nerve that leads from the eye to the brain). However, it also may spread to other organs, such as the bone marrow.

Symptoms and Diagnosis

Symptoms of a retinoblastoma can include a white pupil or strabismus (cross-eyes). Retinoblastomas of sufficient size also may affect vision but tend to produce few other symptoms.

If a doctor suspects a retinoblastoma, the child is given general anesthesia and both eyes are examined by looking at the retina through the lens and iris; general anesthesia is necessary because small children are not able to cooperate during the careful, time-consuming examination required to diagnose retinoblastoma. The cancer can also be identified by computed tomography (CT) or magnetic resonance imaging (MRI). Both tests help determine whether the cancer has spread to the brain. Doctors also look for cancer cells in a sample of cerebrospinal fluid (taken by spinal tap [lumbar puncture]); finding cancer cells is further evidence that the cancer has spread to the brain. Because the cancer can spread to the bone marrow, a sample of bone marrow is obtained for examination.

DID YOU KNOW?

- Retinoblastoma almost always occurs before age 4.
- Retinoblastoma may be hereditary.
- Retinoblastoma can usually be cured.

Prognosis and Treatment

Without treatment, most children with retinoblastoma die within 2 years. However, with treatment, children with retinoblastoma are cured more than 90% of the time. When only one eye is affected and that eye has little or no vision, doctors usually remove the entire eyeball along with part of the optic nerve. When there is significant vision in the affected eye, or the cancer affects both eyes, doctors sometimes give chemotherapy and try to avoid surgery in an attempt to spare the eyeballs. Chemotherapy drugs include etoposide, carboplatin, vincristine, and cyclophosphamide. The chemotherapy may completely eliminate the cancer and often shrinks it enough that the remainder may be removed with lasers, freezing (cryogenic) probes, or patches containing radioactive material. If these treatments do not eliminate the cancer, doctors may remove the eyeball or give radiation therapy. Sometimes, both eyeballs must be removed. Chemotherapy is also used when the cancer has spread beyond the eye or if the cancer returns after initial treatment.

Radiation therapy to the eye has significant consequences, such as cataracts, decreased vision, chronic dry eye, and wasting of the tissue around the eye. The bones of the face may fail to grow normally, resulting in a deformed appearance.

After treatment, doctors re-examine the eyes every 2 to 4 months to determine whether the cancer has returned. Children with the hereditary type of retinoblastoma have a particularly high risk of having the cancer recur. Furthermore, within 50 years from the time of diagnosis, as many as 50% of those with a hereditary retinoblastoma develop a second cancer, such as soft tissue sarcomas, melanomas, and osteosarcomas. Doctors recommend that immediate family members of any child with a retinoblastoma have regular eye examinations. Other young children in the family need to be examined for a retinoblastoma, and adults need to be examined for a retinocytoma, a noncancerous tumor caused by the same gene. Family members who have no evidence of cancer can have their DNA analyzed to see if they carry the retinoblastoma gene.

Acute Lymphocytic Leukemia

Acute lymphocytic (lymphoblastic) leukemia is a life-threatening disease in which the cells that normally develop into lymphocytes (a type of white blood cell) become cancerous and rapidly replace normal cells in the bone marrow.

- Children can develop fever, weakness, paleness, easy bruising and bleeding, infections, and other symptoms.
- Diagnosis is by bone marrow biopsy.
- Treatment is with chemotherapy given intravenously, injection of drugs via a lumbar puncture, and sometimes stem cell transplantation.

White blood cells develop from stem cells in the bone marrow. Sometimes the development goes awry, and pieces of chromosomes get rearranged. The resulting abnormal chromosomes interfere with normal control of cell division, so that affected cells multiply uncontrollably and become cancerous (malignant), resulting in leukemia.

Acute lymphocytic leukemia (ALL) is acute, meaning that it progresses rapidly, and lymphocytic, meaning that it develops from cancerous changes in lymphocytes or in cells that normally produce lymphocytes. ALL occurs in people of all ages but is the most common cancer in children, accounting for 25% of all cancers in children younger than 15 years. ALL most often affects young children between the ages of 2 and 5 years.

In ALL, very immature leukemia cells accumulate in the bone marrow, destroying and replacing cells that produce normal blood cells. The leukemia cells are also carried in the bloodstream to the liver, spleen, lymph nodes, brain, and testes, where they may continue to grow and divide. They can irritate the layers of tissue covering the brain and spinal cord, causing inflammation (meningitis), and can cause anemia, liver and kidney failure, and other organ damage.

Symptoms and Diagnosis

Early symptoms result from the inability of the bone marrow to produce enough normal blood cells. Fever and excessive sweating, which may indicate infection, result from too few normal white blood cells. Weakness, fatigue, and paleness, which indicate anemia, result from too few red blood cells. Easy bruising and bleeding, sometimes in the form of nosebleeds or bleeding gums, result from too few platelets. Leukemia cells in the brain may cause headaches, vomiting, and irritability, and those in the bone marrow may cause bone and joint pain. A sense of fullness in the abdomen and sometimes pain can result when leukemia cells enlarge the liver and spleen.

Blood tests, such as a complete blood count, can provide the first evidence that a child has ALL. The total number of white blood cells may be decreased, normal, or increased, but the number of red blood cells and platelets is almost always decreased. In addition, very immature white blood cells (blasts) are seen in blood samples examined under a microscope. A bone marrow biopsy is almost always performed to confirm the diagnosis and to distinguish ALL from other types of leukemia.

DID YOU KNOW?

- Acute lymphoblastic leukemia, previously highly lethal, can now usually be cured.

Prognosis and Treatment

Before treatment was available, most people who had ALL died within 4 months of the diagnosis. Now, nearly 80% of children with ALL are cured. For most people, the first course of chemotherapy brings the disease under control (complete remission). Children between the ages of 3 and 7 have the best prognosis. Children younger than 2 fare less well than older children. The white blood cell count and particular chromosome abnormalities in the leukemia cells also influence outcome.

Chemotherapy is highly effective and is administered in phases. The goal of initial treatment (induction chemotherapy) is to achieve remission by destroying leukemia cells so that normal cells can once again grow in the bone marrow. The child may need to stay in the hospital for a few days or weeks, depending on how quickly the bone marrow recovers. Blood and platelet transfusions may be necessary to treat anemia and to prevent bleeding, and antibiotics may be needed to treat infections. Intravenous fluids and therapy with a drug called allopurinol may also be used to help rid the body of harmful substances, such as uric acid, that are released when leukemia cells are destroyed.

One of several combinations of chemotherapy drugs is used, and doses are repeated for several days or weeks. One combination consists of prednisone taken by mouth and weekly doses of vincristine given with an anthracycline drug (usually daunorubicin) or asparaginase, and sometimes cyclophosphamide, given intravenously. Other drugs are being investigated.

For treatment of leukemia cells in the meninges (the layers of tissue covering the brain and spinal cord), some combination of methotrexate, cytosine arabinoside, and a corticosteroid is usually injected directly into the cerebrospinal fluid. This chemotherapy may be given in combination with radiation therapy to the brain. Even when there is little evidence that the leukemia has spread to the brain, a similar type of treatment is usually given as a preventive measure because of the high likelihood of spread to the meninges.

A few weeks after the initial, intensive treatment, additional treatment (consolidation chemotherapy) is given to destroy any remaining leukemia cells. Additional chemotherapy drugs, or the same drugs as were used during the induction phase, may be used a few times over a period of several weeks. Further treatment (maintenance chemotherapy), which usually consists of fewer drugs, sometimes at lower doses, may continue for 2 to 3 years. For some children who are at high risk of relapse because of particular chromosomal changes found in their cells, stem cell transplantation is often recommended.

Leukemia cells may begin to appear again (a condition termed relapse), often in the blood, bone marrow, brain, or testes. Reappearance in the bone marrow is particularly serious. Chemotherapy is given again, and although most children respond to treatment, the disease has a strong tendency to come back, especially in children younger than 2. When leukemia cells reappear in the brain, chemotherapy drugs are injected into the cerebrospinal fluid 2 times a week. When leukemia cells reappear in the testes, radiation therapy is given along with chemotherapy.

For children who have relapsed, high-dose chemotherapy along with stem cell transplantation offers the best chance of cure, but this procedure can be performed only if stem cells can be obtained from a person who has a compatible tissue type (HLA-matched). The donor is usually a sibling, but cells from matched, unrelated donors (or occasionally partially matched cells from family members or unrelated donors, as well as umbilical stem cells) are sometimes used.

After relapse, additional treatment for a child who is unable to undergo stem cell transplantation is often poorly tolerated and ineffective, frequently causing the child to feel much sicker. However, remissions can occur.

CHAPTER 30

Miscellaneous Disorders

This chapter describes several miscellaneous disorders that cannot easily be grouped together with other childhood conditions. These include canker sores, infantile spasms, lice infestation, progeroid syndromes, and sickle cell disease.

Canker Sores

Canker sores (aphthous ulcers) are small, painful sores inside the mouth.

- They are common and may recur.
- Rinses and gels can relieve the symptoms.

Canker sores are very common. The cause is unknown, but stress seems to play a role—for example, an adolescent may get canker sores during exam week. A canker sore appears as a round white spot with a red border. The sore almost always forms on soft, loose tissue on the inside of the lip or cheek; on the tongue, the floor of the mouth, or soft palate; or in the throat. Small canker sores (less than $1/2$ inch in diameter) often appear in clusters of two or three; generally, they disappear by themselves within 10 days and do not leave scars. Larger canker sores are less common; they are irregularly shaped, can take many weeks to heal, and frequently leave scars. People with AIDS often have large canker sores that persist for weeks.

Many people who get canker sores get them repeatedly— often several times a year.

Symptoms and Diagnosis

The main symptom of a canker sore is pain—far more than would be expected from something so small. The pain, which lasts 4 to 7 days, worsens if the tongue or food rubs the sore or if hot or spicy foods are eaten. Severe canker sores can cause fever, swollen lymph nodes in the neck, and a generally run-down feeling.

A doctor or dentist identifies a canker sore by its appearance and the pain it causes.

Treatment

Treatment consists of relieving the pain until the sore heals by itself. An anesthetic such as dyclonine or lidocaine may be used as a mouth rinse. However, because these mouth rinses numb the mouth and throat and thus may make swallowing difficult, children using them should be watched to ensure that they do not choke on their food. Also, anesthetics in any form should be taken only in limited amounts, for example, before meals and bedtime. Lidocaine in a thicker preparation (viscous lidocaine) can also be swabbed directly on the canker sore. A protective coating gel of carboxymethylcellulose, often combined with a corticosteroid (such as triamcinolone or betamethasone), may be applied to protect the sore and temporarily relieve pain by reducing inflammation.

If a child older than 8 years has many canker sores, a doctor or dentist may prescribe a tetracycline mouth rinse. Children who have repeated outbreaks of canker sores may start using the tetracycline mouth rinse as soon as they feel a sore developing. Another treatment option, applying silver nitrate directly to the canker sore, destroys the nerves under the sore to relieve pain.

Finally, for the most severe cases, a corticosteroid may be prescribed as a dexamethasone mouth rinse or, rarely, as prednisone tablets taken by mouth. However, before prescribing a corticosteroid, a doctor ensures that the child does not also have oral herpes simplex infection, which can be further spread by corticosteroids.

Corticosteroid rinses and tablets are absorbed into the body more than are corticosteroids given in gel form, so the side effects may be a concern. For example, long-term use in children may disturb growth, impair the immune system, and have psychologic effects.

Infantile Spasms

- Infantile spasms are seizures in which the arms bend, the neck and upper body bend forward, and the legs straighten.
- Spasms are treated with adrenocorticotropic hormone and sometimes clonazepam or nitrazepam.

In infantile spasms (salaam seizures), a child lying on his back suddenly raises and bends the arms, bends the neck and upper body forward, and straightens the legs. These spasms last for only a few seconds, but they may recur many times a day. They are rare but usually occur in children younger than 3 years. In many children, the spasms evolve into another type of seizure disorder later in life. In most children with infantile spasms, neurologic function develops slowly, and mental retardation is present. Usually, adrenocorticotropic hormone (ACTH) or another corticosteroid is used to treat these spasms. Usually, anticonvulsants are not effective in stopping the spasms; however, clonazepam and nitrazepam may have some benefit.

Lice Infestation

Lice infestation (pediculosis) is a skin infestation by tiny wingless insects.

- Eggs of head lice can be seen on hair shafts.
- Infestation may cause intense itching, but children may not notice scalp irritation.
- Prescription and nonprescription drugs can be used to kill lice; however, live eggs must also be removed manually by using a fine-toothed comb.

Lice are barely visible wingless insects that spread easily from person to person by body contact and shared clothing and

A Close-up Look at Lice

Three types of lice infest the body. Lice measure up to $1/8$ inch (3 millimeters) across.

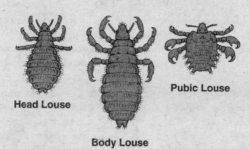

Head Louse

Body Louse

Pubic Louse

personal items. Three species of lice inhabit different parts of the body.

Head lice infest the scalp hair. The infestation is spread by personal contact and possibly by shared combs, brushes, hats, and other personal items. Head lice are a common scourge of school children of all social strata. Head lice are less common among blacks. Body lice and pubic lice can also cause infestations, the latter occurring in adolescents.

DID YOU KNOW?

- Lice infestation occurs in children of all socioeconomic backgrounds.
- Head lice infestation is not a sign of unhygienic conditions.
- The term "nit-picking" originally described the tedious process of removing lice eggs from the scalp.

Symptoms and Diagnosis

Lice infestation can cause severe itching and intense scratching, which may break the skin and lead to bacterial infections. However, children may hardly notice head lice or may have only a vague scalp irritation.

Lice themselves are sometimes hard to find, but their eggs are readily apparent. Female lice lay shiny grayish white eggs (nits) that can be seen as tiny globules firmly stuck to hairs near their base. With chronic scalp infestations, the nits grow out with the hair and therefore can be found some distance from the scalp, depending on the duration of the infestation. Occasionally lice can be seen as tiny insects that jump around the hair or scalp.

Nits are distinguished from other foreign material present on hair shafts by the fact that they are so strongly attached to the hair.

Treatment

Several prescription and nonprescription drugs are available to treat lice. Nonprescription shampoos and creams containing pyrethrins plus piperonyl butoxide are applied for 10 minutes and are then rinsed out. Prescription permethrin, applied as a liquid or as a cream, is also effective. Lindane—a prescription drug that can be applied as a cream, lotion, or shampoo—also cures lice infestation but is not as effective as the other preparations and is not recommended for children younger than age 2 years because of possible neurologic side effects. Prescription malathion, although highly effective at killing both adult lice and eggs, is not considered a first line treatment because it is flammable, has an objectionable odor, and must remain on the skin for 8 to 12 hours. All louse treatments are repeated in 7 to 10 days to kill newly hatched lice. Drugs applied to the scalp are often ineffective; if so, ivermectin, a drug taken by mouth, usually works.

After a drug application, live nits must be removed manually. Nits within $1/4$ inch of the scalp are assumed to be live. Removal requires a fine-tooth comb—which is often packaged with the medication—and careful searching (hence the term "nit-picking"). Because the nits are so strongly stuck to the hair, several nonprescription preparations are available to loosen them.

Sources of infestation (combs, hats, clothing, and bedding) should be decontaminated by laundering or dry cleaning.

Progeroid Syndromes

Progeroid syndromes are disorders characterized by features of premature aging and by shortened life expectancy.

The most striking feature of these rare disorders is extremely accelerated aging. Affected children develop all of the external signs of old age, including baldness, hunched posture, and dry, wrinkled skin. Unlike normal aging, however, progeroid syndromes also include such features as lack of ovarian or testicular activity (including sterility and absence of menstrual periods) and unusually short stature. Thus, progeria is not an exact model of accelerated aging.

Two forms of progeroid syndromes are Hutchinson-Gilford syndrome (commonly referred to as progeria), which begins in early childhood, and Werner's syndrome, which begins in adolescence or early adult life. Both syndromes are caused by genetic mutations. Hutchinson-Gilford syndrome produces scleroderma, baldness, and other conditions normally associated with aging (for example, diseases of the heart, kidneys, and lungs). Similarly, Werner's syndrome produces the skin changes of scleroderma and baldness and a high rate of atherosclerosis. The central nervous system, and therefore daily activities dependent on brain function, is largely spared in both Hutchinson-Gilford syndrome and Werner's syndrome, unless an affected person has a stroke. Other features of Werner's syndrome include premature cataracts, muscle wasting, and a high rate of cancer (including some types that are rare in unaffected people).

Sickle Cell Disease

Sickle cell disease is an inherited condition characterized by sickle (crescent)-shaped red blood cells and chronic anemia caused by excessive destruction of red blood cells.

- A child must inherit the gene for sickle cell disease from both parents in order to develop the disease.
- Symptoms of anemia, such as fatigue and weakness, and yellowish discoloration of the skin and eyes (jaundice) are typical, but there may be few other symptoms unless a crisis occurs.

- Several types of sickle cell crises can occur; a "pain crisis" can cause extreme discomfort.
- The abnormally shaped blood cells can be seen in a blood sample examined under a microscope.
- Treatment is aimed at controlling anemia, relieving symptoms, and preventing crises.

Sickle cell disease is a common hemoglobinopathy. Hemoglobinopathies distort the hemoglobin molecule, which carries oxygen in red blood cells to the tissues. As a result, not enough oxygen may be carried. Other hemoglobinopathies are similar to sickle cell disease but usually not as severe.

Sickle cell disease affects blacks almost exclusively. About 10% of blacks in the United States have one copy of the gene for sickle cell disease (that is, they have sickle cell trait); they do not develop sickle cell disease, although rarely they may notice blood in their urine. About 0.3% of blacks have two copies of the gene; they develop the disease.

Red Blood Cell Shapes

Normal red blood cells are flexible and disk-shaped, thicker at the edges than in the middle. In several hereditary disorders, red blood cells become spherical (in hereditary spherocytosis), oval (in hereditary elliptocytosis), or sickle-shaped (in sickle cell disease).

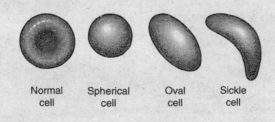

| Normal cell | Spherical cell | Oval cell | Sickle cell |

In sickle cell disease, as in other hemoglobinopathies, the red blood cells contain an abnormal form of hemoglobin (the protein that carries oxygen) that reduces the amount of oxygen in the cells. The reduced oxygen causes some of the red blood cells to become sickle-shaped. Because these deformed cells are fragile, they break apart as they travel through the smallest blood vessels, causing severe anemia, blocked blood flow, and reduced oxygen supply. The deformed cells also damage the spleen, kidneys, brain, bones, and other organs.

Symptoms and Complications

Children who have sickle cell disease always have some degree of anemia (which can cause fatigue, weakness, paleness, fainting, increased thirst, sweating, a weak and rapid pulse, and rapid breathing) and mild jaundice, but they may have few other symptoms. Anything that reduces the amount of oxygen in their blood, such as vigorous exercise, being at high altitudes without sufficient oxygen, or an illness, may bring on a sickle cell crisis. Different types of sickle crises exist, including a sudden worsening of anemia, pain (often in the abdomen or long bones of the arms and legs), and sometimes shortness of breath from a crisis in the lungs. Abdominal pain may be severe, and vomiting may occur during these crises.

One type of cell crisis, called acute chest syndrome, is characterized by severe chest pain and difficulty breathing. The exact cause of acute chest syndrome is unknown but may be related to or produced by an infection or a blocked blood vessel resulting from a blood clot or an embolus (a piece of a blood clot that has broken off and lodged in a blood vessel).

DID YOU KNOW?

- One in 10 black people in the USA carries the gene for sickle cell disease.
- If people want to avoid having children with sickle cell disease, the parents and, if necessary, the fetus can be tested.
- For children with sickle cell disease, obtaining all recommended vaccinations can be life-saving.
- The disease can damage the spleen, causing the child to be susceptible to infections, as well as the liver and heart.

Most children who have sickle cell disease develop an enlarged spleen. By the time the child reaches adolescence, the spleen is often so badly injured that it shrinks and no longer functions. Because the spleen helps fight infection, children with sickle cell disease are more likely to develop pneumococcal pneumonia and other infections. Viral infections, in particular, can decrease blood cell production, so anemia becomes more severe. The liver becomes progressively larger throughout life, and gallstones often form from the pigment of broken-apart red blood cells. The heart usually enlarges because it is pumping harder than normal, and heart murmurs are common.

Children who have sickle cell disease often have short stature. Changes in the bones and bone marrow may cause bone pain, especially in the hands and feet. Episodes of joint pain with fever may occur, and the hip joint may become so damaged that it eventually needs to be replaced.

Poor circulation to the skin may cause sores on the legs, especially at the ankles. Young men may develop persistent, often painful erections (priapism). Blocked blood vessels may cause strokes that damage the nervous system.

Diagnosis

In many states, sickle cell disease is initially diagnosed in newborns because of routine screening tests. In infants and older children who have not yet been diagnosed, doctors may diagnose sickle cell disease when evaluating chronic anemia. Or they may diagnose the disease if the child has a sickle cell crisis from the combination of anemia and bone pain (or another type of crises). Sickle-shaped red blood cells and fragments of destroyed red blood cells can be seen in a blood sample examined under a microscope.

A blood test called hemoglobin electrophoresis can detect abnormal hemoglobin and indicate whether a child has sickle cell trait or sickle cell disease. Discovering the trait may be important for family planning, to determine the risk of having a child with sickle cell disease.

Treatment and Prevention

Sickle cell disease can be a relatively mild disease that requires little treatment or a severe, recurring disease that causes enormous disability and early death. Rarely, a child or adolescent who has sickle cell trait dies suddenly while undergoing very strenuous exercise that has caused severe dehydration, such as during athletic training.

Treatment is aimed at preventing crises, controlling the anemia, and relieving symptoms. Children who have this disease should try to avoid activities that reduce the amount of oxygen in their blood and should receive prompt medical attention for even minor illnesses, such as viral infections. Because they are at increased risk of infection, they should be immunized with pneumococcal, meningococcal, and *Haemophilus influenzae* vaccines. All children and adolescents with sickle cell disease should take penicillin daily to prevent infections. They should also take folic acid daily to prevent folic acid deficiency anemia.

Sickle cell crisis may require hospitalization. The child is given drugs to relieve pain. Blood transfusions and oxygen may be given if a doctor suspects that anemia is severe enough to pose a risk of stroke, heart attack, or lung damage. Conditions that may have caused the crisis, such as an infection, are treated.

Drugs can help control sickle cell disease. Hydroxyurea increases the production of a form of hemoglobin found predominantly in fetuses, which decreases the number of red blood cells becoming sickle-shaped. Therefore, it reduces the frequency of sickle cell crises.

On rare occasions, bone marrow or stem cells from a family member or other donor who does not have the sickle cell gene may be transplanted in a child with the disease. Although such transplantation may be curative, it is risky, and recipients must take drugs that suppress the immune system for the rest of their lives. Gene therapy, a technique in which normal genes are implanted in precursor cells (cells that produce blood cells), is under study.

Prenatal diagnosis and counseling are available for couples who know they are at risk for having a child with sickle cell disease. Fetal cells obtained through amniocentesis can be directly examined, and the presence of one or two copies of the sickle cell gene can be accurately determined.

Part IV

Mental Health and Social Problems

CHAPTER 31

Mental Health Disorders

Several important mental health disorders, such as depression, often develop in childhood. Some disorders, such as autism, develop only in childhood.

With a few exceptions, the symptoms of mental health disorders tend to be similar to feelings that every child experiences, such as sadness, anger, suspicion, excitement, withdrawal, and loneliness. The difference between a disorder and a normal feeling is the extent to which the feeling becomes so powerful as to overwhelm and interfere with the activities of normal life and cause the child to suffer. Because of this, doctors must use a significant degree of judgment to determine when particular thoughts and emotions stop being a normal component of childhood experience and become a disorder.

DID YOU KNOW?

- The symptoms of most mental health disorders tend to be similar to feelings every child experiences.
- The difference between a normal feeling and a disorder is the extent to which the feeling interferes with activities of normal life.

In children, some disorders affect both mental health and the child's overall development. These are called the pervasive developmental disorders, which include autism, Asperger's disorder, pervasive developmental disorder not otherwise specified (PDD-NOS), Rett's disorder, and childhood disintegrative disorder. The pervasive developmental disorders comprise a group of related conditions that all involve some combination of impaired social relationships, stereotyped or ritualistic behavior, abnormal language development and use, and in some cases, intellectual impairment.

Among eating disorders, which include bulimia nervosa and binge eating disorder, anorexia nervosa affects mainly adolescents.

Autism

Autism is a disorder in which a young child cannot develop normal social relationships, uses language abnormally or not at all, behaves in compulsive and ritualistic ways, and may fail to develop normal intelligence.

- Mental retardation and resistance to changes in routines are common.
- Treatment may involve intense behavioral modification techniques and drug therapy.

Autism, the most common of the pervasive developmental disorders (see page 517), occurs in 5 of 10,000 children. Symptoms of autism may appear in the first 2 years of life and always before age 3. The disorder is 2 to 4 times more common in boys than in girls. Autism is different from mental retardation, although many children with autism have both.

The specific cause of autism is not fully understood, although it is clearly a biologically determined disorder. Several chromosomal abnormalities, such as fragile X syndrome, contribute to the development of autism. Prenatal infections, for example, viral infections such as rubella or cytomegalovirus, may also play a role. It is clear, however, that autism is *not* caused by poor parenting, adverse childhood conditions, or vaccination.

DID YOU KNOW?

- Autism is not caused by poor parenting, adverse childhood conditions, or vaccination.
- Autistic children whose IQ is below about 50 are likely to need full-time institutional care as adults.
- No good evidence supports the use of special diets, gastrointestinal therapies, or immunologic therapies.

Symptoms

Autistic children develop symptoms in at least 3 of the following areas: social relationships, language, behavior, and sometimes intelligence. Symptoms range from mild to severe and often keep children from functioning independently in school or society. In addition, about 20 to 40% of autistic children, particularly those with an intelligence quotient (IQ) less than 50, develop seizures before reaching adolescence.

Social Relationships: An autistic infant does not cuddle and avoids eye contact. Although some autistic infants become upset when separated from their parents, they may not turn to parents for security as do other children. Older autistic children often prefer to play by themselves and do not form close personal relationships, particularly outside of the family. When interacting with other children, they do not use eye contact and facial expressions to establish social contact, and they are not able to interpret the moods and expressions of others.

Language: About 50% of autistic children never learn to speak. Those who learn do so much later than normal and use words in an unusual way. They often repeat words spoken to them (echolalia) or reverse the normal use of pronouns, particularly using you instead of I or me when referring to themselves. These children rarely have an interactive dialogue with others. Autistic children often speak with an unusual rhythm and pitch.

Behavior: Autistic children are very resistant to changes, such as new food, toys, furniture arrangement, and clothing. They often become excessively attached to particular inanimate objects. They often repeat certain acts, such as rocking, hand flapping, or spinning objects in a repetitive manner. Some may injure themselves through repetitive behaviors such as head banging or biting themselves.

Intelligence: About 70% of children with autism have some degree of mental retardation (an IQ less than 70). Their performance is uneven; they usually do better on tests of motor and spatial skills than on verbal tests. Some autistic children have idiosyncratic or "splinter" skills, such as the ability to perform complex mental arithmetic or advanced musical skills. Unfortunately, such children are often not able to use these skills in a productive or socially interactive way.

Diagnosis

The diagnosis is made by close observation of the child in a playroom setting and careful questioning of parents and teachers. Standardized tests, such as the Childhood Autism Rating Scale, may help the evaluation. In addition to giving standardized tests, a doctor should perform certain tests to look for underlying treatable or inherited medical disorders (such as hereditary disorders of metabolism—see page 475—and fragile X syndrome—see page 116).

Prognosis and Treatment

The symptoms of autism generally persist throughout life. The prognosis is strongly influenced by how much usable language the child has acquired by age 7. Autistic children with below-normal intelligence—for example, those who score below 50 on standard IQ tests—are likely to need full-time institutional care as adults.

Autistic children may benefit from certain intensive behavioral modification techniques. Children whose IQs are normal may be helped by psychotherapy aimed at correcting social difficulties. Special education is crucial and often includes speech, occupational, physical, and behavioral therapy within a program equipped to manage children with autism.

Drug therapy cannot change the underlying disorder. However, the selective serotonin reuptake inhibitors (SSRIs), such as fluoxetine, paroxetine, and fluvoxamine, are often effective in reducing ritualistic behaviors of autistic children. Antipsychotic drugs, such as risperidone, may be used to reduce self-injurious behavior, although the risk of side effects (such as movement disorders) must be considered.

Although some parents try special diets, gastrointestinal therapies, or immunologic therapies, currently there is no good evidence that any of these therapies helps children with autism.

Asperger's Disorder and Pervasive Developmental Disorder Not Otherwise Specified

These pervasive developmental disorders are closely related to autism but are less severe.

Children with Asperger's disorder have impaired social interactions similar to those of children with autism, as well as stereotyped or repetitive behaviors and mannerisms and nonfunctional rituals. However, language skills are normal and sometimes superior to those of an average child, and IQ is normal.

DID YOU KNOW?

- Children with Asperger's disorder have normal intelligence.

Children who have significantly impaired social interactions or stereotyped behaviors without all of the features of autism or Asperger's disorder are considered to have pervasive developmental disorder not otherwise specified (abbreviated as PDD-NOS). Children with Asperger's disorder or PDD-NOS tend to function at a higher level than children with autism and may be able to function independently. Children with Asperger's disorder often respond well to psychotherapy.

Rett's Disorder

Rett's disorder is a rare genetic disorder occurring in girls that causes impaired social interactions, loss of language skills, and repetitive hand movements.

A girl with Rett's disorder appears to develop normally until some time between the age of 5 months and 4 years. When the disorder begins, the growth of her head slows and her language and social skills deteriorate. Typically, she displays repetitive hand motions resembling washing or wringing. Purposeful hand movements are lost, walking is impaired, and trunk movements are clumsy. Mental retardation develops and is usually severe.

Slight spontaneous improvements in social interaction may occur in late childhood and early adolescence, but the language and behavior problems progress. Most girls with Rett's disorder need full-time care and specialized educational programs. There is no cure.

Childhood Disintegrative Disorder

In childhood disintegrative disorder, an apparently normal child begins to act younger (regress) after age 3.

In most children, physical and mental development occur in spurts. It is common for children to take a step backward; for example, a toilet-trained child occasionally wets himself. Childhood disintegrative disorder, however, is a rare serious disorder in which a child older than age 3 stops developing normally and regresses to a much lower level of functioning, typically following a serious illness, such as an infection of the brain and nervous system.

The typical child with childhood disintegrative disorder develops normally until age 3 or 4, learning speech, becoming toilet trained, and displaying appropriate social behavior. Then, after a period of a few weeks or months during which time the child is irritable and moody, the child undergoes obvious regression. He may lose previously acquired language, motor, or social skills, and he may no longer have control over his bladder or bowels. In addition, the child develops difficulties in social interaction and begins performing repetitive behaviors similar to those that occur in children with autism. Quite often the child gradually deteriorates to a severely retarded level. A doctor makes the diagnosis based on the symptoms and searches for an underlying disorder.

Childhood disintegrative disorder cannot be specifically treated or cured, and most children, particularly those who are severely retarded, need lifelong care.

Childhood Schizophrenia

Childhood schizophrenia is a chronic disorder involving abnormal thought and social behavior.

- Typically, children become withdrawn and lose interest in activities; they develop distorted thinking and perception.
- Diagnosis is based on a doctor's observation of a child over time as well as a determination that no underlying medical condition exists.
- Symptoms can be managed with antipsychotic drugs.

Schizophrenia is quite rare in childhood; it typically develops in late adolescence and early adulthood. When schizophrenia does develop in childhood, it usually begins between the age of 7 and the start of adolescence.

Schizophrenia probably occurs because of chemical abnormalities in the brain. Doctors do not know what causes these abnormalities, although it is clear that there is an inherited vulnerability and that it is not caused by poor parenting or adverse childhood conditions.

Symptoms and Diagnosis

A child with schizophrenia typically becomes withdrawn, loses interest in activities, and develops distorted thinking and perception. These symptoms may continue for some time before progressing. Children with schizophrenia are likely to develop hallucinations, delusions, and paranoia, often fearing that others are planning to harm them or are controlling their thoughts. Children with schizophrenia typically have blunted emotions—neither their voice nor facial expressions change in response to emotional situations. Events that would normally make people laugh or cry may produce no response. In adolescents, use of illicit drugs may mimic symptoms of schizophrenia.

There is no specific diagnostic test for schizophrenia. A doctor bases the diagnosis on a thorough assessment of the symptoms over time, psychologic tests, and lack of evidence of an underlying medical condition, such as drug abuse, a brain tumor, and other disorders.

DID YOU KNOW?

- Childhood schizophrenia is not caused by poor parenting or adverse childhood conditions.

Treatment

Childhood schizophrenia cannot be cured, although hallucinations and delusions may be controlled with antipsychotic drugs, such as haloperidol, olanzapine, quetiapine, and risperidone. Children are particularly susceptible to the side effects of antipsychotic drugs, such as tremors, slowed movements, and movement disorders. Psychologic and educational support for the child and counseling for family members are essential to help everyone cope with the illness and its consequences.

Children with schizophrenia may need to be hospitalized at times when the symptoms worsen, so that drug doses can be adjusted and their safety can be assured.

Depression

Depression is a feeling of intense sadness; it may follow a recent loss or other sad event but is out of proportion to that event and persists beyond an appropriate length of time.

- Children lose interest in activities that normally give them pleasure.
- Appetite and sleep patterns may change, and the child may have little energy.
- Diagnosis is by questioning the child and his parents and sometimes teachers.
- Treatment includes antidepressants and psychotherapy.

Sadness and unhappiness are common human emotions, particularly in response to troubling situations. For children, such situations may include the death of a parent, divorce, a friend moving away, difficulty in adjusting to school, and difficulty making friends. Sometimes, however, feelings of sadness are out of proportion to the event or persist far longer than might be expected. In this case, particularly when the negative feelings cause difficulties in day-to-day functioning, the child may have depression. Like adults, some children become depressed even without unhappy life events. This is more common if there is a family history of mood disorders.

Depression occurs in 1 to 2% of children and as many as 8% of adolescents. Doctors do not know exactly what causes depression, but chemical abnormalities in the brain are probably involved. Some tendency to depression is inherited. A combination of factors, both life experience and genetic vulnerability, appear to contribute. Sometimes, a medical disorder, such as an underactive thyroid, is the cause.

Symptoms and Diagnosis

The symptoms of depression in children relate to feelings of overwhelming sadness, worthlessness, and guilt. The child loses interest in activities that normally give him pleasure, such as playing sports, watching television, playing video games, or playing with friends. Appetite may be increased or decreased, often leading to significant weight changes. Sleep is usually disturbed, with either insomnia or excessive sleeping. Depressed children often are not energetic or physically active. However, particularly in younger children, depression is sometimes masked by seemingly contradictory symptoms, such as overactivity and aggressive, antisocial behavior. Symptoms typically interfere with the child's ability to think and concentrate, and schoolwork usually suffers. Suicidal thoughts, fantasies, and attempts are common. The doctor must always assess the risk of suicide in depressed children.

To diagnose depression, a doctor relies on several sources of information, including an interview with the child or adolescent and information from parents and teachers. Sometimes, structured questionnaires help distinguish depression from a normal reaction to an unfortunate situation. A doctor tries to find out whether family or social stresses may have precipitated the depression and also determines whether a physical disorder, such as an underactive thyroid, is the cause.

DID YOU KNOW?

- Even very young children can have depression.
- Sometimes behavior in depressed younger children is overactive, aggressive, and antisocial.

Treatment

There is a wide range of severity of depression, and the intensity of treatment depends on the severity of the symptoms.

Antidepressant drugs correct chemical imbalances in the brain. Serotonin reuptake inhibitors (SSRIs), such as sertraline, and particularly, fluoxetine, are the drugs most commonly prescribed to depressed children and adolescents. The tricyclic antidepressants, such as imipramine, are much less effective in children than adults and have more side effects, and so are rarely used in children.

Treatment of depression requires more than drug therapy. Individual psychotherapy, group therapy, and family therapy may all be beneficial. Suicidal children must be hospitalized, usually briefly until they are no longer a risk to themselves.

SYMPTOMS OF DEPRESSION IN CHILDREN

- Sad mood
- Apathy
- Withdrawal from friends and social situations
- Reduced capacity for pleasure
- Feeling rejected and unloved
- Sleep disturbance, nightmares
- Self-blame
- Poor appetite, weight loss
- Thoughts of suicide
- Giving away valued possessions
- New physical complaints
- Falling grades

Manic-Depressive Illness

Manic-depressive illness is a disorder in which periods of intense elation and excitation alternate with periods of depression and despair.

Children normally have fairly rapid mood swings, going from happy and active to glum and withdrawn. These swings rarely indicate mental illness of any kind. Manic-depressive illness (also called bipolar disorder) is far more severe than these normal mood changes and is rare in children, but more common than previously thought. More typically, it begins in adolescence or early adulthood.

The cause is unknown, but a tendency to the disorder can be inherited. Rarely, drugs with stimulant effects, such as amphetamines, which are sometimes used for attention deficit/hyperactivity disorder (ADHD—see page 185), produce symptoms in children similar to manic-depressive illness.

DID YOU KNOW?

- Manic-depressive illness is sometimes confused with attention deficit/hyperactivity disorder.
- Manic-depressive illness is also called bipolar disorder.

Symptoms

Many children with manic-depressive illness exhibit a mixture of mania—a state of elation, excitation, racing thoughts, irritability, and grandiosity (in which the child feels he has some great talent or has made an important discovery)—and depression. The mania and depression occur simultaneously or in rapid alteration. During manic episodes, sleep is disturbed, the child may become aggressive, and school performance often deteriorates. Children with manic-depressive illness appear normal between episodes, in contrast to children with hyperactivity, who have a constant state of increased activity. Because ADHD can produce some similar symptoms, differentiating between the two conditions is important.

Treatment

Manic-depressive illness is treated with mood-stabilizing drugs, such as lithium, carbamazepine, and valproate. Individual and family psychotherapy help children and their families cope with the consequences of the disorder.

Suicidal Behavior

Suicidal behavior, an action intended to harm oneself, encompasses both suicide attempts and completed suicide.

- Suicidal behavior usually occurs in a child or adolescent with an underlying mental heath disorder, such as depression or alcohol or illicit drug use, particularly if a stressful event occurs.
- Children and adolescents who are at risk for suicidal behavior should be evaluated by a mental health specialist immediately.

Suicide is rare in children before puberty and is mainly a problem of adolescence, particularly between the ages of 15 and 19, and of adulthood. However, child suicide does occur and must not be overlooked in preadolescents. After accidents, suicide is the leading cause of death in adolescents, resulting in 2,000 deaths per year in the United States. It is also likely that a number of the deaths attributed to accidents, such as from motor vehicles and firearms, are actually suicides.

Many more young people attempt suicide than actually succeed. A survey performed by the Centers for Disease Control and Prevention found that 28% of high school students had suicidal thoughts and 8.3% had attempted suicide.

Among adolescents in the United States, boys outnumber girls in completed suicide by more than four to one. Girls, however, are 2 to 3 times more likely to attempt suicide than boys.

Risk Factors

Multiple factors typically interact before suicidal thoughts become suicidal behavior. Very often, there is an underlying mental health problem and a triggering stressful event. Examples of stressful events include the death of a loved one, loss of a boyfriend or girlfriend, a move from familiar surroundings (school, neighborhood, friends), humiliation by family or friends, failure at school, and trouble with the law. Stressful events such as these are fairly common among children, however, and rarely lead to suicidal behavior if there are no other underlying problems. The two most common underlying problems are depression and alcohol or drug abuse. Adolescents with depression have feelings of hopelessness and helplessness that limit their ability to consider alternative solutions to immediate problems. The use of alcohol or drugs lowers inhibitions against dangerous actions and interferes with anticipation of consequences. Finally, poor impulse control is a common factor in suicidal behavior. Adolescents attempting suicide are commonly angry with family members or friends, are unable to tolerate the anger, and turn the anger against themselves.

Sometimes suicidal behavior results when a child imitates the actions of others. For instance, a well-publicized suicide, such as that of a celebrity, is often followed by other suicides or suicide attempts. Suicides may cluster in families with a genetic vulnerability to mood disorders.

DID YOU KNOW?

- Suicide is rare in children before adolescence, but it does occur.
- Suicide is the second leading cause of deaths in adolescents.
- Among adolescents in the United States, boys attempt suicide less often but complete suicide more often than girls.
- Directly asking an at-risk child about suicide decreases (rather than increases) the risk that suicide will be attempted.
- Any indication that a child may be thinking of suicide should not be dismissed.

Prevention, Diagnosis, and Treatment

Parents, doctors, teachers, and friends may be in a position to identify children who might attempt suicide, particularly those who have had any recent change in behavior. Children and adolescents often confide only in their peers, who must be encouraged not to keep a secret that could result in the tragic death of the suicidal child. Children who express overt thoughts of suicide such as "I wish I'd never been born" or "I'd like to go to sleep and never wake up" are at risk, but so are children with more subtle signs, such as social withdrawal, falling grades, or parting with favorite possessions. Health care professionals have two key roles: evaluating a suicidal child's safety and need for hospitalization, and treating underlying conditions, such as depression or substance abuse.

Directly asking an at-risk child about suicidal thoughts and plans reduces, rather than increases, the risk that the child will attempt suicide because identifying suicidal thinking can lead to interventions. Crisis hot lines, offering 24-hour assistance, are available in many communities, and provide ready access to a sympathetic person who can give immediate counseling and assistance in obtaining further care. Although it is difficult to prove that these services actually reduce the number of deaths from suicide, they are helpful in directing children and families to appropriate resources.

Children who attempt suicide need urgent evaluation in a hospital emergency department. Any type of suicide attempt must be taken seriously, because one third of those who completed suicide had a previous suicidal attempt—sometimes apparently trivial, such as making a few shallow scratches to the wrist or swallowing a few pills. When parents or caretakers belittle or minimize an unsuccessful suicide attempt, children may see this as a challenge, and the risk of subsequent suicide increases.

Once the immediate threat to life has been removed, the doctor decides whether the child should be hospitalized. The decision depends on the degree of risk in remaining at home and the family's capacity to provide support and physical safety for the child. The seriousness of a suicide attempt can be gauged by a number of factors, including whether the attempt was carefully planned rather than spontaneous, whether steps were taken to prevent discovery, the type of method used, and whether any injury was actually inflicted. It is critical to distinguish intent from actual consequences; for example, an adolescent who ingests harmless pills he or she believes to be lethal should be considered at extreme risk. If hospitalization is not needed, families of children going home must ensure that firearms are removed from the home altogether and that drugs and sharp objects are removed or securely locked.

RISK FACTORS FOR CHILD AND ADOLESCENT SUICIDE

- Preoccupation with morbid themes
- Poor hygiene and self care (if an abrupt change)
- Access to firearms and prescription drugs
- Alcohol or drug abuse
- Family history of suicide
- Dramatic changes in mood, peer contact, grades
- Depressed mood, appetite or sleep disturbance
- Previous attempt at suicide

Anorexia Nervosa

Anorexia nervosa is an eating disorder characterized by a distorted body image, an extreme fear of obesity, refusal to maintain a minimally normal body weight, and, in girls, the absence of menstrual periods.

- Anorexia nervosa occurs mostly among psychologically susceptible adolescent girls in middle and upper socioeconomic groups.
- Affected girls usually deny they have a problem.
- Many girls are also depressed.
- Immediate treatment is providing fluids and nutrients.
- Long-term treatment aims to establish a calm, concerned, stable environment and to encourage the consumption of an adequate amount of food.

Hereditary and social factors have been shown to play a role in the development of anorexia nervosa. The desire to be thin pervades Western society, and obesity is considered unattractive, unhealthy, and undesirable. Even before adolescence, children are aware of these attitudes, and two thirds of all adolescent girls diet or take other measures to control their weight. Yet only a small percentage of these girls develop anorexia nervosa. Other factors, such as psychologic susceptibility, probably predispose certain people to developing anorexia nervosa. In areas with a genuine food shortage, anorexia nervosa is rare.

About 95% of people who have anorexia nervosa are female. The disorder usually begins in adolescence, occasionally earlier, and less commonly in adulthood. Anorexia nervosa primarily affects people in middle and upper socioeconomic classes. In Western society, the number of people who have this disorder seems to be increasing: it has been estimated to affect about 1% of girls aged 12 to 18.

DID YOU KNOW?

- Hereditary factors can predispose to anorexia nervosa.
- In populations where food is scarce, anorexia nervosa is rare.
- Many affected people take diuretics or binge on food and then vomit or take laxatives.
- A small percentage of people diagnosed with anorexia nervosa die from its complications, which include fluid and electrolyte disturbances, heart failure, and suicide resulting from depression.

Symptoms

Anorexia nervosa may be mild and transient or severe and persistent. Because many adolescents who develop anorexia nervosa are meticulous, compulsive, and intelligent, with very high standards for achievement and success, an eating disorder may easily go undetected. The first indications of the impending disorder may be a subtle increased concern with diet and body weight. Such concerns seem out of place, because most adolescents who have anorexia nervosa are already thin. Preoccupation and anxiety about weight intensify as the person becomes thinner. Even when emaciated, the person claims to feel fat, denies that anything is wrong, does not complain about weight loss, and usually resists treatment.

Anorexia means "lack of appetite," but adolescents who have anorexia nervosa are actually hungry and preoccupied with food. They study diets and count calories; they hoard, conceal, and deliberately waste food; they collect recipes; and they prepare elaborate meals for others. Half of the people who have anorexia nervosa binge and then purge by vomiting or taking laxatives. The other half simply restrict the amount of food they eat. They also frequently lie about how much they have eaten and conceal their vomiting and their peculiar dietary habits. Many also take diuretics to treat perceived bloating.

Girls with anorexia nervosa stop having menstrual periods, sometimes before losing much weight. Girls and boys with the disorder may lose interest in the opposite sex. Typically, they have a low heart rate, low blood pressure, low body temperature, swelling of tissues caused by fluid accumulation (edema), and fine, soft hair or excessive body and facial hair. People with anorexia nervosa who become very thin tend to remain active, often exercising excessively to control their weight. Until they become emaciated, however, they have few symptoms of nutritional deficiencies. Depression is common.

Hormonal changes resulting from anorexia nervosa include markedly reduced levels of estrogen (in girls) and thyroid hormone and increased levels of cortisol. If a person becomes seriously malnourished, every major organ system in the body is likely to be affected. When weight loss has been rapid or severe—for example, to more than 25% below the ideal body weight—restoring body weight quickly is crucial; such weight loss and the associated changes in electrolytes and fluid balance can be life threatening. Problems with the heart and with fluids and electrolytes (sodium, potassium, chloride) are the most dangerous. The heart gets weaker and pumps less blood through the body. The person may become dehydrated and prone to fainting. The blood may become alkaline (a condition called metabolic alkalosis), and potassium levels in the blood may decrease. Vomiting and taking laxatives and diuretics can worsen the situation. Sudden death, probably from abnormal heart rhythms, may occur.

Diagnosis and Treatment

Anorexia nervosa is usually diagnosed on the basis of severe weight loss and the characteristic psychologic symptoms. The typical person with anorexia nervosa is an adolescent girl who has lost at least 15% of her body weight, fears obesity, stops having menstrual periods, denies being sick, and otherwise appears healthy.

Treatment has two phases: short-term intervention to restore body weight and save the person's life and long-term therapy to improve psychologic functioning and prevent relapse.

The initial treatment of severe or rapid weight loss is best provided in a hospital where experienced staff members firmly but gently encourage the person to eat. Rarely, the person is fed intravenously or by a tube inserted through the nose and passed into the stomach. Sometimes doctors confine those with severe disease in the hospital against their will after obtaining appropriate legal authorization from a parent, guardian, or the court.

When the person's nutritional status is acceptable and stabilized, long-term therapy is begun. Treatment is aimed at establishing a calm, concerned, stable environment while encouraging the consumption of an adequate amount of food. This treatment may include individual, group, and family psychotherapy as well as drug therapy. Combined treatment by the family doctor and a therapist often helps, and consultation with or referral to a specialist in eating disorders is wise.

When depression is diagnosed, antidepressants are prescribed. Certain antidepressants, particularly selective serotonin reuptake inhibitors, are useful for preventing relapse after weight has been restored.

A small percentage of people diagnosed with anorexia nervosa die of it and its complications, which include fluid and electrolyte abnormalities, heart failure, and suicide resulting from depression. However, because mild cases may not be diagnosed, no one knows exactly how many people have anorexia nervosa or what percentage die of it.

Conduct Disorder

A conduct disorder is characterized by a repetitive pattern of behavior in which the basic rights of others are violated.

Although some children are better behaved than others, children who repeatedly and persistently violate rules and the rights of others in ways inappropriate for their age have a conduct disorder. The problem usually begins in late childhood or early adolescence and is more common among boys than girls. Evaluation of conduct must take the child's social environment into account. Misconduct developed by children as an adaptation to life in war-torn areas, settings of civil unrest, or other highly stressed environments is not a conduct disorder.

In general, children with a conduct disorder are selfish, do not relate well to others, and lack an appropriate sense of guilt. They tend to misperceive the behavior of others as threatening and react aggressively. They may engage in bullying, threatening, and frequent fights and may be cruel to animals. Other children with conduct disorder damage property, especially by setting fires. They may be deceitful or engage in theft. Seriously violating rules is common and includes running away from home and frequent truancy from school. Girls with conduct disorder are less likely than boys to be physically aggressive; they typically run away, lie, abuse substances, and sometimes engage in prostitution.

DID YOU KNOW?

- Children with conduct disorder rarely perceive anything wrong with their behavior.
- About half the children with conduct disorder stop such behaviors by adulthood.

About half of the children with conduct disorder stop such behaviors by adulthood. The younger the child is when the conduct disorder began, the more likely the behavior is to continue. Adults in whom such behaviors persist often encounter legal trouble, chronically violate the rights of others, and are often diagnosed with antisocial personality disorder.

Treatment

Treatment is very difficult because children with conduct disorder rarely perceive anything wrong with their behavior. Often the most successful treatment is to separate the child from a troubled environment and to provide a strictly structured setting, in either a mental health or a juvenile justice setting.

Oppositional Defiant Disorder

Oppositional defiant disorder is a recurring pattern of negative, defiant, and disobedient behavior.

Children with oppositional defiant disorder are stubborn, difficult, and disobedient without being physically aggressive or actually violating the rights of others. Many preschool and early adolescent children occasionally display oppositional behaviors, but oppositional defiant disorder is diagnosed only if behaviors persist for 6 months or more and are serious enough to interfere with social or academic functioning. Most often, children develop this disorder by age 8.

DID YOU KNOW?

- Children with oppositional defiant disorder are not physically aggressive.
- Children do know right from wrong and feel guilty if they do something that is seriously wrong.

Typical behaviors of children with oppositional defiant disorder include arguing with adults; losing their temper; actively defying rules and instructions; blaming others for their own mistakes; and being angry, resentful, and easily annoyed. These children do know the difference between right and wrong and feel guilty if they do anything that is seriously wrong.

Oppositional defiant disorder is best treated through behavior management techniques, which include a consistent approach to discipline and appropriate reinforcement of desired behavior. Parents and teachers can be instructed in these techniques by the child's counselor or therapist.

Separation Anxiety Disorder

Separation anxiety disorder is characterized by excessive anxiety about being away from home or separated from people to whom the child is attached.

- Children with separation anxiety disorder may avoid going to school.

Some degree of separation anxiety is normal and occurs in almost all children, especially in very young children (see page 144). In contrast, separation anxiety disorder is excessive anxiety that goes beyond that expected for the child's developmental level. Separation anxiety is considered a disorder if it lasts at least a month and causes significant distress or impairment in functioning. The duration of the disorder reflects its severity.

Some life stress, such as the death of a relative, friend, or pet or a geographic move or change in schools, may trigger the disorder. Genetic vulnerability to anxiety also typically plays a key role.

Symptoms

Children with this disorder experience great distress when separated from home or from people to whom they are attached. They often need to know the whereabouts of these people and are preoccupied with fears that something terrible will happen either to them or to their loved ones. Traveling by themselves makes them uncomfortable, and they may refuse to attend school or camp or to visit or sleep at friends' homes. Some children are unable to stay alone in a room, clinging to a parent or "shadowing" the parent around the house.

Difficulty at bedtime is common. Children with separation anxiety disorder may insist that someone stay in the room until they fall asleep. Nightmares may disclose the children's fears, such as destruction of the family through fire or another catastrophe.

Treatment

Because a child who has this disorder often avoids school, an immediate goal of treatment is enabling the child to return to school. Doctors, parents, and school personnel must work as a team to ensure the child's prompt return to school. Individual and family psychotherapy and anxiety-reducing drugs may play an important role.

EFFECTS OF STRESS ON CHILDREN

A stressful change in a child's life, such as a geographic move, divorce of the parents, or the death of a family member or pet, can trigger an **adjustment disorder.** Adjustment disorder is an acute but time-limited response to environmental stress. The child may have symptoms of anxiety (for example, nervousness, worries, and fears), symptoms of depression (for example, tearfulness or feelings of hopelessness), or behavioral problems. The symptoms and problems abate as the stress diminishes.

Posttraumatic stress disorder is a much more extreme response and may occur after a natural disaster (such as a hurricane, tornado, or earthquake), an accident, death, or a senseless act of violence, including child abuse. The child usually fails in his attempts to avoid remembering the event, suffers a persistent state of anxiety, and may reexperience the traumatic event while awake (flashback) or asleep (nightmares). Crisis intervention is usually necessary, in the form of an extended period of individual, group, or family therapy. Treatment with anxiety-reducing drugs may be needed.

Somatoform Disorders

Somatoform disorders are a group of disorders in which an underlying psychologic problem causes distressing or disabling physical symptoms.

- The child does not fabricate the symptoms.
- Diagnosis is made after a doctor determines that the symptoms are not caused by a physical illness.
- Treatment often involves individual and family psychotherapy.

A child with a somatoform disorder may have a number of symptoms, including pain, difficulty breathing, and weakness, without evidence of a physical cause. Often, a child develops psychologically based physical symptoms when another family member is seriously ill. These physical symptoms are thought to develop unconsciously in response to a psychologic stress or problem. It is clear that the symptoms are not consciously fabricated, and the child is actually experiencing the symptoms he describes.

Somatoform disorders are further classified as conversion disorder, somatization disorder, body dysmorphic disorder, and hypochondriasis. In **conversion disorder,** the child may seem to have a paralyzed arm or leg, become deaf or blind, or have shaking activity resembling seizures. These symptoms begin suddenly, usually in relation to a precipitating event, and may or may not resolve abruptly. A **somatization disorder** is similar to conversion disorder, but the child develops numerous symptoms that are more vague, such as headaches, abdominal pain (see page 392), and nausea. These symptoms may come and go for long periods of time. In **body dysmorphic disorder,** the child becomes preoccupied with an imagined defect in appearance, such as the size of his nose or ears, or develops a markedly excessive concern with a minor abnormality, such as a wart. In **hypochondriasis,** the child has no specific, ongoing symptoms but is obsessed with bodily functions, such as heartbeat, digestion, and sweating, and is convinced that he has a serious disease when nothing is actually wrong.

Somatoform disorders are equally common among young boys and young girls, but they are more common among adolescent girls than adolescent boys.

Diagnosis

Before establishing the diagnosis of a somatoform disorder, the doctor makes sure that the child does not have a physical illness that could account for the symptoms. However, extensive laboratory tests are generally avoided because they may further convince the child that a physical problem exists and unnecessary diagnostic tests may themselves traumatize the child. If no physical illness can be found, the doctor then talks to the child and family members to try to identify underlying psychologic problems or troubled family relationships.

Treatment

A child may balk at the idea of visiting a psychotherapist because to the child his symptoms are purely physical. However, an approach combining individual and family psychotherapy and physical rehabilitation has been shown to be effective in many cases.

CHAPTER 32

Social Issues Affecting Children and Their Families

In order to thrive, a child must experience the consistent and ongoing care of a loving, nurturing caregiver, whether it be a parent or someone else. The security and support that such an adult can provide give a child the self-confidence and resiliency to cope effectively with stress.

In order to mature emotionally and socially, children must interact with people outside the home. These interactions typically occur with close relatives; friends; neighbors; and people at childcare sites, schools, churches, and sports teams or other activities. By coping with the minor stresses and conflicts of these interactions, children gradually acquire the skills to handle more significant ones.

DID YOU KNOW?

- Illness or death in an infant or a child often makes parents feel guilty, even when they are not at fault.
- Sometimes children need to hear the same message about a difficult issue over and over.
- Children who are bullied are often too frightened or embarrassed to tell an adult.

WHAT IS BULLYING?

Bullying is repeated physical or psychologic attacks that are performed to dominate or humiliate. Although it typically involves only two people, bullying can involve groups. Bullying hurts and demeans the victim. In addition, the bully often unknowingly repels his friends and peers, hurting himself.

Although they sometimes tell family members or friends, victims are often too embarrassed and frightened to disclose bullying to an adult. Occasionally, a teacher informs a parent. Victims may refuse to go to school, appear sad or withdrawn, or become moody.

Victims need reassurance that bullying is always unacceptable. Parents can demonstrate ways a victim can respond to the bully—for example, telling an adult, walking away, changing their routines to avoid the bully, or engaging in counseling. Although it is usually not advisable (for safety reasons) to directly confront the bully, teaching the child to ignore and actually not be bothered by the bully will reduce the bully's satisfaction and eventually lessen the bullying. Praising the victim's courage for reporting bullying can begin to rebuild the child's self-esteem.

If bullying occurs at school, parents should inform school officials. The victim's parents should also inform the bully's parents but should avoid confrontation, which could be counterproductive by making the bully's parents defensive. Victims may fear that telling the bully's parents will worsen bullying, but it often stops bullying, particularly if the discussion is positive and not accusatory, but instead focuses on the harmful behavior.

The bully's parents should make it clear to their child that bullying is not acceptable. These parents should insist that the bully apologize and make amends to the victim. Doing so can help the bully learn right from wrong, can make the bully more sensitive to the victim, and can make others see the bully more sympathetically. Adults should watch the child closely to ensure that bullying stops. Counseling can sometimes help the child who is doing the bullying, who often is expressing his or her unmet needs or who is modeling the aggressive behavior of a parent or older sibling.

However, certain major events, such as illness and divorce, may challenge a child's abilities to cope. These events may also interfere with the child's emotional and social development. For example, a chronic illness may prevent a child from participating in activities and also impair performance in school.

Events affecting the child may also have adverse consequences for people close to the child. Everyone who cares for a sick child is under stress. The consequences of such stress vary with the nature and severity of the illness and with the family's emotional and other resources and supports.

TALKING WITH CHILDREN ABOUT DIFFICULT TOPICS

Many life events, including illness or death of someone close, divorce, and bullying, are scary or unpleasant for children. Even events that do not directly affect the child, such as natural disasters, war, or terrorism, may cause anxiety. Fears about all of these, rational or irrational, can preoccupy a child.

Children often have difficulty talking about unpleasant topics. However, open discussion can help the child deal with difficult or embarrassing topics and dispel irrational fears. A child needs to know that anxiety is normal and will get better.

Parents should discuss difficult topics during a quiet time, in a private place, and when the child is interested. Parents should remain calm, present factual information, and give the child undivided attention. Acknowledging what was said with phrases such as, "I understand," or with a quiet nod encourages the child to confide; so does reflecting back what was said. For example, if a child mentions anger about a divorce, one could say, "So, the divorce makes you angry," or "Tell me more about that." Asking how the child feels can also encourage him to discuss sensitive emotions or fears—for example, fear of abandonment by the noncustodial parent during a divorce or guilt for causing the divorce.

By disclosing their own feelings, parents encourage children to acknowledge their fears and concerns. For example, about a divorce, a parent might say, "I am sad about the divorce, too. But, I also know it is the right thing for mommy and daddy to do. Even though we cannot live together anymore, we will both always love you and take care of you." By doing this, parents are able to discuss their own feelings offer reassurance, and explain that divorce is the right choice for them.

them. Sometimes children, particularly younger ones, need to hear the same message repeatedly.

Sometimes a parent must raise a difficult topic with a child, such as telling the child about a serious illness in a relative or friend. If tragedy affects someone else, children may feel more confident, and less helpless, if they can contribute—for example, by picking flowers; writing or drawing a card; wrapping a present; or collecting food, clothing, money, or toys. When a child appears withdrawn or sad, refuses to engage in usual activities, or becomes aggressive, the parent should seek professional help.

A parent may also have to address a difficult aspect of the child's own behavior. For example, a parent who suspects the child or adolescent of using drugs or alcohol should address the issue directly with the child. A parent might say "I am worried that you are using drugs. I feel this way because . . ." The parent should then calmly list the behaviors that concern him, limiting the list to three or four behaviors. If the child denies there is a problem, the parent should restate the concerns calmly and explain to the child that there is a plan of action in place (such as an appointment with a pediatrician or counselor).

Throughout any discussion, the parent should reassure the child that he is loved and will be supported.

Illness and Death in Infants

- Seeing, touching, and interacting with an infant who has a severe illness or birth defect helps parents bond with the infant.

The medical needs of ill or premature newborns and infants often require that these children be separated from their parents temporarily. Although doctors may allow parents to hold their infant some of the time, medical care often sharply limits the opportunity for parents to interact with their infant. In addition, parents are usually emotionally distressed by their infant's condition. The separation and parental distress can interfere with bonding (see page 17), particularly in severely ill infants who are hospitalized for a long time. Parents need to see, hold, and interact with their infant as soon as it is practical. Even with severely ill infants, parents often can help to feed, bathe, and change their infant. Breastfeeding may be possible, even if the infant must be fed through a tube at first.

DID YOU KNOW?

- Seeing and touching an infant who has died helps parents begin to grieve.

If an infant has a birth defect, parents may experience guilt, sadness, anger, or even horror. Many feel even more guilt because they have such feelings. Seeing and touching the child can help the parents look beyond the birth defect and see the infant as a whole person; this helps the bonding process begin. Information about the condition, possible treatments, and the infant's prognosis can help the parents adjust psychologically and plan for the best medical care.

Death of an infant is always traumatic for parents. However, if a newborn dies before being seen or touched by the parents, the parents may feel as though they never had a baby. Although painful, holding or seeing the dead baby can help parents begin to grieve and begin the process of closure. Emptiness, lost hopes and dreams, and fear may overwhelm parents, who may become depressed. Parents tend to feel guilty, blaming themselves even when they are not responsible for the death. The grief and guilt that follow may strain the relationship between parents.

Many families whose infants are severely ill or who have died can benefit from counseling from psychologic or religious personnel. Parent and family support groups also may help; some groups include special sessions for siblings.

Illness in Children

- Severe or chronic illness causes stress and emotional distress for the child, parents, and other family members.
- Illness can interfere with a child's education, self-image, and relationships with other children and family members.

- A child's illness can disrupt the parents' relationship with each other and with their other children.
- Hospitalization should be avoided if possible, or if unavoidable, it should be as brief as possible.
- Learning about the child's illness can help parents deal with the situation and make decisions about care.

Severe illness, even if temporary, can provoke a great deal of anxiety for children. Chronic illness or disability usually causes even more emotional distress.

Coping with illness may require coping with pain, undergoing tests, taking drugs, and changing diet and lifestyle. Chronic illness often interferes with a child's education because of frequent absences from school. The illness as well as side effects from treatments may impair the child's ability to learn. Parents and teachers may have lower academic expectations of ill children; however, it is important for them to maintain the challenges and encouragement children need to achieve their best.

Illness and hospitalization deprive children of opportunities to play with other children. Other children may even reject or taunt an ill child because of physical differences and limitations. A child can become self-conscious if illness changes his body, particularly when the change occurs during childhood or adolescence rather than being present from birth. Parents and family members may overprotect the child, discouraging independence.

Chronic illness places enormous psychologic and physical burdens on parents. Sometimes the parents become closer by working together to overcome these burdens. However, often the burdens can strain the relationship. Parents may feel guilty about the illness, particularly if it is genetic, resulted from complications during pregnancy, or was caused by an accident (such as a motor vehicle collision), or a behavior of a parent (such as smoking). In addition, medical care can be expensive and can cause the parents to miss work. Sometimes, one parent assumes the burden of the care, which can lead to feelings of resentment in the caregiving parent or feelings of isolation in the other. Parents may feel angry with health care providers, themselves, each other, or the child. The emotional distress involved in providing care can also make it difficult to form a deep attachment to a disabled or seriously ill child.

DID YOU KNOW? _____

- Parents and family members may overprotect a child who is ill, discouraging independence.
- Sometimes one parent assumes the burden of the care and later resents it, while the other parent may feel isolated.
- Parents may spend more time or be more lenient with the ill child than with siblings, who may then become resentful and feel guilty about their resentment.

Parents who spend a lot of time with an ill child often have less time to devote to other children in the family. Siblings may resent the extra attention the ill child receives and then feel guilty for feeling that way. The ill child may feel guilty about hurting or burdening the family. Parents may be too lenient with the ill child, or they may enforce discipline inconsistently, particularly if the symptoms come and go.

Hospitalization is a frightening event for children even under the best circumstances, and it should be avoided whenever possible. If hospitalization is needed, it should be as brief as possible, preferably in a part of the hospital used exclusively for children. In many hospitals, parents are able to stay with their children, even during painful or fear-provoking procedures. Despite their parents' presence, children often become clingy or dependent (regress) while in the hospital.

Although a child's illness is always stressful for the entire family, there are several steps a parent can take to help lessen the impact. Parents should learn as much as possible about their child's illness from reliable sources, such as the child's doctors and reliable medical resources. Information obtained from some Internet sources is not always accurate, and parents should check with their doctors about the information they read. A support group or another family that has already faced similar issues can provide information and emotional support; doctors can often refer parents to such people.

Services needed by the child may involve care by medical specialists, nurses, home health personnel, mental health personnel, and personnel from a variety of other services. A case manager may be needed to help coordinate medical care for children with complex chronic illnesses. The child's doctor, nurse, social worker, or other professional can serve as the case manager. The case manager can also ensure that the child receives training in social skills and that the family and child receive appropriate counseling, education, and psychologic and social support, such as respite care.

Divorce

- After a divorce, children may feel insecure, abandoned, anxious, angry, sad, or responsible for the divorce.
- Children's behavior and school performance may deteriorate during a divorce.
- The turmoil felt by children after a divorce subsides as new arrangements are worked out.
- Parents can help children by cooperating with each other and focusing on the children's needs.
- Giving children a say in arrangements that affect them and talking with them openly help children adjust.

Separation and divorce interrupt the stability and predictability that children need. Other than the death of an immediate family member, divorce is the most stressful event that can affect a family. Because the world as they know it has ended, children may feel a great loss as well as anxiety, anger, and sadness. Children may fear being abandoned or losing their parents' love. For many reasons, parenting skills often worsen around the time of the divorce. Parents are usually preoccupied and may be angry and hostile toward each other. Regardless of whether they contributed to the divorce, children may feel guilty about causing it. If parents ignore children or visit sporadically and unpredictably, children feel rejected.

Once parents decide to separate and divorce, family members move through several stages of adjustment. In the acute stage (the period when parents decide to separate, including the time preceding the divorce), turmoil is often maximal. This stage may last up to 2 years. During the transitional stage (the weeks around the actual divorce), the child has more control over change and adjusts to the new relationship between the parents, visitation, and the new relationship with the noncustodial parent. After the divorce (the post-divorce stage), stability usually returns.

During the divorce, schoolwork may seem unimportant to children and adolescents, and school performance often worsens. Children may have fantasies that parents will reconcile. Children aged 2 to 5 years may have difficulty sleeping, temper tantrums, and separation anxiety. Toileting skills may deteriorate. Children aged 5 to 12 years can experience sadness, grief, intense anger, and irrational fears (phobias). Adolescents often feel insecure, lonely, and sad. Some engage in risk-taking behaviors such as drug and alcohol use, sex, theft, and violence. Others may develop eating disorders, become defiant, skip school, or join peers who are engaging in risk-taking behaviors.

Children need to be able to express their feelings to an adult who listens attentively. Counseling can provide children with a caring adult who, unlike their parents, will not be upset by their feelings.

Children adjust best when parents cooperate with each other and focus on the child's needs. Parents must remember that a divorce only severs their relationship as husband and wife, not their relationship as parents of their children. Whenever possible, parents should live close to each other, try not to anger each other, maintain the other's involvement in the child's life, and consider the child's wishes regarding visitation. Older children and adolescents should be given increasing say in living arrangements. Parents should never suggest that their children take sides and should try not to express negative feelings about the other parent to their children. Parents should discuss issues openly, honestly, and calmly with their children; remain affectionate with them; continue to discipline consistently; and maintain normal expectations regarding chores and schoolwork. Most children regain a sense of security and support within about a year after divorce if the parents adjust and work to meet the child's needs.

For a child, remarriage of either parent can restore a sense of stability and permanency but can also create new conflict. Some children feel disloyal to one parent by accepting the other parent's new spouse.

THE CHANGING STRUCTURES OF FAMILIES.

Most people picture a traditional family as a married man and woman and their biological children. However, a family may consist of a gay couple, single parent, or even a group of unrelated adults who live and rear children together.

During the last several decades, increasing numbers of families have deviated from the traditional model. Divorces force many children into single parent families or blended families created by remarriage. About one third of children are born to single mothers; about 10% of children are born to single teenage mothers. Many children are reared by grandparents or other relatives. About one million children live with adoptive parents.

Even traditional families have changed. Often both parents work outside the home, requiring many children to receive regular care outside of the family setting. Because of school and career commitments, many couples postpone having children until their 30s and even 40s. Changing cultural expectations have resulted in fathers spending increasing amounts of time rearing children.

Conflicts develop in every family, but healthy families are strong enough to resolve conflicts or thrive despite them. Whatever their makeup, healthy families provide children with a sense of belonging and meet children's physical, emotional, developmental, and spiritual needs. Members of healthy families express emotion and support for each other in ways consistent within their own culture and family traditions.

Childcare

About 80% of children receive childcare outside the home before they start school. Many children aged 5 to 12 also receive care outside the home before or after school. Sources of care include relatives, neighbors, licensed and unlicensed private homes, and childcare centers. Care can also be provided in the home by a relative or nanny. Childcare centers can be licensed, accredited, or both. Accreditation usually requires that the center meet higher standards than those required for licensing.

Care outside of the home varies in quality; while some is excellent, some is poor. Care outside of the home can also have benefits. Children whose parents—particularly single parents—are not able to spend much time interacting with them can benefit from the social and academic stimulation of quality childcare.

DID YOU KNOW?

- Most preschool children receive care outside the home.
- Childcare outside the home can provide benefits: social interaction, physical and other activities, and opportunities to develop independence.

Early exposure to music, books, art, and language stimulates a child's intellectual and creative development. Group play stimulates social development. Outdoor and occasional vigorous play helps dissipate pent-up physical energy and stimulate muscle development. Opportunities to initiate their own activities help children develop independence. Nutritious meals or snacks should be available every few hours. Television and videos contribute little to the child's development and are best avoided. If they are used, the content should be age-appropriate and supervised by an adult.

Exposure to many other children in childcare settings often results in common viral infections. It is not unusual for parents to complain that their child who is in a childcare setting always seems to have a cold. However, these infections are rarely serious, do not impair a child's development, and are not usually reasons to withdraw the child from the childcare setting.

Foster Care

- Children sometimes need to live with another family temporarily.
- A foster family takes care of the child, but the birth parents usually retain legal responsibility.
- The main reasons for foster care are abuse and neglect.
- Children in foster care may feel anxious, helpless, angry, rejected, or guilty.
- They have more physical and emotional problems than other children.

Foster care is care provided for children whose families are temporarily unable to care for them. The local government determines the process of arranging foster care. Foster care is surprisingly common in the United States; around 750,000 children are in the foster care system each year.

The foster parent assumes day-to-day care for the child. However, the birth parents usually remain the child's legal guardians. This means that the birth parents still make legal decisions for the child. For example, if the child needs an operation, only the birth parents can provide consent.

Most children in foster care are from poor families. About 70% of the children in foster care are put there by child protective services because the child has been abused or neglected (see page 550). Most of the remaining 30% are adolescents placed in care by the juvenile justice system. Very few children are placed voluntarily by their parents. Most children in foster care live with foster families, although many adolescents live in group homes or residential treatment facilities.

DID YOU KNOW?

- About half of children in foster care return to their birth families.

Removal from their family is enormously painful to children. In foster care, children may have frequent visits with their families or only limited, supervised visits. Children in foster care leave behind their neighborhoods, communities, schools, and most of their belongings. Many children and adolescents in foster care feel anxious, uncertain, and helpless to control their lives. Many feel angry, rejected, and pained by the separation, or they develop a profound sense of loss. Some feel guilty, believing that they caused the disruption of their birth family. Peers often tease children about being in foster care, reinforcing perceptions that they are somehow different or unworthy. Children in foster care have more chronic illnesses and behavioral, emotional, and developmental problems than do other children. Yet, most children in foster care adjust well as long as the foster family nurtures the child's emotional needs. Most children in foster care benefit from counseling.

About half of the children eventually return to their birth families. About 20% of children in foster care are eventually adopted, most often by their foster family. Other children return to a relative or become too old for foster care. A small number of children are later transferred to another foster care agency.

Adoption

- Children may legally become part of another family when they are orphans or when their parents give up or lose their parental rights.
- Consulting a lawyer and an expert in adoption can help prospective adoptive parents.
- Birth parents may want to visit their child; the child, when older, or the adoptive parents may wish to connect with the birth parents.

Adoption is the legal process of adding a person to an existing family. Adoption, unlike foster care, is meant to be permanent. The goal of adoption is to provide lifelong security to a child and the family.

Children who are orphaned are obvious candidates for adoption. In the United States, children can be adopted if the parents give up the child voluntarily, or if the child is freed involuntarily through the court process known as termination of parental rights. International adoption (adoption of children from other countries, for example, from foreign orphanages) is also often possible. Depending on the source, international adoption may carry with it specific medical issues such as pre-existing chronic health conditions, infectious diseases, lack of vaccination history, and developmental delays. A comprehensive health care visit is recommended for the child soon after the adoption.

Depending on the type, adoption can sometimes cost tens of thousands of dollars. Having experienced legal representation, often from a lawyer, helps the adoptive parents regardless of the type of adoption.

Sometimes, adoptive parents connect with birth parents. The parties may already be related in some way. For example, a stepparent can adopt a spouse's birth child, or grandparents can adopt their grandchildren. In other cases, parents may connect through word of mouth or newspaper advertisements.

In some cases, birth parents may appreciate the chance to visit the child. Also, knowing the birth parents may make adoptive parents less likely to worry that the birth parents will try to reclaim the child. In addition, sometimes there are benefits for the child. All such issues are often best discussed with an expert (such as a mental health and a legal professional) before making decisions.

DID YOU KNOW?

- Children should be told, ideally at about age 7, that they were adopted.
- Some states have a web site that enables birth parents and adopted children to connect with each other if both parties want to.

Most adopted children, including those previously in foster care or foreign orphanages, adjust well and develop few problems. However, as children age, they may develop feelings of rejection because they were given up by their birth family. During adolescence and young adulthood, in particular, an adopted person may be very curious about his birth parents, even if he does not ask about them. Some adopted people seek information about, or seek out, their birth parents, and some birth parents seek out their birth children.

Withholding the fact that children were adopted can hurt them later. Children adjust best if told by about age 7. If asked, adoptive parents should tell the child about the birth parents in a comforting manner. For example, if the child was abused or neglected, parents can say the child was removed because the birth parent had problems or was ill and could not provide proper care. Children need reassurance that they are loved and always will be loved. If children have contact with their birth families, it helps for parents to tell the child that two sets of parents love them.

If birth parents request anonymity, there is controversy about whether children should be able to find information about them. Some states provide a web site for birth parents and children to post their identity. If both do so, then they will be placed in touch with each other. Contact cannot be initiated unless both parties agree.

CHAPTER 33

Child Neglect and Abuse

- A neglected or abused child may appear tired or dirty or have physical injuries or emotional or mental health problems.
- Abuse is suspected when bruises suggest that the injury was not accidental, when injuries do not match a caregiver's explanation, or sometimes when both healed and new injuries are evident.
- If sexual abuse occurred less than 72 hours before the child is evaluated, doctors obtain legal evidence of sexual contact.
- Treatment of neglect and abuse includes protecting the child from further harm and often assisting the family in providing safe, appropriate care.

Children can be mistreated by having essential things withheld from them (neglect) or by having harmful things done to them (abuse). Neglect involves not meeting children's basic needs: physical, medical, educational, and emotional. Emotional neglect is a part of emotional abuse. Abuse can be physical, sexual, or emotional. The different forms of abuse sometimes occur together. Child neglect and abuse often occur together and with other forms of family violence, such as spousal abuse. In addition to immediate harm, neglect and abuse cause long-lasting problems, including mental health problems and substance abuse. For reasons that are unclear, adults who were physically or sexually abused as children are more likely to abuse their own children.

In the United States, more than 800,000 children are neglected or abused every year, and about 1,100 of them die. Neglect is about 3 times more common than physical abuse.

Neglect and abuse result from a complex combination of individual, family, and social factors. Being a single parent, being poor, having problems with drug or alcohol abuse, or having a mental health problem (such as a personality disorder or low self-esteem) can make a parent more likely to neglect or abuse a child. Neglect is 12 times more common among children living in poverty.

Doctors and nurses are required by law to promptly report cases of suspected child neglect or abuse to a local Child Protective Services agency. In other words, these professionals are mandated to report cases that are suspected, even if the abuse or neglect isn't certain. Depending on the circumstances, the local law enforcement agency may also be notified. Prompt reporting is also required from all people whose job places children younger than 18 in their care. Such people include teachers, childcare workers, and police and legal services personnel. Anyone else who knows of or suspects neglect or abuse is encouraged to report it but is not required to do so.

All reported cases of child abuse are investigated by representatives of the local Child Protective Services agency, who determine the facts and make recommendations. Agency representatives may recommend social services (for the child and family members), temporary hospitalization, temporary foster care, or permanent termination of parental rights. Doctors and social workers provide expert opinion to help the representatives from the Child Protective Services agency who are deciding what to do based on the immediate medical needs of the child, the seriousness of the harm, and the likelihood of further neglect or abuse.

DID YOU KNOW?

- Neglect is 3 times more common than physical abuse.
- Parental factors that make neglect and abuse more likely include poverty, single parenthood, substance abuse, mental health problems, and stress.
- Sexual abuse of girls and boys is common.
- Most perpetrators of physical and sexual abuse are males who are known by the victims.
- Serious internal injuries may be present without any visible clues.
- Abused children may be reluctant to disclose information because of shame or threats of retaliation, or because they believe abuse is a normal part of life or even that they deserve the abuse.

Types

There are a number of different types of child neglect and abuse.

Physical Neglect: Not meeting a child's essential needs for food, clothing, and shelter is the most basic form of neglect. But there are many other forms. Parents may not obtain preventive dental or medical care for the child, such as vaccinations and routine physical examinations. Parents may delay obtaining medical care when the child is ill, putting the child at risk of more severe illness and even death. Parents may not make sure the child attends school or is privately schooled. Parents may leave a child in the care of a person who is known to be abusive, or may leave a young child unattended.

Physical Abuse: Physically mistreating or harming a child, including inflicting excessive physical punishment, is physical abuse. Children of any age may be physically abused, but infants and toddlers are particularly vulnerable. Physical abuse is the most common cause of serious head injury in infants. In toddlers, physical abuse is more likely to result in abdominal injuries, which may be fatal. Physical abuse (including homicide) is among the 10 leading causes of death in children. Generally, a child's risk of physical abuse decreases during the early school years and increases during adolescence.

Most perpetrators of physical abuse are males known by the children. Children who are born in poverty to a young, single parent are at highest risk. Family stress contributes to physical abuse. Stress may result from unemployment, frequent moves to another home, social isolation from friends or family members, or ongoing family violence. Children who are difficult (irritable, demanding, hyperactive, or handicapped) may be more likely to be physically abused. Physical abuse is often triggered by a crisis in the midst of other stresses. A crisis may be a loss of a job, a death in the family, a discipline problem, or even a toileting accident.

Sexual Abuse: Any action with a child that is for the sexual gratification of an adult or a significantly older child is considered sexual abuse. It includes penetrating the child's vagina, anus, or mouth, touching the child with sexual intention but without penetration, exposing the genitals or showing pornography to a child, and using a child in the production of pornography. Sexual abuse does not include sexual play. In sexual play, children who are less than 4 years apart in age view or touch each other's genital area without force or coercion.

By the age of 18, about 12 to 25% of girls and 8 to 10% of boys have experienced sexual abuse. Most perpetrators of sexual abuse are people known by the children, commonly a stepfather, an uncle, or the mother's boyfriend. Female perpetrators are less common.

Certain situations increase the risk of sexual abuse. For example, children who have several caregivers or a caregiver with several sex partners are at increased risk. Being socially isolated, having low self-esteem, having family members who are also sexually abused, or being associated with a gang also increases risk.

Emotional Abuse: Using words or acts to psychologically mistreat a child is emotional abuse. Emotional abuse makes children feel that they are worthless, flawed, unloved, unwanted, in danger, or valuable only when they meet another person's needs.

Emotional abuse includes spurning, exploiting, terrorizing, isolating, and neglecting. Spurning means belittling the child's abilities and accomplishments. Exploiting means encouraging deviant or criminal behavior, such as committing crimes or abusing alcohol or drugs. Terrorizing means bullying, threatening, or frightening the child. Isolating means not allowing the child to interact with other adults or children. Emotionally neglecting a child means ignoring and not interacting with the child; the child is not given love and attention. Emotional abuse tends to occur over a long period of time.

Münchausen by Proxy: In this unusual type of child abuse, a caregiver, usually the mother, exaggerates, fakes, or causes an illness in the child.

Symptoms

The symptoms of neglect and abuse vary depending partly on the nature and duration of the neglect or abuse, on the child, and on the particular circumstances. In addition to obvious physical injuries, symptoms include emotional and mental health problems. Such problems may develop immediately or later and may persist.

Physical Neglect: Physically neglected children may appear undernourished, tired, or dirty or may lack appropriate clothing. They may frequently be absent from school. In extreme cases, children may be found living alone or with siblings, without adult supervision. Physical and emotional development may be slow. Some neglected children die of starvation or exposure.

Physical Abuse: Bruises, burns, welts, or scrapes are common. These marks often have the shape of the object used to inflict them, such as a belt or lamp cord. Cigarette or scald burns may be visible on the arms or legs. Severe injuries to the mouth, eyes, brain, or other internal organs may be present but not visible. Children may have signs of old injuries, such as broken bones, that have healed. Sometimes injuries result in disfigurement.

Toddlers who have been intentionally dunked into a hot bathtub have scald burns. These burns may be located on the buttocks and may be shaped like a doughnut. The splash of hot water may cause small burns on other parts of the body.

Infants who are shaken may have shaken baby (shaken impact) syndrome. This syndrome is caused by violent shaking, often followed by throwing the infant. Infants who are shaken may have no visible signs of injury and may appear to be sleeping deeply. This sleepiness is due to brain damage and swelling, which may result from bleeding between the brain and skull (subdural hemorrhage). Infants may also have bleeding in the retina (retinal hemorrhage) at the back of the eye. Ribs and other bones may be broken.

Children who have been abused for a long time are often fearful and irritable. They often sleep poorly. They may be depressed and anxious. They are more likely to act in violent, criminal, or suicidal ways.

Sexual Abuse: Changes in behavior are common. Such changes may occur abruptly and be extreme. Children may become aggressive or withdrawn or develop phobias or sleep disorders. Children who are sexually abused may behave in sexual ways inappropriate for their age. Children who are sexually abused by a parent or other family member may have conflicted feelings. They may feel emotionally close to the offender, yet betrayed.

Sexual abuse may also result in physical injuries. Children may have bruises, tears, or bleeding in areas around the genitals, rectum, or mouth. Injuries in the genital and rectal areas may make walking and sitting difficult. Girls may have a vaginal discharge. A sexually transmitted disease, such as gonorrhea, chlamydial infection, or sometimes human immunodeficiency virus (HIV) infection, may be present.

Emotional Abuse: In general, children who are emotionally abused tend to be insecure and anxious about their attachments to other people because they have not had their needs met consistently or predictably. Infants who are emotionally neglected may seem unemotional or uninterested in their surroundings. Their behavior may be mistaken for mental retardation or a physical disorder. Children who are emotionally neglected may lack social skills or be slow to develop speech and language skills. Children who are spurned may have low self-esteem. Children who are exploited may commit crimes or abuse alcohol or drugs. Children who are terrorized may appear fearful and withdrawn. They may be distrustful, unassertive, and extremely anxious to please adults. Children who are isolated may be awkward in social situations and have difficulty forming normal relationships. Older children may not attend school regularly or may not perform well when they do attend.

CHILDREN WHO WITNESS DOMESTIC VIOLENCE

Each year, at least 3.3 million children are estimated to witness physical or verbal abuse in their homes. These children may develop problems such as excessive anxiety or crying, fearfulness, difficulty sleeping, depression, social withdrawal, and difficulty in school. Also, children may blame themselves for the situation. Older children may run away from home. Boys who see their father abuse their mother may be more likely to become abusive adults. Girls who see their father abuse their mother may be more likely to tolerate abuse as adults. The perpetrator may also physically hurt the children. In homes where domestic violence is present, children are much more likely to be physically mistreated.

Diagnosis

Neglect and abuse are often difficult to recognize unless children appear severely undernourished or are obviously injured or unless neglect or abuse is witnessed by other people. Neglect and abuse may not be recognized for years. There are many reasons for this difficulty. Abused children may feel that abuse is a normal part of life and may not mention it. Physically and sexually abused children are often reluctant to volunteer information about their abuse because of shame, threats of retaliation, or even a feeling that they deserved the abuse. Physically abused children often describe what happened to them if asked directly, but sexually abused children may be sworn to secrecy or so traumatized that they do not.

When doctors suspect neglect or any type of abuse, they look for signs of other types of abuse. They also fully evaluate the physical, environmental, emotional, and social needs of the child.

Physical Neglect: A neglected child is usually identified by health care practitioners or social workers during evaluation of an unrelated issue, such as an injury, an illness, or a behavioral problem. Doctors may notice that a child is not developing physically or emotionally at a normal rate or has missed many vaccinations or appointments. Teachers may identify a neglected child because of frequent unexplained absences from school. If neglect is suspected, doctors often check for anemia, infections, and lead poisoning, which are common among neglected children.

Physical Abuse: Physical abuse may be suspected when an infant who is not yet walking has bruises or serious injuries. Abuse may be suspected when a toddler or older child has certain types of bruises, such as bruises on the back of the legs, buttocks, and torso. When children are learning to walk, bruises often result, but such bruises typically occur on prominent bony areas on the front of the body, such as the knees, shins, forehead, chin, and elbows.

Abuse may also be suspected when parents appear to know little about their child's health or to be unconcerned about an obvious injury. Parents who abuse their child may be reluctant to describe to the doctor or friends how an injury occurred. The description may not fit the age and nature of the injury or may change each time the story is told.

If doctors suspect physical abuse, they obtain accurate drawings and photographs of the injuries. Sometimes x-rays are taken to look for signs of previous injuries. If a child is younger than 2 years, x-rays of all bones are often taken to check for fractures.

Sexual Abuse: Often, sexual abuse is diagnosed on the basis of the child's or a witness's account of the incident. However, because many children are reluctant to talk about sexual abuse, it may be suspected only because the child's behavior becomes abnormal. If a child has been sexually abused within

72 hours, doctors examine the child to collect legal evidence of sexual contact, such as swabs of body fluids and hair samples from the genital area. Photographs of any visible injuries are taken. In some communities, health care practitioners who are specially trained to evaluate sexual abuse of children perform this examination.

Emotional Abuse: Emotional abuse is usually identified during evaluation of another problem, such as poor performance in school or a behavioral problem. Children who are emotionally abused are checked for signs of physical and sexual abuse.

Treatment

A team of doctors, other health care practitioners, and social workers try to deal with the causes and effects of neglect and abuse. The team helps family members understand the child's needs and helps them access local resources. For example, a child whose parents cannot afford health care may qualify for medical assistance from the state. Other community and government programs can provide assistance with food and shelter. Parents with substance abuse or mental health problems may be directed to appropriate treatment programs. Parenting programs are available in some areas.

All physical injuries and disorders are treated. Some children are hospitalized for treatment of injuries, severe undernutrition, or other disorders. Some severe injuries require surgery. Infants with shaken baby syndrome usually need to be admitted to a pediatric intensive care unit. Sometimes healthy children are hospitalized to protect them from further abuse until appropriate home care can be ensured.

Some children who have been sexually abused are given drugs to prevent sexually transmitted diseases, sometimes including HIV infection. Many children need immediate counseling and support, and most children should have counseling at some time. Sexually abused children, even those who appear unaffected initially, are referred to a mental health care practitioner, because long-lasting problems are common. Long-term psychologic counseling is often needed. Doctors refer other children for counseling if behavioral or emotional problems develop.

The goal of treatment is to return children to a safe, healthy family environment. Depending on the nature of the abuse and the abuser, children may go home with their family or may be removed from their home and placed with relatives or in foster care. This placement is often temporary, for example, until the parents can obtain housing or employment or until regular home visits by a social worker are established. In severe cases of neglect or abuse, the parents' rights may be permanently terminated. In such cases, the child remains in foster care (see page 546) until the child is adopted or becomes an adult.

Resources for Help and Information

AIDS
CDC National AIDS/HIV Hotline
800-342-2437
www.ashastd.org

AIDS Action
Washington, DC
202-530-8030
www.aidsaction.org

The American Foundation for AIDS Research
New York, NY
800-342-2437
212-806-1600
www.amfar.org

ALLERGY & ASTHMA
Allergy and Asthma Network/Mothers of Asthmatics, Inc.
Fairfax, VA
800-727-8462
703-573-7794
www.aanma.org

American Academy of Allergy, Asthma, and Immunology
Milwaukee, WI
414-272-6071
www.aaaai.org

Asthma & Allergy Foundation of America
Washington, DC
800-727-8462
202-466-7643
www.aafa.org

ARTHRITIS
American Juvenile Arthritis Organization
Atlanta, GA
800-283-7800
404-965-7514

Arthritis Foundation
Atlanta, GA
800-283-7800
www.arthritis.org

ASTHMA
(see ALLERGY & ASTHMA)

ATTENTION DEFICIT DISORDER
Attention Deficit Disorder Association
Pottstown, PA
484-945-2101
www.add.org

Children and Adults With Attention Deficit Disorders
Landover, MD
800-233-4050
www.chadd.org

Learning Disabilities Association of America
Pittsburg, PA
412-341-1515
www.ldanatl.org

AUTISM
Autism Research Institute
San Diego, CA
619-563-6840
www.autism.tv

Autism Society of America
Bethesda, MD
800-328-8476
301-657-0881
www.autism-society.org

National Autism Hotline/Autism Services Center
Huntington, WV
304-525-8014

BIRTH DEFECTS
(see also CLEFT PALATE; SPINA BIFIDA)

Federation for Children With Special Needs
Boston, MA
800-331-0688
617-236-7210
www.fcsn.org

March of Dimes Birth Defects Foundation
White Plains, NY
888-663-4637
914-428-7100
www.modimes.org

National Foundation for Jewish Genetic Diseases, Inc.
New York, NY
212-371-1030
www.nfjgd.org

BLOOD DISORDERS

Leukemia Society of America
White Plains, NY
800-955-4572
914-949-5213
www.leukemia.org

**Sickle Cell Disease Association
of America, Inc.**
Culver City, CA
800-421-8453
www.sicklecelldisease.org

CANCER & OTHER TUMORS

American Cancer Society
Atlanta, GA
800-227-2345
404-320-3333
www.cancer.org

Cancer Care, Inc.
New York, NY
800-813-4673
212-712-8080
212-302-2400
www.cancercare.org

National Cancer Institute
Bethesda, MD
800-422-6237
301-496-5583
www.cancer.gov

The Children's Brain Tumor Foundation
New York, NY
866-228-4673 (toll free)
212-448-9494
www.cbtf.org

CEREBRAL PALSY
United Cerebral Palsy Associations, Inc.
Washington, DC
800-872-5827
202-776-0406
202-973-7197 (TTY)
www.ucpa.org

CHILD ABUSE & NEGLECT
American Humane Association,
Children's Division
Englewood, CO
800-227-4645
303-792-9900
www.amerhumane.org

Kempe Children's Center
Denver, CO
303-864-5252
www.kempecenter.org

CLEFT PALATE
Cleft Palate Foundation
Chapel Hill, NC
800-242-5338
www.cleftline.org

Wide Smiles
Stockton, CA
209-942-2812
www.widesmiles.org

CYSTIC FIBROSIS
Cystic Fibrosis Foundation
Bethesda, MD
800-344-4823
301-951-4422
www.cff.org

DEAFNESS & HEARING DISORDERS
Alexander Graham Bell Association for the Deaf and Hard of Hearing
Washington, DC
800-432-7543
202-337-5220
202-337-5221 (TTY)
www.agbell.org

American Association of the Deaf-Blind
Silver Spring, MD
800-735-2258
301-495-4403
301-495-4402 (TTY)
www.aadb.org

American Society for Deaf Children
Gettysburg, PA
800-942-2732 (Parent Hotline)
717-334-7922
www.deafchildren.org

Helen Keller National Center
Sands Point, NY
800-255-0411
516-944-8637 (TTY)
www.helenkeller.org/national

National Association of the Deaf
Silver Spring, MD
301-587-1788
301-587-1789 (TTY)
www.nad.org

DEATH & BEREAVEMENT
Aiding Mothers and Fathers Experiencing Neonatal Death (AMEND)
St. Louis, MO
314-487-7582
www.amendgroup.com

DEPRESSION
Depression and Related Affective Disorders Association (DRADA)
Baltimore, MD
410-955-4647
www.drada.org

National Depressive and Manic-Depressive Association
Chicago, IL
800-826-3632
312-642-0049
www.ndmda.org

Recovery, Inc.
Chicago, IL
312-337-5661
www.recovery-inc.com

DIABETES
American Diabetes Association
Alexandria, VA
800-342-2383
www.diabetes.org

The Juvenile Diabetes Foundation International
New York, NY
800-533-2873
212-785-9500
www.jdrf.org

DIGESTIVE DISORDERS
Crohn's & Colitis Foundation of America
New York, NY
800-343-3637
www.ccfa.org

Digestive Disease National Coalition
Washington, DC
202-544-7497
www.ddnc.org

International Foundation for Functional Gastrointestinal Disorders
Milwaukee, WI
889-964-2001
414-964-1799
www.iffgd.org

DOWN SYNDROME
Association for Children With Down Syndrome
Plainview, NY
516-933-4700
www.acds.org

National Down Syndrome Congress
Atlanta, GA
800-232-6372
770-604-9500
www.ndsccenter.org

National Down Syndrome Society
New York, NY
800-221-4602
www.ndss.org

DRUG ABUSE
Cocaine Anonymous World Service
Los Angeles, CA
800-347-8998
310-559-5833
www.ca.org

Hazelden
Center City, MN
800-257-7810
651-213-4000
www.hazelden.org

Narcotics Anonymous
Van Nuys, CA
818-997-3822
www.na.org

EATING DISORDERS
National Association of Anorexia Nervosa and Associated Disorders
Highland Park, IL
847-831-3438
www.anad.org

GAUCHER'S DISEASE
National Gaucher Foundation
Rockville, MD
800-925-8885
800-428-2437
www.gaucherdisease.org

GENERAL
American Academy of Family Physicians
Leawood, KS
www.familydoctor.org

American Academy of Pediatrics
Elm Grove, IL
847-434-4000
www.aap.org

American Medical Association
Chicago, IL
312-464-5000
www.ama-assn.org

Centers for Disease Control and Prevention
Atlanta, GA
800-311-3435
404-639-3311
www.cdc.gov

The Merck Manuals
Merck & Co, Inc.
West Point, PA
www.merckmanuals.com

National Institutes of Health
Bethesda, MD
301-496-4000
www.nih.gov

U.S. Department of Health and Human Services
Washington, DC
877-696-6775
202-619-0257
www.os.dhhs.gov

U.S. Food and Drug Administration
Office of Consumer Affairs Inquiry Information Line
Rockville, MD
888-463-6332
www.fda.gov

GENETIC DISEASES
Alliance of Genetic Support Groups
Washington, DC
202-966-5557
www.geneticalliance.org

LEARNING DISABILITIES
(see ATTENTION DEFICIT DISORDER)

American Association on Mental Retardation
Washington, DC
800-424-3688
202-387-1968
www.aamr.org

Learning Disabilities Association
Pittsburgh, PA
412-575-7373
www.ldanatl.org

National Center for Learning Disabilities
New York, NY
888-575-7373
212-545-7510
www.ncld.org

MENTAL RETARDATION
The ARC of the United States (formerly Association for Retarded Citizens of the United States
Silver Spring, MD
301-565-3842
www.thearc.org

FRAXA Research Foundation
Newburyport, MA
978-462-1866
www.fraxa.org

The Joseph P. Kennedy, Jr. Foundation
Washington, DC
202-393-1250
www.jpkf.org

National Association of Developmental Disabilities Councils
Washington, DC
202-347-1234
www.naddc.org

Voice of the Retarded
Rolling Meadows, IL
847-253-6020
www.vor.net

MUSCULAR DYSTROPHY
Muscular Dystrophy Association-USA
Tucson, AZ
800-572-1717
www.mdausa.org

PRADER-WILLI SYNDROME
Prader-Willi Syndrome Association (USA)
Sarasota, FL
800-926-4797
941-312-0400
www.pwsausa.org

PSYCHIATRIC DISEASE
National Alliance for the Mentally Ill
Arlington, VA
800-950-6264
703-524-7600
www.nami.org

National Institute of Mental Health
Bethesda, MD
301-443-4513
www.nimh.nih.gov

National Mental Health Association
Alexandria, VA
800-969-6642
800-443-5959 (TTY)
703-684-7722
www.nmha.org

Metanoia
800-784-2433
www.metanoia.org/suicide

Survivors of Suicide
www.thewebpager.com/sos

RARE DISORDERS
National Organization for Rare Disorders
Danbury, CT
800-999-6673
203-744-0100
www.rarediseases.org

RESPIRATORY (LUNG) DISORDERS
American Lung Association
New York, NY
800-586-4872
212-315-8700
www.lungusa.org

Asthma & Allergy Foundation of America
Washington, DC
800-727-8462
202-466-7643
www.aafa.org

REYE'S SYNDROME
National Reye's Syndrome Foundation
Bryan, OH
800-233-7393
419-636-2679
www.reyessyndrome.org

SPINA BIFIDA
Spina Bifida Association of America
Washington, DC
800-621-3141
202-944-3285
www.sbaa.org

STUTTERING & OTHER SPEECH DISORDERS
**National Council on Stuttering & Foundation
for Fluency**
Dekalb, IL
815-756-6986

National Stuttering Association
Anaheim Hills, CA
800-364-1677
www.nsastutter.org

Stuttering Foundation of America
Memphis, TN
800-992-9392
901-452-7343
www.stuttersfa.org

SUDDEN INFANT DEATH SYNDROME
SIDS Network
Ledyard, CT
www.sids-network.org

Sudden Infant Death Syndrome Alliance
Baltimore, MD
800-221-7437
410-653-8226
www.sidsalliance.org

TAY-SACHS DISEASE
National Tay-Sachs & Allied Diseases Association
Brighton, MA
800-906-8723
www.ntsad.org

Index

Note: Page numbers in *italics* refer to illustrations, sidebars, or tables.